Managing the Menopause

21st Century Solutions

Edited by

Nick Panay BSc MRCOG MFSRH
Consultant Gynaecologist, Specialist in Reproductive Medicine, Queen Charlotte's and Chelsea & Chelsea and Westminster Hospitals, Honorary Senior Lecturer, Imperial College London, and Director, International Centre for Hormone Health, London, UK

Paula Briggs FRCGP FFSRH
Consultant in Sexual and Reproductive Health for Southport and Ormskirk Hospital NHS Trust, Southport, UK

Gab Kovacs MD FRANZCOG FRCOG
Professor of Obstetrics and Gynaecology, Monash University, Melbourne, VIC, Australia

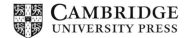
CAMBRIDGE
UNIVERSITY PRESS

CAMBRIDGE
UNIVERSITY PRESS

University Printing House, Cambridge CB2 8BS, United Kingdom

Cambridge University Press is part of the University of Cambridge.

It furthers the University's mission by disseminating knowledge in the pursuit of education, learning and research at the highest international levels of excellence.

www.cambridge.org
Information on this title: www.cambridge.org/9781107451827

© Cambridge University Press 2015

First published 2015
Reprinted 2016
4th printing 2016

Printed in the United Kingdom by TJ International Ltd. Padstow Cornwall

A catalogue record for this publication is available from the British Library

Library of Congress Cataloguing in Publication data
Managing the menopause : 21st century solutions / [edited by] Nick Panay, Paula Briggs, Gab Kovacs.
    p. ; cm.
Includes bibliographical references and index.
ISBN 978-1-107-45182-7 (pbk.)
I. Panay, Nick, editor. II. Briggs, Paula, 1964–, editor. III. Kovacs, Gabor, 1947 April 6–, editor.
[DNLM: 1.   Menopause–physiology. 2.   Female Urogenital Diseases–complications. 3.   Hormone Replacement Therapy–contraindications. 4.   Osteoporosis, Postmenopausal.   WP 580]
RG186
618.1'75–dc23   2015006507

ISBN 978-1-107-45182-7 Paperback

....

BMA
Managing the Menopause

21st Century Solutions

Contents

Contributors

Panagiotis G. Anagnostis MD
Diabetes Endocrinology and Metabolic
Medicine, Faculty of Medicine, Imperial
College London, St. Mary's Campus,
London, UK

**Richard A. Anderson MD PhD FRCOG
FRCP(Ed)**
Elsie Inglis Professor of Clinical
Reproductive Science, MRC Centre for
Reproductive Health, Queens Medical
Research Centre, University of Edinburgh,
Edinburgh, Scotland, UK

**David H. Barlow BSc MD FRCOG FRCP
FMedSci FRSE**
Emeritus Professor, University of Glasgow;
Director of Women's Services, Hamad
Medical Corporation, Qatar

Paula Briggs MRCGP FFSRH
Consultant in Sexual and Reproductive Health
Southport and Ormskirk Hospital NHS
Trust, Southport, UK

Mark P. Brincat PhD MRCP FRCOG
Consultant Obstetrician and Gynaecologist;
Chairman and Head of Department,
Department of Obstetrics and
Gynaecology, Mater Dei Hospital,
Birkirkara, Malta

**Jean Calleja-Agius PhD MRCOG
MRCPI(Irel)**
Obstetrician and Gynaecologist, Lecturer,
Department of Obstetrics and
Gynaecology, Mater Dei Hospital,
Birkirkara, Malta

**Malcolm E. Carruthers MD
FRCPath MRCGP**
Medical Director, Centre for Men's Health,
London, UK; Adjunct Professor,

Department & Alzheimer's Research, Edith
Cowan University, WA, Australia

Elena Cecchi MD
Department of Clinical and Experimental
Medicine, Division of Obstetrics and
Gynecology, University of Pisa, Pisa, Italy

Michael C. Craig PhD FRCOG FRCPsych
Female Hormone Clinic, Maudsley
Hospital, London; Institute of Psychiatry,
Psychology and Neuroscience, Kings
College London, London, UK

David Crook PhD
Research Methodologist, Clinical
Investigation and Research Unit, Royal
Sussex County Hospital, Brighton, UK

Susan R. Davis PhD FRACP
Director, Women's Health Research
Program, School of Public Health and
Preventive Medicine, Monash University,
Melbourne; Consultant Endocrinologist,
Cabrini Medical Centre, Melbourne; Head
of the Women's Specialist Clinic, Alfred
Hospital, Melbourne, VIC, Australia

Claudine Domoney MA MRCOG
Consultant Obstetrician and Gynaecologist,
Chelsea & Westminster Hospital,
London, UK

Philip J. Dutton MBChB MRes
King's College School of Medicine,
London, UK

John Eden MD FRCOG FRANZCOG
Associate Professor of Reproductive
Endocrinology, University of New South
Wales; Director at the Barbara Gross
Research Unit and Clinical Academic at the
Royal Hospital for Women, New South

Wales; Director of Women's Health and Research Institute of Australia, Sydney, Australia

Edzard Ernst MD PhD FAcadMedSci FRCP
Professor Emeritus, University of Exeter, Exeter, UK

Barbara Gardella MD
Research Center for Reproductive Medicine, Gynecological Endocrinology and Menopause, IRCCS S. Matteo Foundation, Department of Clinical, Surgical, Diagnostic and Pediatric Sciences, University of Pavia, Pavia, Italy

Andrea R. Genazzani MD PhD HcD FRCOG
Professor, Department of Clinical and Experimental Medicine, Division of Obstetrics and Gynecology, University of Pisa, Pisa, Italy

Franco Guidozzi FRCOG FCOG
Professor and Chief Specialist, Department of Obstetrics and Gynecology, Faculty of Health Sciences, University of Witwatersrand, Johannesburg, South Africa

Tim Hillard FRCOG
Consultant Obstetrician & Gynaecologist, Poole Hospital NHS Foundation Trust, Poole, UK

Myra S. Hunter PhD CPsychol AFBPS
Professor of Clinical Health Psychology, Institute of Psychiatry, King's College London, London, UK

Jay Iyer MD MRCOG FRANZCOG
Department of Obstetrics and Gynaecology, James Cook University, Townsville, Australia

Jessica W. Kiley MD MPH
Assistant Professor of Obstetrics and Gynecology, Department of Obstetrics and Gynecology, Feinberg School of Medicine of Northwestern University, Chicago, IL, USA

Gab Kovacs MD FRCOG FRANZCOG
Professor of Obstetrics and Gynaecology, Monash University, Melbourne, VIC, Australia

Rossella E. Nappi MD PhD MBA
Research Center for Reproductive Medicine, Gynecological Endocrinology and Menopause, IRCCS S. Matteo Foundation, Department of Clinical, Surgical, Diagnostic and Pediatric Sciences, University of Pavia, Pavia, Italy

Tatijana Nikishina MRCOG
Specialist Registrar, Department of Obstetrics and Gynaecology, Poole Hospital NHS Foundation Trust, Poole, UK

Nick Panay BSc MRCOG MFSRH
Consultant Gynaecologist, Specialist in Reproductive Medicine, Queen Charlotte's & Chelsea and Chelsea & Westminster Hospitals; Honorary Senior Lecturer, Imperial College London; Director of the International Centre for Hormone Health, London, UK

JoAnn V. Pinkerton MD
Professor of Obstetrics and Gynecology, Division Director Midlife Health, University of Virginia Health System, Charlottesville, VA, USA

Paul Posadzki PhD MSc
Researcher in Alcohol Synthesis, The Centre for Public Health, Liverpool John Moores University, Liverpool, UK; Honorary Research Fellow, Plymouth University Peninsula Schools of Medicine and Dentistry, Plymouth, UK

Ajay Rane PhD FRCOG FRANZCOG
Professor and Director of Urogynecology, Department of Obstetrics and Gynecology,

James Cook University, Townsville,
Australia

Anthony J. Rutherford FRCOG
Honorary Senior Lecturer, University of
Leeds; Consultant in Reproductive
Medicine and Gynaecological Surgery,
Leeds Teaching Hospitals NHS Trust,
Leeds, UK

Janice M. Rymer MD FRCOG FRANZCOG
Professor of Obstetrics and Gynaecology
and Dean of Undergraduate Medicine,
King's College School of Medicine,
London, UK

Jenifer Sassarini MBChB
Clinical Lecturer, Obstetrics and
Gynaecology, University of Glasgow,
Scotland, UK

Lee P. Shulman MD
The Anna Ross Lapham Professor in
Obstetrics and Gynecology, Chief, Division
of Clinical Genetics, Department of
Obstetrics and Gynecology, Feinberg
School of Medicine of Northwestern
University, Chicago, IL, USA

Tommaso Simoncini MD PhD
Department of Clinical and Experimental
Medicine, Division of Obstetrics

and Gynecology, University of Pisa,
Pisa, Italy

Sven O. Skouby MD DMSc
Professor of Gynecologic Endocrinology
and Director, Division of Reproductive
Endocrinology, Department of Gynecology
and Obstetrics, Herlev Hospital, Faculty
of Health and Medical Sciences, University
of Copenhagen, Copenhagen, Denmark

John C. Stevenson FRCP
Consultant Metabolic Physician and
Reader, National Heart and Lung Institute,
Imperial College London, Royal Brompton
Hospital, London, UK

John D. Wark FRACP PhD
Professor of Medicine, University of
Melbourne; Department of Medicine
(Royal Melbourne Hospital); Head, Bone
and Mineral Medicine, Royal Melbourne
Hospital, Melbourne, Australia

Barry G. Wren MD FRCOG FRANZCOG
Sydney Menopause Centre, Royal Hospital
for Women, Sydney, NSW, Australia

Christopher J. Yates FRACP PhD
Endocrinologist and General Physician,
Royal Melbourne Hospital; Endocrinologist,
Western Hospital, Melbourne, Australia

Foreword

For the past 12 years, the topic of menopause has been the subject of much controversy – fueled by the initial announcement, by way of a press conference in July 2002, that the US Women's Health Initiative randomized controlled trial of continuous combined hormone replacement had shown a 26% increase in breast cancer risk after 5.6 years of follow-up. Not emphasized was the fact that the results were barely statistically significant and were equivalent to an annual risk of <1 extra case of breast cancer per 1000 women treated per year – and then only in women who had previously taken hormone replacement. Much time and effort have been expended in the past 12 years to analyze this initial result in much greater detail – including the documentation that estrogen-only treatment actually reduced breast cancer risk overall. This in turn has led the International Menopause Society and various national societies to publish guidelines summarizing current practice in menopause management. The guidelines are generally directed to a discussion of benefits and risks of hormone therapy with recommendations regarding standard management of women in their late 40s and 50s.

The present volume is much broader in its scope and deals with many aspects not readily available to the general practitioner, gynecologist or endocrinologist involved in the care of mid-life women.

The last chapter is a somewhat surprising addition to the book – andrologists in general do not accept the concept of the male menopause and many of the opinions expressed by Carruthers would be strongly disputed by them.

This is an interesting book with many contributions in areas not generally covered. It is recommended for both a general and a specialist readership and will be a very useful reference source in a number of areas.

Henry Burger
Hudson Institute of Medical Research, Monash University, Clayton, VIC, Australia

Preface

During the 1990s the treatment of menopausal symptoms with hormone replacement therapy (HRT) became widespread practice. Its benefits on bone metabolism were well accepted and it was suggested that HRT may have beneficial effects on the cardiovascular system and long-term cognitive function.

In 2002 the Women's Health Initiative (WHI) study reported an increased risk of cardiovascular disease and breast cancer in long-term users of combined HRT. Although the design of the study was heavily criticized, this resulted in many women giving up their HRT and in many doctors refusing to prescribe. Since the WHI, the care of many menopausal women has been neglected, resulting in a devastating effect on their quality of life and possibly their longevity.

In this book, the editors have assembled a group of international experts to update health professionals on all aspects of the menopause and specifically the benefits and risks of HRT and alternatives. By referring to the relevant chapters, readers will be empowered to individualize their management of women with menopause-related problems and to prescribe with confidence once again.

Nick Panay, Paula Briggs and Gab Kovacs

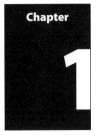

Physiology of the menstrual cycle and changes in the perimenopause

Philip J. Dutton and Janice M. Rymer

Introduction

The menopause marks the permanent cessation of menstruation and heralds the transition in a woman's life from a reproductive state to a non-reproductive one. Whilst the average age of this landmark varies slightly across the world, the menopause generally occurs in the early 50s, and is only truly affected by factors such as smoking, and medical and surgical induction of the menopausal state. However, clinical symptoms may precede this, and the physiological changes which occur with the menopausal transition may begin several years prior to the onset of any manifestations. At the heart of the clinical and biochemical changes associated with the perimenopausal period is the depletion of ovarian follicles to a critical level [1–8].

Although the physiology of the normal menstrual cycle has been studied extensively, research concerning the physiological changes of the menopause and their relationship to menopausal symptoms has only begun to make significant advances in the last two decades. The development of a validated staging system has been immensely beneficial in standardizing nomenclature surrounding the menopause, as well as characterizing the changes at each stage in the transition. Despite these developments, there remain considerable gaps in the literature which require further investigation [1–8]. This chapter outlines current knowledge surrounding the staging and physiology of reproductive aging and its relationship to the troublesome symptoms experienced by the majority of women at this challenging stage of their lives. Before discussing this, however, it is important to have a firm grasp of the concepts surrounding the normal menstrual cycle.

Premenopausal hormonal regulation of ovarian function

The menstrual cycle is controlled by the hypothalamic-pituitary-ovarian axis, which apart from its mid-cycle gonadotropin surge, acts as a negative feedback system, whereby peptide gonadotropins stimulate steroid hormone production in the ovaries, which in turn inhibits gonadotropin secretion, thus allowing cycles to occur [1, 2, 9].

The hypothalamus secretes gonadotropin-releasing hormone (GnRH). This acts on the pituitary gland in a pulsatile manner, which leads to the secretion of the gonadotropins follicle-stimulating hormone (FSH) and luteinizing hormone (LH) [1, 2, 9]. It is the frequency and amplitude of these pulses which determine the quantity of each hormone

Managing the Menopause: 21st Century Solutions, ed. Nick Panay, Paula Briggs, and Gab Kovacs.
Published by Cambridge University Press. © Cambridge University Press 2015.

ultimately secreted. Slower frequencies appear to precipitate FSH secretion, whereas LH secretion has a predilection for higher frequencies of GnRH stimulation [2].

At the start of the menstrual cycle, the ovary contains several antral follicles. These follicles consist of an oocyte, which is separated from a fluid-filled sac called the antrum, both of which are surrounded by a layer of granulosa cells (cumulus cells and mural cells respectively). These cells are surrounded by a basal membrane, around which lies another layer of theca cells. Theca cells develop LH receptors if they are part of the dominant follicle and produce androgens (progesterone or testosterone) from cholesterol. Conversely, granulosa cells have FSH receptors; androgens are absorbed by these cells and metabolized to estradiol (E2) [1, 9]. Granulosa cells also produce the peptide hormone inhibin, which includes two isoforms, A and B [1, 2].

In the late luteal phase (prior to menstruation) and the early follicular phase, levels of circulating FSH rise. This in turn stimulates follicular development and leads to selection of a dominant follicle. Whilst it is not known exactly how a dominant follicle is selected, it is thought that through varying follicular sensitivity, the most sensitive follicle goes on to mature, whilst the other follicles undergo atresia (degeneration). With its development, the dominant follicle secretes increasing levels of E2; this acts on the endometrium to stimulate proliferation. At the pituitary gland, rising levels of E2 and inhibin B act to reduce FSH secretion through a negative feedback mechanism [1, 2, 9].

During the early and mid-follicular phases, E2 also exerts negative feedback on LH secretion, which ensures basal levels during this period. However, about 36 hours prior to ovulation (i.e. in the late follicular phase), E2 reaches levels in the circulation which switch this negative feedback effect to a positive feedback effect. This leads to a surge in LH (which is accompanied by a smaller surge in FSH) over a 24-hour period in the 24 hours prior to ovulation. This LH surge leads to rupture of the dominant follicular wall and release of the oocyte [2, 9].

Following ovulation, there is an abrupt fall in E2 production from the ruptured follicle. The follicle undergoes a series of changes which convert it into an endocrine structure called the corpus luteum ("yellow body"). This produces E2 and progesterone which act on the endometrium to promote implantation. LH maintains the corpus luteum in the week following ovulation, but if pregnancy does not occur, then this begins to degenerate, leading to a gradual reduction in the production of steroid hormones. With falling E2 and progesterone levels, the loss of negative feedback leads to a subsequent rise in FSH, heralding the start of a new menstrual cycle. A summary of these processes is shown in Figure 1.1 [1, 2, 9].

Definitions and staging in reproductive aging

In order to understand the context in which the physiological changes of the menopausal transition are happening, it is necessary to consider the definitions and stages associated with reproductive aging.

The premenopause is typically defined as the phase of a woman's life from the menarche (onset of menstruation) until the beginning of the perimenopausal stage. The perimenopause comprises the time from a woman's mature reproductive state at the point when she begins to experience variability in the length of her cycle or characteristic symptoms of the menopausal transition, to the year following her final menstrual period (FMP). It is only

Menstrual cycle regulation

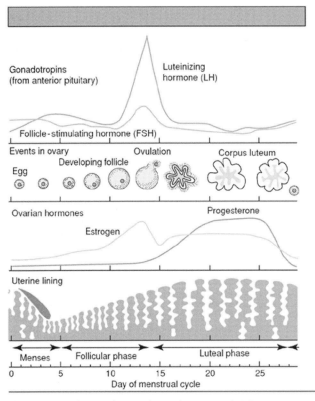

1. Hypothalamus releases GnRH, stimulating the pituitary

2. FSH secreted from pituitary stimulates follicle

3. Follicles produce oestrogen-negative feedback, turning off FSH release

4. Critical level of E_2 stimulates LH peak-positive feedback ovulation

5. Corpus luteum secretes E_2 and P_4, lifespan 12–14 days

Figure 1.1. Endocrine changes during the menstrual cycle.

following this 12-month period of amenorrhea that a diagnosis of menopause can be made. The terms "menopause" and "postmenopause" are often used interchangeably to describe the phase of a woman's life from this point [1–8].

In 2001, the Stages of Reproductive Ageing Workshop (STRAW) met to propose criteria for defining the stages of reproductive life. They generated a staging system which provided guidance on ovarian aging in women. Prior to this, there was no generally accepted staging system. The aim of this was to improve research in women transitioning from a reproductive to a non-reproductive state by standardizing nomenclature and outlining the characteristic changes of each stage to aid consistency across studies. In a clinical context, the STRAW staging system provides health-care providers and women with a guide in the assessment of fertility and contraceptive requirements. In 2006, the ReSTAGE collaboration assessed the validity and reliability of STRAW's criteria and made several recommendations [2–8]. Ten years later, this collaboration and a greater understanding of ovarian aging have led to a revision of the STRAW staging system. The STRAW + 10 staging system is shown in Tables 1.1 and 1.2 [3].

The STRAW + 10 staging system is divided into three phases: the reproductive phase; the menopausal transition; and the postmenopausal phase. The reproductive phase is

Table 1.1. The reproductive phase as outlined in the STRAW + 10 Classification.

Stage	−5	−4	−3b	−3a
Terminology	Reproductive phase			
	Early	Peak	Late	
Duration	Variable			
Menstrual pattern	Variable to regular	Regular	Regular	Some changes in cycle length and flow
FSH			Low	Variable[1]
Inhibin B				Low
AMH			Low	Low
AFC			Low	Low

FSH, follicle-stimulating hormone; AMH, anti-Müllerian hormone; AFC, antral follicle count.
[1] Based on blood samples taken at days 2–5 of cycle.

Table 1.2. The menopausal transition and postmenopausal phase as outlined in the STRAW + 10 Classification.

Stage	−2	−1	+1a	+1b	+1c	+2
Terminology	Menopausal transition		Postmenopausal phase			
	Early	Late	Early			Late
	Perimenopause ———————————————					
Duration	Variable	1–3 years	2 years (1+1)		3–6 years	Remainder of life
Menstrual pattern	Persistent ≥7 day difference in cycle length	Cycles ≥60 days				
FSH	↑ Variable[1]	↑ >25 IU/L[2]	↑ Variable		Stabilizes	
Inhibin B	Low	Low	Low		Very low	
AMH	Low	Low	Low		Very low	
AFC	Low	Low	Very low		Very low	
Symptoms		Vasomotor symptoms likely	Vasomotor symptoms most likely			Increasing urogenital symptoms

FSH, follicle-stimulating hormone; AMH, anti-Müllerian hormone; AFC, antral follicle count; ↑, elevated.
[1] Based on blood samples taken at days 2–5 of cycle.
[2] Based on assays using current international pituitary standard.

subdivided into three stages (−5 to −3). The early reproductive stage (−5) refers to the period immediately following the menarche, before menstrual cycles become regular. During the peak reproductive stage (−4), menstrual cycles are regular. The late reproductive stage (−3) marks the time when fertility begins to go into decline; it is subdivided into two stages [3]. During stage −3b, menstrual cycles are regular but anti-Müllerian hormone (AMH) levels continue to fall (a process which starts from the menarche) as a result of a gradual depletion in the antral follicle count [1, 3, 4]. Stage −3a is characterized by subtle changes in menstrual cycle length and flow. Cycles tend to become shorter and periods heavier [1, 5, 6]. FSH levels rise with increasing variability, whilst levels of antral follicles, AMH and inhibin B are low [3].

From the onset of the early menopausal transition, also known as the perimenopause (−2), cycle variability increases with a persistent difference of 7 days or more in the length of consecutive cycles. Anatomical and biochemical changes are similar to those of stage −3a, but with increasing variability in FSH levels. The late menopausal transition (−1) is characterized by an interval of amenorrhea lasting at least 60 days [3]. There is an increased prevalence of anovulation and further variability in cycle length and hormonal levels [3, 5–7]. Indeed, during this stage, FSH levels are typically defined as being greater than 25 IU/L, and are often associated with high E2 levels. However, E2 does start to fall [3, 4, 6, 7]. This stage is expected to last between 1 and 3 years, and it is during this time that menopausal symptoms, and in particular vasomotor symptoms, usually arise [3].

The late menopausal transition concludes with the final menstrual period (FMP) (0), and gives way to the postmenopausal phase (+1 to +2). Stage +1 is defined as the early postmenopausal stage, and is subdivided into three stages. Stage +1a lasts 1 year following the FMP and the end of this stage is defined as the menopause (a period of amenorrhea lasting 12 months). The end of this stage marks the end of the perimenopause, and 1 year into the postmenopausal phase, although this diagnosis can only be made retrospectively [3]. During stages +1a and +1b (which also lasts 1 year), FSH levels continue to rise, whilst E2 levels continue to fall [3, 4, 6, 7]. Thereafter, levels of these hormones stabilize. Menopausal symptoms, and particularly VMS, are most likely to occur during these stages. Stage +1c marks a period of stabilization in levels of FSH and E2 which lasts between 3 and 6 years. The late postmenopausal stage (+2) lasts for the remaining lifespan of a woman, during which FSH levels tend to fall gradually. Generalized somatic aging processes rather than reproductive aging characterize this period. However, the prevalence of urogenital symptoms increases at this time [3].

Physiological changes in the menopausal transition

At the root of the physiological changes taking place in the menopausal transition is a gradual reduction in the number and quality of ovarian follicles to critical levels [1, 2, 4, 5, 7, 8]. During fetal development, oocyte production occurs until approximately 20 weeks of gestation, at which levels reach between 6 and 7 million [1, 2]. Thereafter, there is no further oocyte production and levels begin to decline through a combination of follicular atresia and oocyte release, until fewer than 100 follicles remain in each ovary at the onset of the perimenopause [1, 2, 5, 7]. In addition, the oocyte and its surrounding layer of granulosa cells are thought to become increasingly incompetent with age [2, 6].

With the declining antral follicle count in the late reproductive stage and early menopausal transition, there is a reduced amount of inhibin B production by the granulosa cells [5, 6, 8]. As discussed earlier, inhibin B normally acts on the pituitary gland in a negative feedback mechanism to reduce rising levels of FSH. Lower levels of inhibin B fail to keep this mechanism in check, which leads to higher levels of FSH during the early follicular phase [5–8]. This in turn leads to increased activity of a single dominant follicle, or the recruitment of multiple dominant follicles, and thus higher levels of E2 production [1, 5]. As E2 levels rise to a critical level at an earlier stage, the LH surge occurs earlier and the follicular phase is shortened, which in turn reduces the overall cycle length [1, 6]. It should be noted that the luteal phase does not change in duration until later in the transition [1]. This shortened menstrual cycle length does not occur in all women entering the perimenopause.

As women move into the late menopausal transition, menstrual cycles become progressively longer in duration. The proportion of cycles which are anovulatory also increases. This may be due to a variety of reasons. Concerning the hypothalamic-pituitary-ovarian axis, there appears to be progressive deregulation of positive and negative feedback mechanisms. Indeed, high levels of E2, which would normally elicit an LH surge during the middle of the cycle have been found to fail in this, whilst a fall in E2 in the luteal phase has failed to lower levels of circulating LH. Thus there may be an element of hypothalamic or pituitary insensitivity. In the ovary, high levels of FSH may also prevent ovulation from occurring, even in the presence of the LH surge. Whilst data are sparse, progesterone levels appear to fall steadily throughout the menopausal transition. This may be in part due to reduced progesterone production by the corpus luteum, as well as an increase in the frequency of anovulatory cycles [5–7].

Levels of E2 only appear to fall in the 2 years preceding the FMP (this has been noted in prolonged ovulatory cycles), whilst levels of FSH continue to rise [4, 6, 7]. Only following the 12-month period of amenorrhea which is defined as the menopause are E2 levels persistently low [1, 5]. In postmenopausal women, it is estrone (E1) which predominates in the circulation. This is generated through the conversion of androgens (secreted by the adrenal glands and postmenopausal ovaries) in the adipose tissue and liver [1]. FSH levels undergo a slow decline in the late menopausal transition [6]. Whilst there is little change in circulating testosterone concentrations across the transition, levels of sex hormone binding globulin fall, leading to an increased proportion of free testosterone [7].

Anti-Müllerian hormone is a glycoprotein produced by antral follicles which differs from the other hormones of the menstrual cycle as it does not appear to be directly involved in feedback mechanisms. Interestingly, the number of antral follicles appears to reflect the size of the primordial pool [2, 5]. Thus, its levels are high at the menarche and decline thereafter [1, 4]. It is for this reason that AMH is of interest as a potential biomarker of reproductive aging and fecundity [2, 4, 5, 7]. However, in order to be used in this context, it would require further validation, as well as the development of more sensitive assays, as it is almost undetectable in the 5 years preceding the menopause [4]. This is discussed in more detail in Chapter 2.

Menopausal symptoms

The menopausal transition and postmenopausal period are characterized by a broad range of physical and psychological symptoms, which can prove extremely debilitating to women undergoing the physiological changes of this period. Physical symptoms comprise vasomotor symptoms, urogenital symptoms, headaches, palpitations, breast tenderness, menorrhagia, musculoskeletal pain, restless leg syndrome, sleep disturbance and fatigue. Psychological symptoms include depression, irritability, poor concentration and memory loss. Sexual dysfunction appears to have somatic and psychogenic origins. Of these symptoms, vasomotor and urogenital symptoms appear to have the most profound effect on quality of life, and it is for these symptoms that women generally seek medical assistance [1, 5, 8].

Physical symptoms

Vasomotor symptoms

Vasomotor symptoms are the most common manifestation of the menopausal transition and postmenopausal period, and present as either hot flashes or night sweats. According to the STRAW + 10 staging system, VMS generally arise in the late menopausal transition and early postmenopausal period, and whilst symptoms generally last up to 5 years after the FMP, they can last as long as 15 years [1, 3, 8].

The exact physiology of VMS is not fully understood, but hot flashes and night sweats are thought to arise as a result of central thermostatic deregulation originating in the hypothalamus; this is supported by findings of VMS in those with pituitary insufficiency and following hypophysectomy (removal of the pituitary gland). There appears to be an association with low E2. Indeed, the increased prevalence of symptoms in the late menopausal transition and early postmenopausal period when E2 levels are falling, and the improvement of these symptoms with estrogen therapy, provides support to this notion. Supplementary progestogens have also been shown to have a beneficial effect on VMS [1, 8].

A hot flash or night sweat is typically characterized by vasodilatation and sweating of the head, neck and chest. Other cardiovascular changes include an increase in heart rate and baseline electrocardiographic changes. Whilst the skin temperature rises by several degrees celsius, the core body temperature appears to fall. Symptoms generally last about 5 minutes, but can last up to an hour, and several episodes occur each day [1, 8]. There also appears to be a predilection for night-time symptoms, which in turn leads to insomnia, and psychological symptoms including depression, irritability, poor concentration and memory loss [1, 5, 8].

Several factors affect the frequency and severity of VMS. African-American women experience VMS more frequently than their white counterparts. Women who have undergone a sudden-onset medically or surgically induced menopause experience significantly worse symptoms than those who have undergone a natural menopause [1, 8].

Urogenital symptoms

Whilst VMS occur in the late menopausal transition and early postmenopausal period as outlined in the STRAW + 10 staging system, urogenital symptoms appear to be a predominating issue in the late postmenopause and worsen in severity over time [1, 3].

At the root of this are estrogen and progesterone receptors which line the urogenital tract. With deficiencies in E2 and progesterone, a number of physiological changes take place including a reduction in vascularity, epithelial cover and musculature, as well as increased adiposity [1].

In the vaginal tract, a loss of elasticity leads to dyspareunia, whilst epithelial deficiency causes traumatic bleeding. Moreover, the pH of the vaginal tract becomes more alkaline in postmenopausal women, and this can lead to a heightened susceptibility to infections. Other symptoms arising from vaginal changes include dryness and irritation. In the urological tract, the onset of the postmenopausal period can lead to urinary frequency, urgency and incontinence. Women are also at an increased risk of urinary tract infections [1].

Other physical symptoms

Little is known about the physiological mechanisms which give rise to other physical symptoms characteristic of the menopausal transition. Concerning headaches, migraines can be a problematic feature of the perimenopause. However, it is not known whether increased or reduced levels of estrogen are a precipitating factor in migraines. Palpitations are a common occurrence in perimenopausal women, and are thought to be related to increased sympathetic activity. During the early menopausal transition, women commonly report breast tenderness, although symptom frequency and severity falls with advancing age. High levels of exogenous estrogen or progestogen have both been found to induce breast tenderness [1]. With progressive ovarian follicular depletion and an increase in anovulatory cycles, women often report menorrhagia [1, 5]. Back pain and joint stiffness are common debilitating features of the perimenopausal period [1]. Many women also report sleep disturbance. This can be attributed to physical symptoms including VMS and restless leg syndrome, but it may also be the result of psychological symptoms and external factors. Disturbed sleep patterns can lead to weakness and tiredness [1, 8].

Psychological symptoms

Psychological symptoms are a common feature of the menopausal transition and include depression, irritability, poor concentration and memory loss. Estrogen, progesterone and testosterone receptors have all been located in several brain centres, whilst estrogen has been shown to have an effect on several neurotransmitters including serotonin, glutamate and gamma-amino butyric acid (GABA), so it is possible that changes in these hormones may play a role in inducing psychological symptoms [1]. To date, there is limited evidence that the endocrine changes of the perimenopausal period are responsible for these symptoms, and external factors may play a significant role [1, 8]. Despite this, hormone replacement therapy (HRT) does appear to improve symptoms of depression in the menopausal transition [1].

Sexuality

Ascertaining the cause of changes in sexuality during the menopausal transition and post-menopause is extremely challenging due to the complex interplay of physical and psychological factors. Many women report a loss of libido, as well as changes in sensitivity during this period. This may be directly due to hormone deficiency; falling levels of estrogen and progesterone directly affect the urogenital tract leading to dyspareunia and other symptoms as described above. Complications associated with aging may play a role; with advancing age, people are increasingly prone to chronic disease processes which may impede their ability to have sexual intercourse, and they may be on medications which may adversely affect their libido. Women can also experience a change in self-image at the time of the menopausal transition. The loss of reproductive capacity, age-related changes and surgical processes such as mastectomies may affect a woman's confidence. Most likely, a combination of these factors attributes to an increased prevalence of diminished sexual activity in the menopausal transition and postmenopausal phase [1].

Other physiological consequences of the menopausal transition
Metabolic syndrome and cardiovascular disease

Presently, the effect of the menopausal transition on a woman's risk of subsequent metabolic syndrome and cardiovascular disease (CVD) is not fully understood. Postmenopausal women have a significantly increased risk of metabolic syndrome, which is defined as a group of clinical disorders including hypertension, insulin resistance, glucose intolerance, dyslipidemia and obesity. Premenopausal women rarely have CVD, but its incidence is equal across the sexes by the eighth decade [5, 8]. This is discussed further in Chapter 5.

To date, there are no longitudinal data available on the relationship between endogenous estrogen levels and subsequent metabolic syndrome and CVD. Furthermore, data concerning progesterone are sparse [5]. However, estrogen is known to have an impact on blood pressure, lipid metabolism and insulin action [8].

Whilst the effect of the menopausal transition on blood pressure is unclear, estrogen is known to reduce blood pressure in several ways. It induces vasodilatation through activation of endothelial nitric oxide synthase, reduces the sensitivity of angiotensin receptors, and impedes angiotensin II formation, which is a potent vasoconstrictor. With falling estrogen levels following the menopausal transition, these protective mechanisms are lost [8].

Weight gain is a common feature of the menopause [5, 8]. Estrogen deficiency appears to be associated with weight gain, whilst treatment with estrogen therapy can reduce the degree of weight gain or lead to weight loss. With the menopausal transition, the distribution of fat also appears to change. This can in part be explained by estrogen, which has a predilection to promote gluteofemoral adipose tissue accumulation. With the loss of estrogen at the time of the menopause, women start to store their fat abdominally, and this can lead to increased insulin resistance [8].

Loss of bone mineral density

Although osteoporosis and increased fracture risk are common features in postmenopausal women, it appears that rapid bone loss occurs during the menopausal transition through a combination of increased bone resorption and reduced bone formation. Bone resorption appears to result from a downward swing in estrogen levels [5]. Indeed, estrogen therapy leads to an improvement in bone mass and a reduction in the risk of vertebral and hip fractures, whilst its cessation causes a reversal of these changes [8]. Falling progesterone levels reduce the rate of bone formation [5]. This is discussed in detail in Chapters 9 and 10.

Breast and endometrial cancer

The menopausal transition has been identified as a time of increased risk for the development of both breast and endometrial cancer. Indeed, perimenopausal women (in their 40s) are more likely to develop breast cancer than their menopausal counterparts (in their 50s). In this period, higher levels of endogenous E2 and lower levels of progesterone are a common finding [5].

Conclusion

In this chapter, we have provided a grounding in the physiology of the normal menstrual cycle, and its dynamic changes through the late reproductive stage, menopausal transition and the postmenopausal period. The STRAW + 10 staging system provides an excellent means of defining and characterizing these changes, and with more research, these stages can be delineated further. Whilst the nature of menopausal symptoms and complications is well understood, the processes which give rise to these changes still require extensive study.

References

1. Bruce D, Rymer J. Symptoms of the menopause. *Best Pract Res Clin Obstet Gynaecol* 2009; **23**: 25–32.

2. Devoto L, Palomino A, Céspedes P, Kohen P. Neuroendocrinology and ovarian aging. *Gynecol Endocrinol* 2012; **28 Suppl 1**: 14–7.

3. Harlow SD, Gass M, Hall JE, *et al*. Executive summary of the Stages of Reproductive Aging Workshop + 10: addressing the unfinished agenda of staging reproductive aging. *J Clin Endocrinol Metab* 2012; **97**: 1159–68.

4. Su HI, Freeman EW. Hormonal changes associated with the menopausal transition. *Minerva Ginecol* 2009; **61**: 483–9.

5. Prior JC, Hitchcock CL. The endocrinology of perimenopause: need for a paradigm shift. *Front Biosci (Schol Ed)* 2011; **3**: 474–86.

6. Butler L, Santoro N. The reproductive endocrinology of the menopausal transition. *Steroids* 2011; **76**: 627–35.

7. Burger HG, Hale GE, Robertson DM, Dennerstein L. A review of hormonal changes during the menopausal transition: focus on findings from the Melbourne Women's Midlife Health Project. *Hum Reprod Update* 2007; **13**: 559–65.

8. Edwards BJ, Li J. Endocrinology of menopause. *Peridontol 2000* 2013; **61**: 177–94.

9. Billings EL, Brown JB, Billings JJ, Burger HG. Symptoms and hormonal changes accompanying ovulation. *Lancet* 1972; **1**: 282–4.

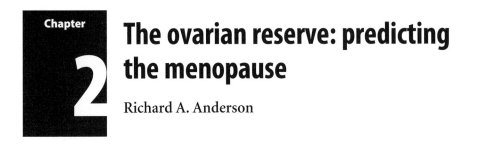

Chapter 2

The ovarian reserve: predicting the menopause

Richard A. Anderson

Sarah is 34. She is a stockbroker. She has worked hard to establish her career and consequently, she has had little time for men. Her friends have pointed out that her "biological clock" is ticking. She read an article about the possibility of social fertility preservation. She comes to see you and asks if you can tell her how long she will be fertile for? She also asks if she should consider social fertility preservation.

The essential cause of the existence of the menopause is that the ovary contains a finite number of follicles: these are progressively lost with time until insufficient remain to support menstrual cyclicity. Ovarian follicles are both the source of the female gamete, and the key site of reproductive hormone production. Depletion of follicle numbers therefore results in both loss of fertility and gonadal estrogen production, and thus differs substantially from the situation in the male where the two functions of the gonad are anatomically and functionally more independent, and loss of one does not necessitate loss of the other.

Establishment and loss of the ovarian reserve

Ovarian follicles are formed during fetal life, with primordial follicles first seen in the ovary from about 18 weeks of gestation. Prior to this, the female germ cells have been specified, migrated to the gonadal ridge where they have proliferated, before they exit mitosis and enter meiosis only to arrest at diplotene of meiosis 1. During this process they reorganize their interactions with surrounding somatic cells to form primordial follicles. This process is complete by birth and indeed some newly formed follicles start growing immediately so that during later fetal life and throughout childhood the ovary contains follicles at a range of stages of development, although the later development of antral follicles to ovulatory stages does not, of course, occur until after puberty when there is sufficient gonadotropic stimulation to support them through to completion of growth and maturation.

Ovaries from different women contain a very wide range of numbers of follicles. This is demonstrated in histologic studies, which have also led to the development of models showing the decline in the primordial follicle pool with age (Figure 2.1) [1]. These studies show that there is a range of at least 50-fold in the number of follicles in the ovaries of women of the same age. The various models that have demonstrated this have tended to present their data on a logarithmic scale which promotes the view that the decline in follicle number accelerates with age. While this may be true when presented as a percentage of the number of follicles present, a very different perspective is gained when the number of follicles is presented on a linear scale (Figure 2.2). This highlights how the vast majority of follicles are

---

Managing the Menopause: 21st Century Solutions, ed. Nick Panay, Paula Briggs, and Gab Kovacs. Published by Cambridge University Press. © Cambridge University Press 2015.

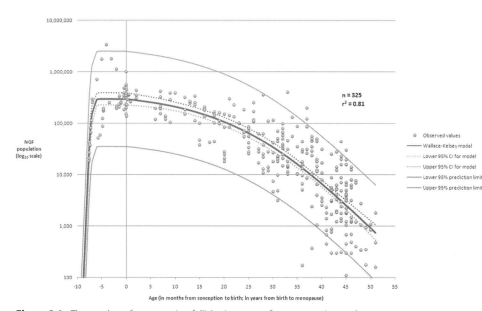

Figure 2.1. The number of non-growing follicles in women from conception to the menopause.
The figure shows the dataset (n = 325), the model, the 95% prediction limits of the model, and the 95% confidence interval for the model.
Reproduced from [1] doi:10.1371/journal.pone.0008772

lost during the early years of life, even before reproductive maturity is achieved. These data can also be used to calculate the number of follicles being lost to either growth or atresia per month in women with a larger or smaller follicle complement. Such analysis indicates that in the ovaries of the "average" woman, with expected age of menopause of 51 years, some 900 follicles will start to grow each month at the peak of this activity (which is at age 14 years), declining to 200 per month at age 35. In women with a high number of follicles, this number is approximately 1900 follicles a month at age 35, whereas in women at the lower end of the still normal range (i.e. with expected age of menopause 42 years) it is approximately 26 follicles a month at the same age, thus less than one a day. This has implications for understanding the range of normality across the major milestones of reproductive life. In this context it has been proposed that women become essentially sterile some 10 years before the menopause and sub-fertile a further 10 years before that [2]. If one considers the range of age at menopause, it will rapidly become clear that the age at which a women may become sub-fertile will also vary considerably, and this also highlights that the reproductive lifespan, i.e. the interval between puberty and this proposed time of sub-fertility, will be relatively brief in women destined to go through a menopause in their early 40s.

Measurement of the ovarian reserve

From these considerations, the size of the remaining follicle pool is clearly a major determinant of age at menopause and indeed of time to menopause, although the rate of loss is also an essential consideration. The size of the ovarian reserve is starting to become clinically assessable. Analysis of the rate of loss cannot be determined from single measurements, although it can be extrapolated with repeated measures over time. Data are starting

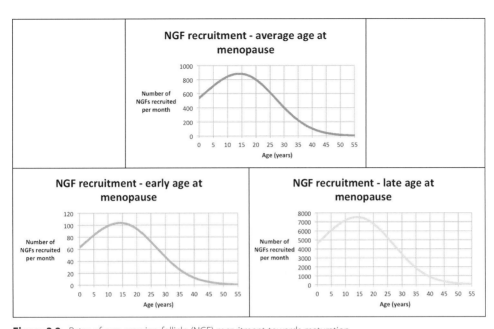

Figure 2.2. Rates of non-growing follicle (NGF) recruitment towards maturation.
Each sub-figure describes the absolute number of NGFs recruited per month, for ages from birth to 55 years, based on population decline predicted by the model shown in Figure 2.1. The red curve denotes recruitment for "average" women with menopause aged 51; maximum recruitment of 880 follicles per month occurs at 14 years 2 months, falling to 221 per month at age 35. The green and yellow curves denote recruitment for women who will have an early or late menopause respectively (42 and 58 years respectively). These indicate maximum recruitment of 104 follicles vs 7,520 follicles per month, at 14 years 2 months, falling to 26 and 1,900 per month at age 35.
Reproduced from [1] doi:10.1371/journal.pone.0008772

to emerge as to the value of measuring the ovarian reserve in the context of predicting the menopause, although this field remains in its infancy. It is therefore not possible to predict "how long Sarah will be fertile for."

Before addressing how one might measure the ovarian reserve, it is important to discuss what is meant by the term. In essence, it is used to mean two separate although related aspects of ovarian biology. Most commonly in the literature, and generally in the context of studies involving assisted reproduction, the ovarian reserve is used to mean the number of follicles that can be recruited to grow by supraphysiological doses of FSH, i.e. as administered during superovulation for IVF. This is a very valuable measure as it will predict the number of oocytes that will be obtained after superovulation, and can be used to identify women either at risk of over response and therefore ovarian hyperstimulation syndrome, or conversely those whose response is less than their age or other markers of ovarian function would have otherwise predicted. The follicles identified through this usage are already at an advanced, antral stage of gonadotropin-dependent growth and probably have been in the growth phase for many weeks already. The second usage of the term ovarian reserve is used to mean the size of the primordial follicle pool. This is a more purist biological usage and thus while perhaps ultimately more correct, its usage in clinical practice is limited as the primordial follicle pool can only be determined at present by histologic analysis, and not *in vivo*. The size of the two follicle pools is related under normal circumstances, although the relationship between the two may well vary in different physiological and pathological states, for example in childhood versus post-pubertally, and in normal ovaries versus common disorders such as hypothalamic amenorrhea, polycystic ovary syndrome as well as for example during hormonal contraceptive use.

The assessment of the ovarian reserve has long been a goal in reproductive medicine, particularly in assisted reproduction, to optimize the prediction of the response of an individual woman. It can be used to improve the safety and effectiveness of superovulation regimes, and in the development of new regimes. As the ovarian reserve declines with age, then age is itself a measure of the ovarian reserve. It also includes an aspect of the quality of the oocytes within that reserve, reflected clinically in the increasing risk of non-conception, miscarriage and chromosomally abnormal conceptions with age. It does not, of course, allow individualization and therefore a range of biochemical and biophysical tests have been explored over the years. It has long been recognized that serum FSH increases with age and a high FSH is one of the diagnostic tests of the menopause, i.e. loss of the ovarian reserve. The biological function of FSH, however, is to regulate antral stages, follicle growth and selection such that only a single follicle emerges as dominant and mono-ovulation occurs, and the early stages of follicle growth are gonadotropin independent. Follicle stimulating hormone remains a useful screening test in that a high FSH predicts a poor ovarian response at IVF, but the accuracy of this prediction is poor and the marked cycle-to-cycle variation within a single woman (as well as variation through the menstrual cycle) has led to a search for more robust indices. Measuring Sarah's FSH would be of little value in predicting her fertile life, although a high value would indicate that it is short. Estradiol is even less use as its production largely reflects the function of the pre-ovulatory follicle of that particular menstrual cycle and not any measure of the ovarian reserve. Inhibin B was identified as a product of the granulosa cells of smaller follicles and indeed is of predictive value in assisted reproduction. It also declines prior to the menopause although this decline is relatively late. The key physiological role of inhibin B is the negative regulation of FSH secretion particularly in the early follicular phase, so the two hormones are functionally interrelated. The identification of anti-Müllerian hormone (AMH) as a product of smaller preantral as well as early antral follicles has led to dramatic development in our ability to clinically assess the ovarian reserve and it has become of routine use in many IVF clinics around the world [3]. AMH is produced by granulosa cells of the follicles as soon as they start to grow, although not by primordial follicles (Figure 2.3). While the concentration of AMH in blood reflects the size of the true as well as the functional ovarian reserve, the relationship with the true ovarian reserve is therefore indirect. As it is produced by smaller and therefore less gonadotropin-dependent follicles, its concentration through the menstrual cycle is much less variable than that of the aforementioned reproductive hormones. While there is some variability, this is generally regarded as not clinically significant as relatively few women will be misclassified; this is a very substantial practical clinical advantage particularly where transvaginal ultrasound (to measure antral follicle count) is not immediately available.

Predicting the menopause

There have now been several studies which have assessed the role of AMH in predicting the menopause. These initially demonstrated that AMH declines to undetectable concentrations some 5 years before the menopause and that it was a more accurate predictor of time to an age at final menstrual period than either FSH or inhibin B. Subsequent studies have

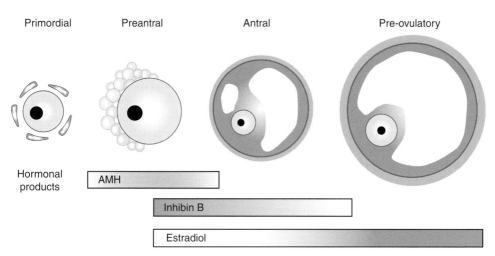

Figure 2.3. Illustration of changing hormone production by the developing follicle. AMH is produced by follicles as soon as they start to grow, but declines sharply at approximately 8–10 mm diameter. Inhibin B is predominantly produced by smaller antral follicles, whereas estradiol production increases through the antral stages to ovulation.

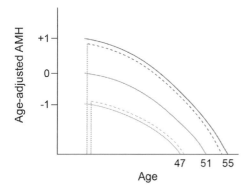

Figure 2.4. Schematic representation of the relationship between AMH and time to menopause. The lines represent the decline in age-adjusted AMH (depicted in standard deviations from the mean) with increasing age, with the menopause occurring when the line crosses the abscissa (indicative values only for mean ± 1 SD). The black, gray and light gray lines indicate the trajectory of women with high, average and low age-adjusted AMH respectively. The dotted lines represent two women of similar age but different age-adjusted AMH: plotting their age against age-adjusted AMH shows which line they are predicted to follow and hence anticipated age at menopause.

confirmed and strengthened this finding and although they show a clear relationship between AMH measured at any adult age and subsequent age at menopause, the predictive ability is relatively modest [4, 5]. It has also been demonstrated that interpretation of AMH concentration is not independent of age, thus a given AMH concentration predicts different age at menopause according to the age of the woman. AMH therefore needs to be age-adjusted (Figure 2.4). This relationship appears to be very clear on a population basis, but while the published studies are promising, the data show very substantial variability and do not appear sufficiently robust to allow an individual woman to have her AMH measured and derive from that a clear and accurate prediction of the age at which she will become menopausal. This may reflect variability in the relationship between AMH and the true ovarian reserve between individual women, but perhaps less explored is the impact of variation in the rate of decline of AMH (and indeed of the ovarian reserve) which may well vary with time within an individual woman, as well as between different women.

An additional problem in this area has been the assays that are available. The current generation of AMH assays are not sufficiently sensitive to detect AMH in the last 5 years before the menopause, although new assays are becoming available that address this. There are also issues of standardization, and no internationally accepted calibration standard exists. It is clear, however, that AMH has substantial promise in this regard and that technical improvements and further large prospective studies will clarify how accurately AMH can be used to predict the menopause. Similar considerations apply to the use of AMH in diagnosing the menopause: normal women currently have undetectable AMH for several years before the menopause, and there are only scant data available regarding AMH in other conditions that present with amenorrhea, other than in polycystic ovary syndrome where AMH levels are high. Thus while measuring Sarah's AMH would be indicative, its accuracy is very unclear.

Biophysical, i.e. ultrasound, markers of the ovarian reserve have also been developed. Both ovarian volume and antral follicle count (AFC) decline with age and both predict the response in assisted reproduction. AFC in particular is of routine value in this context, promoted by its wide availability in the reproductive medicine clinic. Outwith that, and particularly in general practice, ultrasound is less immediately available and biochemical tests may be more useful. There is a close relationship between AFC and AMH and indeed the two markers can be regarded as essentially measuring the same thing, i.e. the population/activity of the small antral follicle pool, as AMH is produced by the granulosa cells of the small follicles that are being counted by ultrasound. Although in skilled hands AFC is as accurate a predictor of ovarian response as AMH, there is much larger opportunity for inter-individual variation and the results obtained are also dependent on the technical quality of the instrument, which is changing with time. Consequently an AFC count carried out by transvaginal ultrasound is of limited value in answering Sarah's question.

Prediction in special circumstances

The above discussion relates primarily to the value of currently available markers in normal healthy women. Specific considerations may apply in certain pathological states; these include women whose ovarian reserve may be damaged iatrogenically either by surgery or chemotherapeutic agents, or in other diseases. Of particular importance in the latter are women who are either identified as being at risk of premature ovarian insufficiency (POI), for example on the basis of family history or risk factors such as having anti-ovarian antibodies, and potentially in the future on the basis of identification of genetic susceptibility.

Anti-Müllerian hormone declines rapidly during chemotherapy, and recovery thereafter is dependent on the gonadotoxicity of the regimen administered. Thus, women treated with alkylating agent-based therapies show much less recovery than those with non-alkylating regimes [6]. More importantly, AMH measured before the administration of chemotherapy has been shown to predict long-term ovarian function post chemotherapy, thus women still menstruating several years after chemotherapy have markedly higher AMH concentrations pretreatment than those who become and remain amenorrheic after chemotherapy [7]. In this context AMH seems a more accurate predictor than age (Figure 2.5) although larger studies are required to fully explore this relationship. These data therefore support the contention that AMH may become valuable in predicting the risk of menopause after cancer therapy. It may also have application in the pediatric oncology context. Prior to puberty, current reproductive hormones are very low but AMH is readily detectable in serum of all healthy girls, and indeed rises steadily through childhood [8]. As in adults, chemotherapy results in a marked decline in serum AMH in girls and adolescents, with very

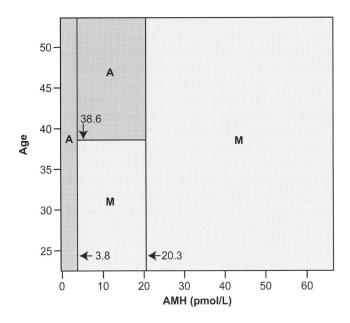

Figure 2.5. Classification mosaic chart for ongoing menses (M) or chemotherapy-related amenorrhea (A) using pre-chemotherapy serum AMH and chronological age as predictor variables, in women with early breast cancer.
The primary cut-off values are both for AMH. Between these AMH levels there is an age threshold, above which amenorrhea is predicted and below which ongoing menses are predicted. The classification schema has a sensitivity of 98.2% and specificity of 80.0%. Reprinted with permission from Anderson *et al.* 2013, *Eur J Cancer* [7].

variable recovery reflecting the predicted gonadotoxicity of the administered regimen [9]. This may well be of use in identifying girls who have suffered POI at a very early age and in whom endocrine therapy to induce puberty can then be started at an earlier age than might previously have been the case. There are as yet no data linking pretreatment AMH with early menopause in childhood cancer survivors. Such a relationship would be expected, but will be complicated by the fact that AMH rises during childhood (as opposed to the steady fall during adulthood), with peak levels at approximately 24 years. During puberty AMH shows a plateau or even slight fall before rising further, thus there are changing relationships between AMH and the ovarian reserve during these periods of development, which are as yet incompletely understood.

Women at risk of POI provide a particularly challenging context in which to address these markers. While there are a wide range of genes that have been identified in animal studies to cause POI, with very few exceptions these have not entered clinical practice. Mother's age at menopause remains a guide, but although this is widely recognized, there are few data assessing its accuracy. Furthermore, in most cases the diagnosis of POI by definition indicates loss of the ovarian reserve that has already happened, and it is a much rarer situation when a woman is identified who is at risk of POI while still having a relatively normal ovarian reserve. Anti-Müllerian hormone in particular may be of value in identifying women whose ovarian reserve is very low, and in the presence of another factor indicating a risk of POI it would seem likely that this would be of clinical use. However, as discussed above, the predictive value of measurement of AMH under these circumstances is of unknown accuracy.

Insuring against oocyte loss

The question arises as to whether one can effectively insure against the inevitable age-related loss of oocyte quality and quantity. For a single woman like Sarah, this essentially means oocyte vitrification, often termed "social egg freezing." The other potential option would be embryo cryopreservation (of course requiring sperm from either a partner or a donor to fertilize the oocytes) or ovarian tissue cryopreservation. The latter is not used in this context, although it is becoming increasingly widely used for young women and indeed prepubertal girls facing chemotherapy-induced ovarian failure. Previously, slow oocyte cryopreservation was possible but relatively ineffective, but with modern vitrification techniques the oocyte viability is essentially as good as that of unfrozen oocytes. Indeed vitrified oocyte banks are increasingly used in IVF centres with large oocyte donation programs. Vitrification involves the extremely rapid freezing of tissue by immersion in liquid nitrogen, with high concentrations of cryoprotectants. This is, however, a still-developing technology with many technical issues still potentially to be optimized, and very limited data on outcomes of infants born as a result of it [10]. Most of the literature refers to embryo outcome after oocyte vitrification in optimal circumstances, i.e. from oocytes donated by young women, and the most important determinant will be the woman's age. Oocyte vitrification is, however, no longer considered experimental by the European Society of Human Reproduction and Embryology and the American Society of Reproductive Medicine. These organizations' guidelines however, highlight the lack of published data on age-specific success rates in terms of live births achieved and the possibility that this technique may have limited success in those older women who are most interested in it.

Calculating the probability of live birth after egg freezing is related to the patient's age and freezing method. An online "egg freezing success calculator" has been developed based on data from 2,265 cycles from 1,805 patients [11], where one enters the patient's age at freezing, number of oocytes frozen, whether with vitrification or slow freezing, and predicts the probability of live birth as a percentage (i-fertility.net). This indicates that if Sarah has 10 eggs frozen by vitrification at her current age of 34, then her probability of live birth is a modest 21.7%.

References

1. Wallace WH, Kelsey TW. Human ovarian reserve from conception to the menopause. *PLoS ONE* 2010; **5**: e8772.

2. Broekmans FJ, Soules MR, Fauser BC. Ovarian aging: mechanisms and clinical consequences. *Endocr Rev* 2009; **30**: 465–93.

3. Dewailly D, Andersen CY, Balen A, *et al.* The physiology and clinical utility of anti-Mullerian hormone in women. *Hum Reprod Update* 2014; **20**: 370–85.

4. Freeman EW, Sammel MD, Lin H, *et al.* Anti-Mullerian hormone as a predictor of time to menopause in late reproductive age women. *J Clin Endocrinol Metab* 2012; **97**: 1673–80.

5. Tehrani FR, Solaymani-Dodaran M, Tohidi M, *et al.* Modeling age at menopause using serum concentration of anti-Mullerian hormone. *J Clin Endocrinol Metab* 2013; **98**: 729–35.

6. Decanter C, Morschhauser F, Pigny P, *et al.* Anti-Mullerian hormone follow-up in young women treated by chemotherapy for lymphoma: preliminary results. *Reprod Biomed Online* 2010; **20**: 280–5.

7. Anderson RA, Rosendahl M, Kelsey TW, *et al.* Pretreatment anti-Mullerian hormone predicts for loss of ovarian function after chemotherapy for early breast cancer. *Eur J Cancer* 2013; **49**: 3404–11.

8. Kelsey TW, Wright P, Nelson SM, *et al.* A validated model of serum anti-Müllerian hormone from conception to menopause. *PLoS ONE* 2011; **6**: e22024.

9. Brougham MF, Crofton PM, Johnson EJ, *et al.* Anti-Mullerian hormone is a

marker of gonadotoxicity in pre- and postpubertal girls treated for cancer: a prospective study. *J Clin Endocrinol Metab* 2012; **97**: 2059–67.

10. Edgar DH, Gook DA. A critical appraisal of cryopreservation (slow cooling versus vitrification) of human oocytes and embryos. *Hum Reprod Update* 2012; **18**: 536–54.

11. Cil AP, Bang H, Oktay K. Age-specific probability of live birth with oocyte cryopreservation: an individual patient data meta-analysis. *Fertil Steril* 2013; **100**: 492–9.

The history and politics of menopause

Barry G. Wren

Introduction

The history and management of the menopause has, for thousands of years, been bound up in the mystique surrounding the presence or absence of the regular loss of vaginal blood from a woman [1, 2].

Early accounts that mentioned the role of menstruation appear to suggest that the regular loss of blood was regarded as nature's mechanism to purge the female body of foul and poisonous fluids. As a result, menstrual blood was regarded as being unclean, revolting and toxic, and to be avoided whenever possible. This fear of menstrual blood influenced and dictated the social and political role that women were allocated in a community and eventually resulted in many unnecessary and cruel treatments [1]. Equally, the absence of regular menstruation with a resultant failure to rid the body of toxins was regarded as the reason some women went "mad" or developed antisocial behavior.

From the pre-Christian era to the 19th century, knowledge about a woman's menstrual activity and its causes was dominated by a male perception of how it came about, what was its purpose and what happened when a woman stopped menstruating.

Early Greek and Roman physicians felt that menstrual blood was necessary to rid the female body of "bad humors" and that the symptoms of the menopause came about because the accumulated toxins in the menstrual blood were not being released.

The symptoms of menopause – episodes of heat, emotional mood swings, depression, sexual dysfunction and even osteoporotic fractures have been mentioned in early texts by the ancient Hippocratic and the Aristotle schools of health and hygiene, both of which postulated that as a woman aged, she was no longer capable of producing the nourishment necessary to form menstrual blood [1, 2]. For that reason these physicians prescribed special diets including spices, fungi and herbs to treat those women who suffered from psychological and vasomotor symptoms.

Later physicians postulated that a man sweats to rid himself of his impurities whereas a woman bleeds. The absence of blood at the menopause was regarded as a "negative" as the impurities and toxins were thought to be retained within the body and to wreak havoc in it. To rid the body of accumulated toxins, it was the advice of some physicians to treat women by bleeding, sometimes by venesection but sometimes by incisions in the vagina.

The Biblical description of menstruation and its effect suggests it was regarded with repellence. In Leviticus 15, menstrual discharge is described "when a woman has a discharge

Managing the Menopause: 21st Century Solutions, ed. Nick Panay, Paula Briggs, and Gab Kovacs. Published by Cambridge University Press. © Cambridge University Press 2015.

of blood which is her regular discharge from her body, she shall be in her impurity for 7 days, and whoever touches her shall be unclean until the evening."

Early education regarding human physiology was taught by monks and philosophers, and one of the earliest written records of their interpretation of menstruation is found in the *Aberdeen Bestiary* in the 12th century. The following is a description by these monks of their understanding of menstruation [2]:

> The menstrual flow is the superfluous blood of a woman. It is called menstrua from the cycle of the light of the moon, which regularly brings about this flow. For the Greek word for 'moon' is mene; menstruation is also called muliebria, 'womanly business'. For the woman is the only creature which menstruates. When they come into contact with menstrual blood, crops do not put forth shoots, wine turns sour, grasses die, trees lose their fruit, iron is corrupted by rust, copper blackens, if dogs eat it they become rabid. Asphalt glue, which cannot be melted by fire or dissolved by water, when it is tainted by this blood, disintegrates by itself.

With such a stigma associated with menstruation, it is little wonder that women looked forward to reaching that time in life when they no longer were afflicted with the "curse." But their travails were not over. In 1597, when Sir William Monson's wife consulted Simon Forman, "she had not had her curse and the menstrual blood runneth to her head." He recorded, that she was "much subject to melancholy and full of fancies" [2].

One of the first gynecologic handbooks, written by a woman, described the menopause as a major cause of ill health "because there are many women who (have) numerous diverse illnesses, some of them almost fatal."

After the 12th century, it was also noted in many parish and town records that older women were being set upon because they were perceived as being responsible for some of the misfortunes to their neighbors. Most were widows or single women who apparently had no gainful occupation, or who lacked family support and who frequently were suffering major physical and health problems, who had lost most (if not all) of their teeth, a number who had developed osteoporotic crush fractures of their spine (resulting in the development of a dowager's hump), and who may have unfortunately developed marked psychological or mental disturbance. These were the crones who barely found sufficient food and shelter to survive in villages and towns during the Middle Ages. If a disaster occurred in a village or a crop failed, it was common for the disaster to be blamed on a witch. When identifying a witch in those medieval times one of the crones was frequently nominated as the culprit. In the 400 years between the 14th and 18th century, it is estimated that some 40,000–60,000 women were burnt at the stake after being accused of witchcraft.

Almost 90% of witches suffering this horrendous fate were women over the age of 65 years! Being accused of witchcraft was almost universally reserved for postmenopausal women and it is easily understood why women were anxious to find some cure for the effects of estrogen deficiency. It is interesting to note that very few men developed the physical stigmata that resulted in the necessity of being tied to a stake in a bonfire.

During 2,000 to 3,000 years, extending from recorded historical times to the 20th century, a variety of therapy programs were prescribed to treat some of the individual symptoms which a woman had been experiencing, all with varying degrees of success.

Chamomile, vitex (chaste tree), sage leaf, panax ginseng, licorice, tribulus, motherwort, dandelion and hypericum perforatum (St. John's wort) were just some of the plants used extensively by Chinese and Indian herbalists in pre-Christian times, while others mixed various combinations of herbs, mushrooms and plant roots to treat the "instability" experienced by an older woman. The first pharmacopeia (the Shennong Bencao Jing) was written during the Han Dynasty (about 200 years BC) and described a variety of plant and fungal extracts to maintain and improve the body equilibrium [1]. Lingzhi was the fungus of choice for treating most women with what could be considered menopausal symptoms. Even today, extracts of these plants and fungi are often the preferred treatment regimens by a very large number of women, not only in Asian countries but also in Western society.

Other cultures (including American Indians who used an extract of black cohosh to reduce fever, sweats and flashes) used a variety of herbs and plant extracts to relieve symptoms of menopause and, in recent times, extracts of these plants have been studied in order to determine if any contain chemicals that can be applied in "modern" medicine.

Dong Quai, Bupleurum, Atractylodes, ginger and Salvia roots have all been used in various combinations to produce Chinese herbal medicines to treat menopause symptoms but no single substance has been identified as having a major and sustained influence on reducing the distressing symptoms of estrogen deficiency.

These plant and herbal preparations were the only medications available for symptoms peculiar to older women during this time in history, but unfortunately they do not relieve the complaints of the vast majority of contemporary women who continue to experience the severe or disabling effects of hormone deficiency. It is only in the last 150 years that a concerted effort has been made to understand the menopause and to determine the cause so that a program of treatment, which would control the symptoms, could be developed.

History of the menopause in the 19th century

In the early 19th century French physicians observed a connection between the development of flashes and the menopause, and appear to have been the first to clinically note that the failure of ovarian activity and the cessation of menstruation coincided with the onset of menopausal symptoms.

The English physician John Tilt, who had studied in France in the 1820s, was responsible for nominating the ovary as being the source of "substances" that caused menstruation, pregnancy and menopause, and believed that the ovaries caused "any madness" that afflicted women during the peri menopause. He promoted the hypothesis that most disabilities suffered by women were ovarian in origin and could be cured by surgical removal of the ovaries, an operation in which he and other surgeons became adept. This surgical "cure" of psychological misbehavior in women, which had a high death rate, showed little evidence of improved behavior, no relief of symptoms and worst of all, created a marked loss of a woman's sexual desire [1, 2].

Fortunately, by 1880, this barbarous operation had been totally abandoned as a treatment of hysteria and female psychiatric disorders.

In spite of evidence that these bizarre interventions were cruel and unnecessary, a woman of the 19th century, entering her menopause, continued to be treated in a shameful way by doctors and it was not until social changes and feminine pressure encouraged doctors to investigate and view the menopause as a life event requiring "treatment," that advances and understanding occurred.

The 20th century introduced the beginning of detailed investigations into hormones and their importance in maintaining the health of the individual, with the initial major breakthrough in endocrinology taking place in understanding the cause and treatment of diabetes, of thyroid function and finally in the 1930s, also of the menopause.

The influence of sexuality in postmenopause

For hundreds of years, when a woman became menopausal and her vagina became dry or tight, lacking the normal elasticity necessary for sexual intercourse – when she became osteoporotic or when she developed mental or psychological dysfunction – it became acceptable in some societies for a married man to take a younger mistress in order to satisfy his sexual desires and inclination.

During the 16th, 17th and 18th centuries unconstrained sexual activity between consenting adults was accepted as normal; to be enjoyed by both men and women, with plays and books being written regarding the pleasure to be obtained by such indulgence both within and outside marriage.

It was not until the Victorian era that such "licentious" attitudes began to change and extramarital relationships were frowned upon. So censorious was the attitude of these puritanical guardians that even within marriage, sexual enjoyment was regarded as a sign of wanton behavior [1].

Sexual enjoyment or promiscuity, particularly by a postmenopausal woman, was regarded as being un-Godly and required both surgical and spiritual intervention. The promiscuous behavior of some women was regarded as "an ominous sign of national decay."

It was not until the later stages of the 19th century that women began to express their desire to contribute to, and enjoy, a different role in society. Some women even declared their desire to participate in sexual activity purely for pleasure! Unfortunately because of atrophic changes in their vagina this became impossible for a large number of them who, having run out of eggs in their ovaries, had entered their menopause and were lacking estrogen.

Women not only joined suffragette groups, but began demanding some medical therapy to prevent hot flashes, sweats and insomnia, as well as to improve the dry, inelastic lining of their vagina. Sexual intercourse for postmenopausal women had become a painful and distressing event and this not only resulted in loss of libido but also accentuated marital conflict and their partner's infidelity. The need to improve the quality of life and the sexual anatomy of postmenopausal women had become not only a medical issue but a social issue as well.

As a result, by the 1940s the role of estrogen in maintaining a woman's health became evident and the development of modern hormone replacement therapy was initiated. Treatment regimens using various estrogen formats all achieved a reliable reputation after undergoing intense research involving detailed scrutiny to ensure the integrity of results.

A woman of the 21st century usually decides to begin estrogen-based hormone therapy because she is experiencing hot flashes, sweats, insomnia or marked vaginal discomfort as she enters the menopause.

However, a series of adverse reports in 2002 and 2003 suggesting that estrogen therapy caused breast cancer [3, 4] has achieved prominence, and as a result a "climate of fear" has developed regarding the use of hormone therapy.

Because of the fear that hormone therapy is responsible for adverse events such as breast cancer, thrombosis and heart attacks, a number of women have turned once again to the use of plant extracts to treat the distressing symptoms of menopause and to avoid the perceived risks.

To take advantage of the fears related to the use of regular HRT, various fungal, herbal and other plant extracts have been extensively promoted and proclaimed as being viable alternative therapies. Some of the claims have been based on the knowledge that the plants contain large amounts of phyto estrogens which are frequently recommended as having a beneficial effect on symptoms, while others have relied on the fact that some plant extracts have been used in traditional medicine for generations. For many individuals suffering severe symptoms, the success of these plant extracts has been less than expected or as advertised, but in spite of negative findings, a large number of women have continued to buy and use these alternative plant therapies instead of using synthesized human hormones.

Estrogens

Estrogen is the name given to a group of *natural* hormones that include estradiol, estrone and estriol. Estradiol is the primary estrogen produced by the ovary. It is the most potent estrogen and is the estrogen most used in HRT. Estradiol is reduced by enzymes in the body to the weaker estrogen *estrone* and then to the even weaker estrogen *estriol.*

Initially the production and administration of natural (bio-identical) estrogen proved expensive and unreliable because of the rapid degradation of the hormone by enzymes in the gut and the liver. For that reason scientists devoted considerable effort in designing synthetic stable hormones that could be employed in managing the menopause.

In 1936 in the UK Professor Dodds invented a stable synthetic estrogen called diethyl-stilboestrol (DES), followed soon after by the German scientists Inhoffen and Hohlweg who, in 1938, invented *ethinyl estradiol* [2].

In the late 1930s, it was recognized that pregnant mares produced copious amounts of equine estrogens, of which the major portion was the biologically inert estrone sulfate. The Ayerst/Wyeth Pharmaceutical Company extracted the conglomerate of equine estrogens from pregnant mares' urine, and by 1942, it was marketing the complex of estrogens as Premarin.

Bio-identical estradiol, now readily synthesized in a laboratory, has been used in most commercial pharmaceutical preparations of hormone therapy for over 50 years. However, because oral estradiol is rapidly metabolized in the gut to the less active molecule estrone, scientists have developed a method to inhibit the degradation of the molecule by esterifying the estradiol molecule (estradiol valerate, estradiol hemihydrate, etc.). This esterification allows for the administration of a lower dose of an estradiol that lasts longer (for between 10 and 16 hours) and is more effective, providing a safer level of estradiol to be taken by mouth.

In 1965, Professor Diczfalusy in Sweden discovered estetrol, a fetal estrogen that is produced only in the liver of a fetus. Estetrol is a potent estrogen that has the ability to protect bone from osteoporosis as well as inhibiting symptoms of the menopause. In research using animals, estetrol also appeared to be capable of protecting against breast cancer. Estetrol may prove to be the most effective estrogen for the treatment of a post-menopausal woman, but this requires further research to determine its full potential.

Progesterone/progestogens

Bio-identical progesterone

In 1937, a biochemical scientist, Russell Marker, described the chemical process that allowed him to synthesize and manufacture bio-identical progesterone from a substrate called diosgenin. Diosgenin is found in many plants but the Mexican wild yam contained the highest quantity and from this Marker was able provide clinicians with a plentiful supply of bio-identical progesterone for clinical use.

Unfortunately oral progesterone is very rapidly metabolized by enzymes in the gut and liver, to excretory metabolites that have no protective effect on the endometrium.

Therefore the development of stable chemicals with a progesterone-like action became a necessity to enable doctors to safely treat a post menopausal woman with estrogen [2].

Progestogen is the name applied to any chemical which induces a progesterone-like effect on the uterine endometrium. Over the past 60 years a large number of progestogens have been developed and used in oral contraceptives as well as in the majority of commercially designed menopause therapy programs.

The history of hormone replacement therapy

Initially, when developing therapies to treat menopausal symptoms, bio-identical progesterone was not considered because prior research had demonstrated poor results when determining the amount required to inhibit the endometrium. The availability of more stable and cheaper synthesized progestogens resulted in these compounds being employed to protect the endometrium.

By the late 1960s, hormone therapy was widely accepted and women were told that their menopause problems could be solved. Dr. Robert A. Wilson published his book *Feminine Forever* [5] and women of the world embraced the use of HRT.

Substantial clinical evidence from studies designed to observe the effect of estrogen on the health of postmenopausal women had begun to accumulate, suggesting that estrogen therapy, begun at the time of the menopause, not only controlled symptoms but reduced the risk of osteoporosis and fractures in a woman, and appeared to reduce the incidence of atherosclerosis and heart attacks.

Pharmaceutical companies competed to produce better and more varied therapeutic regimens, but the plethora of treatment options was dramatically interrupted in 2002 following the publication of the Women's Health Initiative (WHI) Study with the associated hysteria and fear engendered by claims that hormones caused breast cancer.

The Women's Health Initiative Study

Early in life, I had noticed that no event is ever correctly reported in a newspaper

George Orwell

In 1991, the Director of the National Institutes of Health in the USA, Dr. Bernadine Healy, initiated a large project, The Women's Health Initiative (WHI), with a view to analyzing and reporting on the risks and benefits of a variety of strategies that were used to influence the health of women after they had passed the menopause. This study is believed to be the largest and most expensive clinical research ever conducted into women's health.

The results from this study have been of immense value in increasing an understanding and appreciation of the events that influence the health and welfare of postmenopausal women, as well as the factors that have a beneficial or an adverse effect on longevity. Part of the WHI Study involved observing the effect of hormone therapy on the health of postmenopausal women, and the results obtained from the studies based on this group of women have been the focus of much controversy and confusion in deciding how to manage the menopause.

Between 1993 and 1998 the WHI Study enrolled 161,809 women. Of these, 16,608 who still had their uterus intact were allocated to receive either Premarin plus Provera (medroxyprogesterone acetate) or a placebo, while a further 10,739 who had had their uterus removed by hysterectomy, were to receive Premarin only or a placebo.

On July 17, 2002, the first of many articles written by the WHI Writing Group responsible for collating and reporting on the outcome of the WHI Study investigating the effect of Premarin and Provera on the long-term health of postmenopausal women was published in the *Journal of the American Medical Association* (*JAMA*) [3].

Unfortunately the Writing Group, in an extraordinary decision, released their results to a select group of health reporters on July 10, 2002, one week prior to publication of the scientific evidence in the *JAMA*. The headlines, using terminology provided by the Writing Group, caused consternation and panic among women around the world when the media reported a 26% increase in breast cancer, a 29% increase in heart attacks and a 41% increase in stroke among women using the combined Premarin/Provera therapy.

When clinicians were able to read and critically review the paper in the *JAMA* one week after its extraordinary release to the media, it was obvious the results had been deliberately reported in relative values rather than absolute figures. The actual numbers were not considered to be alarming when it was realized that over 65% of women recruited to the study were over the age of 60 years (10–30 years after their menopause), 70% were overweight, 36% were being treated for hypertension and about 15–20% were being treated for other medical problems including diabetes, hypercholesterolemia and prior heart disease. None of the women had hot flashes, sweats or complained of dyspareunia.

When clinicians reviewed the actual number of adverse events it was found that there was only eight extra cases of breast cancers in 10,000 women, seven extra heart attacks in 10,000 and eight cases of thrombosis in 10,000.

The consensus review of the WHI report in 2002 was that it appeared to have been a deliberate attempt to magnify the adverse events and to strike fear into the minds of those women and their clinicians who were using HRT. Although the increase in individual adverse events was not statistically significant, the manner of presentation to the media resulted in a major blow to the use of estrogen therapy used to improve the quality of life for postmenopausal women.

In a related article published in *The Lancet* in August 2003, the senior author of the Million Women Study (MWS) claimed that 20,000 new cases of breast cancer had occurred in Britain as a result of the use of HRT [4]. This claim was based on an analysis of self-reported data from a cohort of women attending for their regular mammogram in the UK and the data were reviewed and published by a group of epidemiologists. As with the WHI Study 1 year previously, the MWS attracted a large amount of adverse comments about HRT.

In 2011 a highly critical review of the series of MWS papers was published [6]. The authors of this critical review wrote:

> In spite of the massive size of the Million Women Study the findings for the estrogen plus progestogen, and for the unopposed estrogen therapy, did not satisfy the criteria of time order, information bias, confounding, statistical stability and strength of association, duration-response, internal consistency, external consistency or biological plausibility. If selection bias had altered the identification of breast cancer by as little as 0.3/1,000 per year, the apparent risks associated with hormone therapy would have been nullified.

Initially estrogen was blamed for the spurious increase in breast cancer, despite a WHI Study in 2004 involving 10,700 women, showing that women using unopposed Premarin for almost 7 years had a 23% decrease in the risk of breast cancer (a fall from 33 to 26 per

10,000 per year) [7]. Because of that study, blame for breast cancer was then directed towards the progestogen/progestin (medroxyprogesterone acetate–Provera) being used.

But the stigma that breast cancer was caused by estrogen as claimed in the original WHI paper, was not absolved. Women, and even some doctors, were still convinced that estrogen actually caused breast cancer. It has taken more than 10 years for some clinicians to realize that promotion of growth is different to initiation of breast cancer.

In 2011 the women involved in the WHI Premarin-only study were reviewed for possible adverse events. It was found that after almost 11 years the risk of stroke was not increased, the risk of deep venous thrombosis was decreased, the reduction in the risk of heart attacks, bowel cancer and hip fracture was not altered while the risk of a woman developing breast cancer was still reduced by 23%.

Professor Henry Burger, past Director of the Prince Henry's Institute of Medical Research, and Professor of Endocrinology at Monash University, Melbourne, commented on the unusual circumstances in which the initial WHI results were released at a press conference held a week before any health professionals or the general community had an opportunity to examine the data that had led to the dramatic and frightening media headlines. He expressed his opinion "that the original announcements lacked objectivity and appeared motivated by a strong wish to cast hormone therapy in the worst possible light" [2].

Professor Bluming from the USA, who wrote in *The Cancer Journal*, supported this point of view [2]:

> It is difficult to resist the conclusion that the WHI investigators have been doing everything they could to wring the bleakest possible interpretation from their recalcitrant data ... reports attributing an increased risk of breast cancer, cardiac events and Alzheimer's disease to the administration of HRT required critical review, not blind acceptance.

Consequences of the WHI Study

When the WHI Study was published in 2002 and estrogen therapy received such adverse publicity, a very large number of women immediately stopped using HRT in the belief that by avoiding estrogen therapy, they would avoid developing breast cancer.

Ten years later, research confirms what was feared may occur when a woman stops her HRT. The Kaiser Permanente Health Organization in Southern California carried out a longitudinal study of 80,955 postmenopausal women. During a mean of 6.5 years of follow-up after the release of the WHI findings it was found that hip fracture increased by 55% among those who ceased HRT compared with those who continued on their estrogen therapy [8].

As estrogen therapy begun at the time of the menopause and during the "window of opportunity" is known to reduce the risk for a woman developing cardiovascular disease, osteoporosis and possibly also of dementia, a similar increase in these events is expected to be recorded among women who ceased their HRT because of the scare tactics associated with WHI and the MWS.

One of the major consequences of the WHI Study and the resulting furore and confused debate is that most discussion and argument has centred on the 5–10 years surrounding the actual menopause rather than how therapy can be safely administered to prevent the onset of osteoporosis, cardiovascular disease, dementia and pelvic tissue atrophy in women over the age of 65 years. Women wish to maintain their femininity, their beauty and their sexuality into advanced age, but because various groups and individuals have extrapolated data from inappropriate studies in order to alarm both doctors and their female patients, the women who would otherwise be able to choose whether they wished to use hormone therapy to avoid adverse changes as they age are now being denied this opportunity. The reason some research reports are expressed as negative or fixed opinions is likely to be related to individual biases rather than altruism.

Conclusion

Menstruation and the changes that occur because of the menopause have long been a mystery to philosophers and males in general. For over 2,000 years, men have hypothesized as to why women menstruated and as a consequence some distressing, useless and cruel therapies were administered to women in order to relieve both postmenopausal and menstrual adverse symptoms.

It was not until the 20th century that scientific research identified the hormonal changes involved in menstruation, and the benefit achieved by beginning estrogen therapy during the menopause, in order to develop and maintain the health of women. The introduction of hormone replacement therapy has improved the long-term health of women [9] but there are still many questions to be answered, particularly regarding the ideal route of delivery of estrogens and the development of synthesized steroids (progestogens) and selective estrogen receptor modulators (SERMs) capable of inhibiting abnormal endometrial response as well as maintaining bone, brain and cardiovascular activity.

References

1. Foxcroft L. *Hot Flushes, Cold Science: A History of the Modern Menopause.* London: Granta Books; 2009.

2. Wren BG and Stephenson MM. *Menopause: Change, Choice and HRT.* Sydney: Rockpool Publishing; 2013.

3. Rossouw JE, Anderson GL, Prentice RL, et al. Risks and benefits of estrogen plus progestin in healthy postmenopausal women: principal results from the Women's Health Initiative randomized controlled trial. *JAMA* 2002; **288**: 321–33.

4. Beral V. for the Million Women Study Collaborators. Breast cancer and hormone replacement therapy in the Million Women Study. *Lancet* 2003; **362**: 419–27.

5. Wilson R. *Feminine Forever.* London: WW Allen; 1966.

6. Shapiro S. The million women study: potential biases do not allow uncritical acceptance of the data. *Climacteric* 2004; 7: 3–7.

7. Anderson GL, et al. for the Writing Group for the Women's Health Initiative Study. Effects of conjugated equine estrogen in postmenopausal women with hysterectomy. The Womens Health Initiative randomized controlled trial. *JAMA* 2004; **291**: 1701–12.

8. Karim R, Dell RM, Greene DF, et al.. Hip fracture in post-menopausal women after cessation of hormone therapy: results from a prospective study in a large health management organisation. *Menopause* 2011; **18**: 1172–7.

9. Paganini-Hill A, Corrada MM, Kawas CH. Increased longevity in older users of postmenopausal estrogen therapy: The Leisure World Cohort Study. *Menopause* 2006; **13**: 12–18.

Clinical features of the menopause transition

Paula Briggs and Gab Kovacs

Denise is 47 years old. Recently her periods have become irregular and heavier. She is having hot flashes several times a day and she has been feeling tired and emotional, which she puts down to a poor sleep pattern. She has had to take time off work due to frequent migraine. She has four children and the youngest has just gone to university. She has been crying a lot. Her best friend has advised her to see her general practitioner as she thinks that Denise might be in "the change."

Before considering the various symptoms potentially attributable to the "menopause," some of which Denise may be suffering from, a better understanding of the changes taking place can be gained by reviewing the physiology. This will help define the terminology.

Whilst "menopause" means the "end of menstruation," "menopausal symptoms" refer to a number of different symptoms associated with the climacteric, the transition from mature reproductive function, through the perimenopause to no ovarian follicular function.

Postmenopause is the period a woman enters once she has not menstruated for at least 12 months. However, the hormonal changes leading up to this stage commence several years earlier, and this period is called the "perimenopause" or "menopause transition."

The physiological basis of these changes relates to the changes in a woman's ability to ovulate (Chapter 1). Normal ovulation is the culmination of a complex interaction between the various elements of the hypothalamic-pituitary-ovarian axis. Loss of regulation of these complex hormonal changes results in widely fluctuating levels of estrogen. The loss of a predictable cycle at this time is associated with the development of menopausal symptoms.

Before menopause transition, estrogen and progesterone circulate throughout the body, and have many different effects on various systems, some of which we do not necessarily understand as yet. The development of the Graafian follicles with maturation of the oocyte, ovulation, and then subsequent formation of the corpus luteum is a complex process. Should any component of the menstrual cycle not function properly, there will be changing levels of circulating hormones, which can have deleterious effects.

A woman has about 400,000 potential oocytes in the ovary at menarche, and she loses these at a rate of about 1,000 per month, regardless of whether she takes the combined oral contraceptive pill, which inhibits ovulation but does not spare oocytes, or not. It is well recognized that with aging, there are fewer and fewer potential oocytes, and less effective ovulation. Therefore ovulatory cycles frequently have a deficient corpus luteum function, with lower levels and/or a shortened period of progesterone secretion, and many cycles are anovulatory with no progesterone secreted at all. The consequent imbalance in

Managing the Menopause: 21st Century Solutions, ed. Nick Panay, Paula Briggs, and Gab Kovacs.
Published by Cambridge University Press. © Cambridge University Press 2015.

estrogen and progesterone is thought to be responsible for some of the symptoms during the perimenopause, especially those associated with menstrual problems. Once a woman becomes postmenopausal, ovarian function ceases completely, and the symptoms of the postmenopause relate to an estrogen deficiency syndrome. This chapter focuses on the menopause transition, also known as the climacteric.

As these symptoms and signs are usually reported as a continuum, we usually consider them together, and classify them into several types:

1. Vasomotor – these include "hot flashes," palpitations, night sweats, an altered sleep pattern and fatigue.
2. Neuromuscular – these include headaches and joint and muscle pain. Other degenerative changes may occur such as hair and skin changes, which can include a crawling sensation (formication) and itchy skin.
3. Psychogenic – these include poor concentration, forgetfulness, depression, anxiety, claustrophobia, agoraphobia, irritability, difficulty coping, tearfulness and lack of drive, including sex drive.
4. Urogenital – symptoms of vaginal dryness, uterovaginal prolapse and urinary symptoms of urge incontinence/overactive bladder. Although stress incontinence is more common in postmenopausal women, the etiology of this is probably not due to estrogen deficiency (Chapter 6).
5. Indirect symptoms of menopausal osteoporosis – repeated fractures.

There is huge variation in the frequency and severity of menopausal symptoms between different women. About 20% of women have no significant symptoms, 60% have mild-to-moderate symptoms and 20% have very severe symptoms.

Women who have menopause induced by surgery (oophorectomy) or chemo/radio-therapy usually have more severe symptoms.

Vasomotor symptoms

These are the classic symptoms heralding the onset of the menopause. About 75% of women in the USA report experiencing troublesome flashes – or flushes as they are called in the UK [1]. Hot flashes adversely affect the quality of life and the day-to-day functioning of many women during the "peri menopause." Data on the duration of these symptoms are available from the Melbourne Womens' Midlife Health Project [2]. The researchers found that out of 205 women who never used hormone replacement therapy (HRT) and were followed up for 13 years, the mean duration of troublesome symptoms was 5.2 years (median 4 years and standard deviation of 3.8 years). Interestingly, even in women who used HRT (total sample 438 women) the duration did not change, with a mean of 5.5 years, standard deviation of 4.0 years and a median of 4 years.

Thus it appears that vasomotor symptoms in a cross-section of women persist for about 5 years on average.

The mechanism of hot flashes

The basic physiological mechanism for hot flashes is an activation of the heat dissipation response most likely due to a hypothalamic mechanism triggered by decreasing estrogen levels [1]. It is thought that estrogen deprivation results in a loss of negative feedback for hypothalamic noradrenaline synthesis [3].

Peripheral changes that result in altered vascular activity, and a narrowed thermoneutral zone, have also been implicated [4]. Consequently, fluctuations in temperature that would not normally trigger vasodilatation and sweating (cooling down mechanisms) result in inappropriate flashing due to narrowing of the thermoneutral zone. Women suffering from hot flashes lose the ability to respond to an ice stimulus with vasoconstriction. It is thought likely that the α-adrenergic system, specifically noradrenaline, is the chemical trigger.

Flashes can be aggravated by stress and anxiety, and even by diet, lifestyle and other medications.

The intensity of hot flashes can be measured by the increase in finger blood flow, respiratory exchange ratio, core body temperature and skin temperature. In laboratory studies, sternal skin conductance is usually measured with good reproducibility [1].

Although night sweats can keep women awake at night, insomnia associated with the menopause is likely to be due to a separate mechanism (loss of neuronal modulation of energy metabolism), and one can occur without the other [5].

Neuromuscular symptoms

Joint pain is a common complaint in perimenopausal women and was reported by 77% of participants in the WHI Study at baseline. When estrogen-only HRT use was compared with placebo, pain was reported less commonly in the estrogen group than the placebo group (76.3% vs. 79.2%, $P=0.0001$) at 1 year and 72.5% of women in the estrogen group reported joint pain whereas 81.7% of those in the placebo group ($P=0.006$) reported joint pain after 3 years. Estrogen is thought to attenuate inflammation and promote cartilage turnover [6].

Headache and migraine are also common symptoms in the perimenopause, although the exact nature of the association between estrogen levels and headache are unknown and in some women treated with estrogen, symptoms remit, whilst in others there is a deterioration in symptom control [7]. In women with migraine, continuous hormone replacement therapy should be considered, preferably using a non-oral route and the lowest effective dose. For women who have contraindications to estrogen therapy or do not wish to use it, preparations that inhibit serotonin reuptake, such as venlafaxine, fluoxetine and paroxetine, have all shown efficacy [8]. In addition to the above treatment options, lifestyle changes, alone or combined with isoflavones, may be considered for the prevention of migraine associated with the menopause transition, although evidence of efficacy is limited. Gabapentin is an additional non-hormonal option to reduce frequency and severity of migraine. Although clonidine is licensed in several countries for migraine prophylaxis and treatment of vasomotor symptoms, any benefit from treatment is often offset by side effects [8].

Psychogenic symptoms

Emotions are the result of the interaction of many environmental factors. During the perimenopausal period, there are many life factors operating, such as fear of aging (and wrinkles!), changing body shape, financial pressures, relationship issues, a changing role with children becoming independent and of course estrogen imbalance may aggravate any or all of these. Women who have a past history of depression, or have a history of premenstrual syndrome are more likely to experience psychogenic changes during the perimenopause.

Providing HRT will alleviate estrogen deficiency, but cannot compensate for many of the factors which may be responsible for low mood. However, certain types of depression, which are due to estrogen deficiency, are best treated by HRT [9].

Urogenital symptoms

Pelvic organ prolapse (POP) and urinary incontinence are described in full in Chapter 6.

Vaginal problems are common and under-reported. Vaginal dryness, as a result of estrogen deficiency, can cause sexual problems due to lack of lubrication and loss of tissue elasticity. Loss of normal vaginal secretions can also be associated with an overgrowth of vaginal commensal organisms, resulting in vaginal discharge. In addition to the vagina, the urogenital tract is also affected by lack of estrogen and this may present as urgency or urge incontinence. Urogenital problems respond best to local estrogen therapy. This may need to be used in conjunction with systemic therapy for vasomotor symptoms. There are several options available for local estrogen therapy including creams, tablets and vaginal rings, although only Vagifem® 10 micrograms, inserted into the vagina twice a week, is licensed to be used without additional progestogen lifelong in women with an intact uterus.

Osteoporosis

Whilst osteoporosis is not a symptom, it is a very important part of female aging, especially after ovarian failure. We know women lose 1% of their bone mass each year after ovarian failure, and that estrogen replacement can inhibit this. Because of the importance of bone mineral density in relation to the care of women in the perimenopause, we have allocated two chapters to this topic – Chapter 9: Osteoporosis recognition and assessment in the menopause, and Chapter 10: Hormonal management of osteoporosis during the menopause. The reader is directed to those chapters for discussion of bone density, its investigation and available therapeutic measures.

Quantifying symptoms

To document the severity of symptoms, a quantitative score sheet has been developed. This enables women to self-score symptoms on a scale of 0 to 3, and for the total score to be calculated. Not only does this allow the severity of symptoms to be more accurately assessed but it also allows follow-up of any change/improvement as a result of therapy. An example of a score sheet used by the authors is shown in Table 4.1.

Differential diagnosis

Before we ascribe a woman's symptoms as being due to the climacteric, we need to be sure that we are not missing a medical problem. The three commonest problems which can be confused with menopausal symptoms are hypothyroidism, anemia and depression. Depression is particularly difficult, as this is far more common in women during the perimenopause.

Conclusion

Denise is likely to be perimenopausal, on account of her age alone, bearing in mind that the average age of the perimenopause is 46.

Table 4.1. Menopausal symptomatology scoring sheet.

Symptom	Score: 0 = nil 1 = mild, 2 = moderate, 3 = severe
Vasomotor symptoms Hot flashes Night sweats Crawling feelings under the skin (formication) Dry skin	
Neuromuscular symptoms Muscle pains Backache Headaches Joint pains	
Psychological symptoms Depression Irritability Mood swings Anxiety Inability to sleep Tiredness Loss of sex drive Unloved feelings Tearfulness	
Urogenital symptoms Dry vagina Painful sex Urinary frequency/urgency	

At baseline, take a medical history and establish a baseline blood pressure and body mass index (BMI). Blood pressure ideally should be within normal limits or controlled prior to commencing HRT.

Measuring gonadotropin levels will be of very little help in her management, as values often vary widely during the menopause transition.

Fortunately, as with many endocrine deficiency disorders (e.g. underactive thyroid), estrogen deficiency in the menopause transition can be managed with estrogen replacement therapy. For healthy women, below the age of 60, provision of hormone replacement therapy carries no increase in risk, but results in control of symptoms and has other potential benefits such as maintenance of bone health.

What else do you need to know?

Does she have an intact uterus?

If the answer to this question is no, she can be provided with estrogen alone. There are a number of delivery route options including oral, transdermal – gels or patches, and subcutaneous (implants).

Non-oral delivery does not increase the risk of VTE over and above the individual's inherent risk, based upon their individual risk factors (Chapter 23), but if there are no underlying risk factors then the choice of delivery rests with the patient and this will influence compliance and symptom control.

If she has an intact uterus, does she use hormonal contraception?

This may influence the type of HRT provided should she wish to proceed with therapy.

Women using combined hormonal contraception (CHC) are unlikely to develop menopausal symptoms. Women using progestogen-only methods can do.

Mirena® has a license to provide endometrial protection in addition to contraception and it also has a license for the management of heavy menstrual bleeding. This makes it an ideal solution to many of the issues in the perimenopause. Women using Mirena® for endometrial protection can have a choice of estrogen delivery in the same way as women who have had a hysterectomy.

If Denise does not wish to proceed with the option of Mirena® for endometrial protection and she does not require contraception e.g. her husband has had a vasectomy, she might opt for Uterogestan®, a micronized progesterone preparation taken either continuously or sequentially, or she may prefer a commercially available sequential HRT preparation with predictable, usually light, withdrawal bleeds.

Recommendations

Take a good history especially about symptoms relating to the menopause. Using the score sheet shown in Table 4.1 is a valuable way to record symptoms and their severity. Take a detailed history with respect to risk factors for breast cancer, thromboembolic disorders and osteoporosis.

Ordering a series of expensive hormone tests (estradiol, progesterone, follicle stimulating hormone (FSH), luteinizing hormone (LH), androgens, sex hormone binding globulin etc.) is not indicated for women who are having a physiological menopause. Firstly, FSH levels are variable and a single raised level is not meaningful. Secondly, estrogen levels vary a lot from day-to-day, and the blood levels of the hormone bear no relationship to the symptoms experienced. Thirdly, the results of hormone tests will not change the management of the patient – this should be determined by the woman's symptoms.

The initial prescription of HRT is a "therapeutic trial." If the woman's symptoms and quality of life improve, then she will continue with the prescribed treatment. If there is no improvement, a different preparation of HRT can be tried. Using the "score sheet" from Table 4.1 will facilitate a more objective evaluation of any improvement in symptoms.

A total score is then obtained by adding together all the scores. The maximum possible score is $20 \times 3 = 60$.

References

1. Sievert LL. Subjective and objective measures of hot flashes. *Am J Hum Biol* 2013; **25**: 573–80.

2. Col NF, Guthrie JR, Politi M, Dennerstein L. Duration of vasomotor symptoms in middle-aged women: a longitudinal study. *Menopause* 2009; **16**: 453–7.

3. Vilar-Gonzales S, Perez-Rozos A, Cabarillas-Farpon R. Mechanism of hot flashes. *Clin Trans Oncol* 2011; **13**: 143–7.

4. Sassarini J, Fox H, Ferrell W, Sattar N, Lumsden MA. Hot flushes, vascular reactivity and the role of α-adrenergic system. *Climacteric* 2012; **15**: 332–8.

5. Bourey RE. Primary menopausal insomnia: definition, review, and practical approach. *Endocr Pract* 2011; **17**: 122–131.

6. Kaunitz AM. Should new-onset arthralgia be considered a menopausal symptom? *Menopause* 2013; **20**: 591–3.

7. Tassorelli C, Greco R, Allena M, Terreno E, Nappi RE. Transdermal hormonal therapy in perimenstrual migraine: why, when and how? *Curr Pain Headache Rep* 2012; **16**: 467–73.

8. MacGregor EA. Headache and hormone replacement therapy in the postmenopausal woman. *Curr Treat Options Neurol* 2009; **11**: 10–17.

9. Studd J. Personal view: hormones and depression in women. *Climacteric* 2014 Jul 21: 1–3. [Epub ahead of print].

Chapter 5

Hormone replacement therapy and cardiovascular disease

Tommaso Simoncini, Elena Cecchi and Andrea R. Genazzani

Menopause as a cardiovascular risk factor

Coronary heart disease is the leading cause of death and infirmity amongst women in Western countries; yet, the health impact of heart disease is underestimated. In addition, heart attacks and other major cardiovascular events are under-detected in women notwithstanding their higher in-hospital mortality. There are several reasons for this: for instance, myocardial infarction in women often reveals itself with atypical signs, which make diagnosis more difficult.

Aging and the presence of risk factors such as smoking, hypertension, hypercholesterolemia and diabetes significantly increase the risk of cardiovascular disease (CVD), particularly in women. Management of risk factors has proved to decrease female CVD mortality as much as improved treatment. However, recent data indicate an increase of CVD among women, whereas incidence amongst men has declined. This could be partially explained by the high levels of obesity in the female population.

Since CVD is rare in young women, it is commonly believed that during their premenopausal years women are protected against heart disease by endogenous estrogens. The annual incidence of cardiovascular disease increases according to menopausal status. During the menopausal transition, women undergo changes in their cardiovascular system.

Perimenopausal women commonly gain weight. This is mainly attributed to an increase in body fat, which is concentrated in the abdomen (android) rather than subcutaneously (gynoid). Increased body fat decreases insulin sensitivity and increases systolic blood pressure, particularly in women. This is particularly true for increased visceral accumulation of fat, and in women, the waist-to-hip ratio has a higher correlation with CVD incidence and mortality than body mass index (BMI).

Menopause is also associated with an increase in triglycerides (TGs), total cholesterol (TC) and low-density lipoprotein cholesterol (LDL-C) and lipoprotein A concentrations. The levels of high-density lipoprotein cholesterol (HDL-C) gradually fall after the menopause, even though concentrations remain relatively higher in women than in men. The drop in HDL-C and the increase of LDL-C are stronger predictors of cardiovascular risk in women than in men.

Insulin resistance and diabetes have been noted to be associated with a higher cardiovascular risk among women in clinical trials, with a greater predictive value than in men. Data from a meta-analysis suggest that the risk for fatal coronary heart disease associated with diabetes is 50% higher in women. The results also show that diabetes and hypertension represent the two most important cardiovascular risk factors in women, particularly when they occur simultaneously. Estrogens seem to influence glucose homeostasis through

Managing the Menopause: 21st Century Solutions, ed. Nick Panay, Paula Briggs, and Gab Kovacs. Published by Cambridge University Press. © Cambridge University Press 2015.

increased glucose transport into the cells, whereas lack of estrogens has been associated with a progressive decrease in glucose-stimulated insulin secretion and insulin sensitivity as well as with insulin resistance. These may explain why HRT administration to postmenopausal women is associated with a significant decrease in the incidence of type II diabetes.

Identification of CVD risk factors is important before embarking on HRT and, thereafter, patients should be regularly monitored to identify the emergence of any cardiovascular risk factor. All perimenopausal women that seek medical help to control menopausal symptoms should be evaluated for the risk of developing CVD and for the risk of complications in the presence of existing disease. Specific attention should be devoted to the development of high blood pressure, central obesity, dyslipidemia, fasting hyperglycemia or impaired glucose tolerance, particularly in women with a family history of CVD.

Role of estrogens in cardiovascular risk

Estrogens are the predominant sex hormones in women, affecting the development and function of the female reproductive system. A common clinical application of estrogen is its use as a component of hormone replacement therapy (HRT) for hot flashes, night sweats and vaginal dryness.

Natural estrogens include estrone (E1), estradiol (E2) and estriol (E3). The ovaries are the main source of circulating E2 in premenopausal women. E1 and E3 are mostly formed in the liver from E2 or in peripheral tissues from androstenedione. The source and plasma levels of estrogens change with age. In fact, in postmenopausal women, E1 is the predominant estrogen, produced in peripheral tissues from androstenedione.

Estrogens bind to estrogen receptors (ERs) with high affinity and specificity. ERα is expressed in the uterus, vagina, ovaries, breasts and the hypothalamus. ERβ is highly expressed in the lung, brain and bone. Remarkably, ERα and ERβ have distinct roles in the cardiovascular system. Estrogens modulate vascular function by targeting estrogen receptors in endothelial cells (ECs) and in vascular smooth muscle cells (VSMC). Pleiotropic functions are exerted by estrogens on the cardiovascular system through genomic and non-genomic signaling pathways. Estrogens enhance the release of the vasodilators nitric oxide (NO) and prostacyclin (PGI2) and decrease the production of the vasoconstrictors endothelin (ET-1) and angiotensin II (AngII), maintaining an efficient endothelial function. The rapid effects of estrogens in cardiovascular cells are achieved through complex interactions with membrane-associated signaling ERs leading to activation of downstream cascades such as mitogen-activated protein kinase (MAPK) and phosphatidylinositol 3-OH kinase (PI3K). These cascades play crucial roles in regulating the expression of target proteins implicated in cell proliferation, apoptosis, differentiation, movement and homeostasis.

Animal and human studies have shown that the vascular benefits of estrogen are mediated by ERs and that these benefits depend upon the integrity of vascular endothelium and its functional status. Aging and atherosclerosis result in vascular wall damage and loss of estrogen receptors and/or function compromising the functional status of the endothelium. Since estrogen receptor expression is dependent upon circulating estrogen levels, estrogen receptors in vascular endothelium and vascular smooth cells begin to disappear soon after the menopause when circulating estrogen levels drop. Function of ERs may also be lost through methylation of the promoter site of the ERα throughout aging, and particularly in diseased areas of the vasculature. So, maintaining premenopausal circulating levels of estrogens may be useful to preserve estrogen receptors after menopause and their actions in the cardiovascular system [1].

Moreover, estrogens modulate inflammation and its mediators in atherosclerosis, and this also seems to be a key feature of estrogen actions in the cardiovascular system. Estradiol, through ERs, reduces the synthesis of a series of a pro-atherogenic cytokines and monocyte-endothelial cell adhesion factors. For instance, plasma levels of inflammatory molecules, such as C-reactive protein, cytokines (TNF-α), interleukins (IL-6) and several endothelial-leukocyte adhesion molecules are increased in patients with hypertension and atherosclerosis. E2 counteracts these changes, by decreasing TNF-α secretion and increasing prostaglandin I_2 production, therefore reducing both oxidative stress and platelet activation. Reductions of circulating levels of vascular adhesion molecules have also been identified in postmenopausal women receiving HRT.

Menopausal complaints and cardiovascular risk

Loss of ovarian follicular activity explains the fall in estrogen production at menopause. These hormonal changes have profound neuroendocrine implications, resulting in hot flashes, night sweats, insomnia, mood changes, anxiety, irritability, poor memory and concentration (Figure 5.1). The urogenital tract is also affected, with the progressive development of urogenital atrophy and eventually urinary incontinence and dyspareunia. These features lead many women to seek medical help, but patients and physicians are generally unaware of the growing evidence that those women who are most symptomatic at the menopausal transition may also be at increased risk for CVD throughout aging.

Interventions that mitigate menopausal complaints through lifestyle modifications are an appropriate first step to consider in any woman before initiating or in addition to pharmacologic or hormonal treatments. Increasing physical activity, avoiding smoking, moderating alcohol intake are measures associated with improvement in vasomotor symptoms and other menopausal symptoms. However, they are also the mainstay of any intervention that mitigates against cardiovascular risk later in life. Thus, the menopause

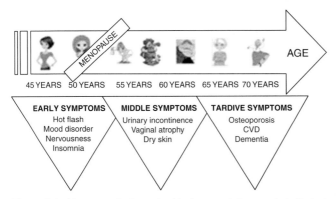

Figure 5.1. Menopause is determined by hormonal changes that affect a large series of body targets, causing atrophy of tissues, metabolic modifications, along with psychological and sexual changes that are experienced by women in different ways. The first signs include vasomotor symptoms, nocturnal sweats and mood disorder. Soon after these first manifestations, atrophic changes and body composition changes occur. Cardiovascular disease and osteoporosis are the main long-term consequences of the hormonal changes at time of menopause.

transition is a key time in a woman's life to start or to reinforce a healthy lifestyle, that will improve the aging process and decrease the incidence of CVD.

Added to this, the introduction of HRT after the menopause also has profound implications in terms of future cardiovascular risk.

Cardiovascular effects of hormone replacement therapy
Observational studies

Cardiovascular diseases are less common in premenopausal as compared with postmenopausal women, implying vascular benefits of estrogens. For this reason 40 years ago the use of HRT became widespread in Western countries. In the mid-1970s, evidence from observational studies, such as the Nurses' Health Study (NHS), showed that estrogen therapy in postmenopausal women was associated with a reduction of CVD by 35–50%. Also, meta-analyses of observational studies showed a 33% reduction of fatal CVD among users as compared with non-users [2].

Based on these observations, large-scale clinical trials have been performed to assess the impact of estrogen and/or progestogen administration on the risk of developing cardiovascular and other diseases in postmenopausal women.

Randomized controlled trials (RCTs)

Based on the assumption that estrogens effectively protect the heart and the vessels, trials were performed to explore whether individuals with recent coronary events may benefit from initiation of estrogen administration. The Heart and Estrogen Replacement Study (HERS) remains the main secondary prevention trial ever performed. This randomized, double-blinded, placebo-controlled trial included 2,763 postmenopausal women with an intact uterus, who received either 0.625 mg of conjugated equine estrogens (CEE) plus 2.5 mg of medroxyprogesterone acetate (MPA) or placebo. The mean age of participants was 66.7 years and all of them had suffered a recent coronary event. Initiation of HRT in this population did not prove to provide a protective effect on the heart, but rather increased the incidence of recurrent coronary heart disease (CHD) during the first year of treatment [3].

Lack of beneficial effects by HRT in preventing recurrent CHD was confirmed by the Estrogen in the Prevention of Reinfarction Trial (ESPRIT) that explored different types of estrogens. In this study 1,017 postmenopausal women, aged between 50–69, who had survived a first myocardial infarction were enrolled in the trial. For 2 years, women received 2 mg of estradiol valerate or placebo daily. Frequency of re-infarction did not differ between the two groups.

The Women's Estrogens for Stroke Trial (WEST) was designed as a randomized, placebo-controlled trial of estrogen replacement (1 mg of 17β-estradiol per day) for the secondary prevention of cerebrovascular diseases. The trial included 664 postmenopausal women who had recently had an ischemic stroke or transient ischemic attack (TIA). The mean age of participants was 71 years. No significant difference was observed between the two groups in terms of incidence of non-fatal myocardial infarction.

Thus a number of well-conducted trials support that HRT should not be started for the secondary prevention of cardiovascular diseases [4], and it may have a detrimental effect on the long-term outcome.

The Women's Health Initiative (WHI) trial is a landmark study in this field. This trial was initiated in 1992 and was planned to continue until 2007. A total of 16,608 postmenopausal women aged 50–79 with an intact uterus were recruited to receive 0.625 mg/day of CEE plus 2.5 mg/day of MPA or placebo (WHI-EP) [5]. The parallel WHI estrogen-only trial (WHI-E) was performed to evaluate the effect of estrogen administration in women having had a prior hysterectomy, enrolling 10,739 postmenopausal women to receive either 0.625 mg/day of CEE or placebo [6].

In 2002, after an average follow-up of 5.2 years, the WHI-EP was stopped because the interim analysis performed by the study data safety monitoring board showed an excess risk of breast cancer and CHD in women receiving hormone therapy. In 2004, after an average follow-up of 6.8 years, the WHI-E was also terminated a year earlier than planned due to an increased risk of stroke in hormone therapy users.

The WHI trial had a huge negative impact on the adoption of HRT amongst postmenopausal women. The publication of the data was followed by a rapid decline in the number of HRT users, due to fear of breast cancer and cardiovascular disease. However, after a 10-year debate, the initial interpretation of the WHI trial results have been reviewed, highlighting that WHI and the secondary prevention trials do not necessarily conflict with the wealth of existing information generated by the earlier observational studies.

A modern view on the effect of postmenopausal hormone therapy on cardiovascular disease

Reinterpretation of the results from the studies performed in the field of hormonal therapies and menopause has led to the view that the different outcome of the observational vs. the most recent randomized trials is mostly due to the notable differences in the populations enrolled.

In the observational studies the women who used HRT were healthier than non-users. Additionally, the observational studies looked at women who started HRT around the time of the menopause transition, with the indication of controlling climacteric symptoms. Conversely, women in HERS and WHI were much older with the vast majority of the participants commencing HRT several years after the menopause [4].

This major difference in the characteristics of the populations reflects findings in experimental and animal data [7] that identify estrogens as hormones that can maintain healthy vascular tissue in a good functional state, but there is little or no protective effect on atherosclerotic vessels. Therefore common sense suggests that the benefit derived from HRT is maximized in younger women with minimal atherosclerotic lesions, and there is no benefit seen in older women with CVD risk factors or pre-existing CVD.

This concept is currently identified as the "timing hypothesis," which suggests that the cardiovascular effects of HRT strongly depend on individual vascular health and that administration of the same compounds at different stages in a woman's life have markedly different effects (Figure 5.2). In line with this hypothesis, a major meta-analysis including 23 RCTs with a total of 39,049 participants followed for 191,340 patient-years [2] and including the WHI population, showed that HRT significantly reduced CHD events in younger women (odds ratio (OR) 0.68, 95% confidence interval (CI) 0.48–0.96), but not in older women (OR 1.03, CI 0.91–1.16).

Data that support the timing hypothesis are reflected in all the recent randomized trials. For instance, in the WHI-E study a significant reduction in CVD risk in women who were

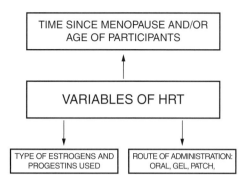

Figure 5.2. In accordance with the timing hypothesis, the moment when the HRT is commenced, jointly with its composition or preparation, crucially determines its effectiveness.

administered HRT within 10 years of menopause was found [6]. The WHI-EP study did not show a cardiovascular benefit in younger women receiving hormones, but in women aged 50–59 years there was no increased risk of CVD, while the risk was increased in women 60 years and older at enrollment [5]. While these latter data do not confirm a protective effect, it should be noticed that the baseline characteristics of the WHI participants identify a population at moderate-high cardiovascular risk, due to the prevalence of obesity, hypertension and diabetes. Thus even the finding of a neutral effect on cardiovascular risk in younger women confirms the view that the vascular system has to be free from disease to benefit from continued estrogen exposure after the menopause. This also fits with the finding of the Cancer Prevention Study II, a 12-year observational study of 290,823 women. In this cohort, CHD death was lowest among HRT users with a BMI <22 while there was no association between HRT use and CHD in women with BMI >30. The CHD outcome according to BMI from the WHI-E trial showed a similar pattern.

More recently, the timing hypothesis has been tested in the Early versus Late Intervention Trial with Estradiol (ELITE), in which 643 postmenopausal women without a history of CVD were classified for time-since-menopause (<6 years and >10 years) and were randomized to receive placebo or oral estradiol 1 mg/day with progesterone vaginal gel for 10 days each month. Subclinical atherosclerosis progression was determined every month using carotid intima-media thickness (CIMT). Enrollment started in 2004 and the preliminary results have been so far disclosed at congresses, but not yet published. According to the preliminary reports, CIMT progression was significantly slower in women starting estrogen treatment early as compared with those initiating therapy later in life, in agreement with the timing hypothesis.

The effect of HRT on cardiovascular risk in postmenopausal women also seems to be affected by the type of estrogen used, dose and route of administration. Estrogens can be administered orally, as a percutaneous gel, transdermal patch or subcutaneous implants. Other trans-mucosal preparations have been tried in the past. A number of hormone preparations are available (Table 5.1) and newer delivery systems and hormone combinations are currently in developement. The route of administration of estrogens has a significant influence on cardiovascular effect. Transdermal estrogens, in contrast to oral preparations, are not associated with an increased risk of venous thrombosis. This is because oral estrogens are subject to first-pass hepatic metabolism, promoting prothrombotic hemostatic changes in factor IX, activated protein resistance C and tissue plasminogen activator [8], thereby favoring deep vein thrombosis, pulmonary embolism and possibly thrombotic complications of atherosclerotic plaques.

Table 5.1. Most common formulations available as hormone therapy for postmenopausal women. Patients with an intact uterus require a combined therapy (estrogen plus progestin). Women with previous hysterectomy do not need the addition of a progestin.

Route of administration	Women with uterus	Women without uterus
Transdermal patch	estradiol-17β + NETA estradiol-17β + LNG	estradiol-17β
Transdermal gel		estradiol-17β
Oral	Conjugated equine estrogens + MPA estradiol-17β + DRSP estradiol-17β + NOMAC estradiol-17β + DYD estradiol-17β + CYP estradiol emihydrate + NETA estradiol valerate + MPA	Conjugated equine estrogens estradiol valerate

DRSP, drospirenone; MPA, medroxyprogesterone acetate; NOMAC, nomegestrol acetate; DYD, didrogesterone; CYP, cyproterone acetate; NETA, norethisterone acetate; LNG, levonorgestrel.

Oral conjugated equine estrogens (CEE) is the most widely used estrogen preparation in HRT, particularly in North America; it is a mix of estrogenic compounds including estrone sulfate and at least 10 other hormones, some of which are not found in humans. It is understood that some of the estrogen receptor ligands comprised in CEE act as partial agonist/antagonists, or as selective estrogen receptor modulators (SERMs). Thus the overall effect on tissues depends on the unique mix of compounds found in CEE, rather than on one of the components.

The alternate compound used for HRT, particularly in European countries, is 17β-estradiol, the most potent and natural form of estrogen in premenopausal women. The estrogen receptor binding potency of estrone is approximately 2/3 the affinity of estradiol for ERα, and about 1/3 the affinity of estradiol for ERβ. Estradiol is available as transdermal or trans-mucosal preparations, or as an oral form, in its valerate or emihydrate forms, to make it resistant to gastric passage.

The Kronos Early Estrogen Prevention Study (KEEPS) was performed to compare the effect on CIMT progression of oral CEE vs. transdermal 17β-estradiol or placebo. KEEPS was a multicenter, randomized, double-blind, placebo-controlled trial, designed to test the hypothesis that HRT in recently postmenopausal women reduces the progression of subclinical atherosclerosis over a period of 4 years. The trial began in 2005 with complete enrollment of 727 women in June 2008. The participants were aged 42–58 years, at least 6 months but not more than 36 months postmenopausal and in good general health. The trial failed to show any difference in the progression of CIMT in the three groups, and was not sufficiently powered to compare the rate of cardiovascular events [9].

The Danish Osteoporosis Prevention Study (DOPS) is possibly the best available evidence that looks at the effects of HRT on cardiovascular risk. This was an open-label trial evaluating the effects of estradiol and norethisterone acetate (NETA) on CVD [10]. In this trial 1,006 healthy, recently postmenopausal women aged 45–58 were randomized to receive a cyclic sequential treatment with 1–2 mg/day of estradiol combined with

NETA 1 mg/day, continuous estradiol 2 mg/day for hysterectomized women, or no treatment. After 10 years of randomized treatment, women receiving HRT commenced early after the menopause had a significantly reduced risk of cardiovascular mortality, heart failure or myocardial infarction, without any apparent increase in risk of cancer, venous thromboembolism or stroke.

An emerging variable that may also affect cardiovascular risk during HRT is the progestin component. A number of studies in this area have been performed upon the publication of the two WHI trials, showing a better cardiovascular performance at any given age in women receiving estrogens only as compared with those also receiving medroxyprogesterone acetate (MPA). While all progestins seem to have unique actions on vascular cells and tissues, MPA seems to have a particularly unfavorable profile on items such as vasodilatation, vasoconstriction, metabolic changes, lipid changes and hemostatic parameters. In general, MPA antagonizes many of the beneficial actions of estrogens in experimental, animal and clinical systems. Conversely, natural progesterone seems to be neutral on most of these processes, thereby suggesting that the choice of the progestin used to protect the endometrium after the menopause during HRT influences the future CV risk.

Should HRT be prescribed to prevent CVD?

The decision to start HRT in a woman transitioning toward menopause requires a personalized discussion on the unique balance of risks and benefits in that particular individual. The long-term impact of HRT is often a matter of interest to women seeking consultation. The potential benefits regarding reducing the risk of fracture and cardiovascular risk are still perceived by many women as one of the reasons to consider HRT.

Thorough counseling on the relevance of improving lifestyle, dietary habits and implementing physical activity should be provided. Menopause physicians should appropriately stress how these behavioral changes are far more important to prevent cardiovascular risk than any pharmacologic or hormonal intervention.

Within this frame, the available evidence shows that the balance of benefits and risks for HRT is most favorable within the first 10 years of menopause. When started during this "window of opportunity" HRT has long-term protective effects on the cardiovascular system, reflected in an approximate 40–50% reduction in cardiovascular events in most clinical studies. While this decrease is clinically relevant, expert agreement is that HRT should still be primarily initiated for the management of climacteric symptoms to improve quality of life. Long-term preventive strategies, particularly cardiovascular protection, should not be a primary goal. However, based on the wealth of information available now, it is no longer in dispute that in this population the benefit/risk profile is favorable and if HRT is continued for a few years, no cardiovascular harm, but rather benefit will ensue [11].

References

1. Fu XD, Simoncini T. Extra-nuclear signaling of estrogen receptors. *IUBMB Life* 2008; **60**: 502–10.

2. Salpeter SR, Walsh JM, Greyber E, Salpeter EE. Brief report: coronary heart disease events associated with hormone therapy in younger and older women. A meta-analysis. *J Gen Intern Med* 2006; **21**: 363–6.

3. Hulley S, Grady D, Bush T, *et al.* Randomized trial of estrogen plus progestin for secondary prevention of coronary heart disease in postmenopausal women. Heart and Estrogen/Progestin Replacement Study (HERS) Research Group. *JAMA* 1998; **280**: 605–13.

4. Genazzani AR, Simoncini T. Pharmacotherapy: benefits of menopausal

hormone therapy – timing is key. *Nature Rev Endocrinol* 2013; **9**: 5–6.

5. The Writing Group for the Women's Health Initiative Investigators. Risks and benefits of estrogen plus progestin in healthy postmenopausal women: principal results from the Women's Health Initiative randomized controlled trial. *JAMA* 2002; **288**: 321–33.

6. The Women's Health Initiative Steering Committee. Effects of conjugated equine estrogen in postmenopausal women with hysterectomy: the Women's Health Initiative Randomized Controlled Trial. *JAMA* 2004; **291**: 1701–12.

7. Mikkola TS, Clarkson TB. Coronary heart disease and postmenopausal hormone therapy: conundrum explained by timing? *J Womens Health (Larchmt)* 2006; **15**: 51–3.

8. Olie V, Canonico M, Scarabin PY. Postmenopausal hormone therapy and venous thromboembolism. *Thrombosis Research* 2011; **127 Suppl 3**: S26–9.

9. Harman SM, Black DM, Naftolin F, *et al.* Arterial imaging outcomes and cardiovascular risk factors in recently menopausal women: a randomized trial. *Ann Intern Med* 2014; **161**: 249–60.

10. Schierbeck LL, Rejnmark L, Tofteng CL, *et al.* Effect of hormone replacement therapy on cardiovascular events in recently postmenopausal women: randomised trial. *Br Med J* 2012; **345**: e6409.

11. Hodis HN, Mack WJ. Hormone replacement therapy and the association with coronary heart disease and overall mortality: clinical application of the timing hypothesis. *J Steroid Biochem Mol Biol* 2014; **142**: 68–75.

Pelvic organ prolapse and incontinence in association with the menopause

Ajay Rane and Jay Iyer

Joanne is a symptomatic 57-year-old, para 5, who had "big babies," two of which were delivered by forceps extraction. She is 5 years postmenopause (her LMP was age 52). She comes for help regarding her hot flashes, emotional lability, vaginal dryness causing dyspareunia and decreased libido. She is most concerned that she has recently noticed a lump in her vagina. In addition to this, she complains of a dragging sensation "down below" at the end of a tiring day at the office.

Recently she has noticed that she "wets" herself during high-impact activities like jogging and aerobic exercise.

Joanne has become incontinent of urine whilst having sex.

All of this is very embarrassing for Joanne and she is deeply distressed.

Her close friend has suggested that she see a doctor.

Introduction

Pelvic organ dysfunction may be associated with significant morbidity that can affect quality of life. It may manifest as pelvic organ prolapse, lower urinary tract symptoms, voiding and defecatory problems, and sexual dysfunction.

The effect of age on the anatomy and function of the pelvic floor is well recognized. However, the exact pathophysiological mechanisms remain elusive. Pelvic floor disorders result from a combination of causative influences including anatomic, physiologic, genetic, lifestyle and reproductive factors [1]. The role of the menopause on pelvic floor dysfunction is unclear, but there is not thought to be any association.

The Womens' Health Initiative (WHI) studies indicated a prevalence of some degree of pelvic organ prolapse (POP), based on examination, to be 41.1% for women aged between 50 and 79 years. A US study of women over the age of 80 years found a prevalence of incontinence of 31.7%, compared with women aged 40–59 years, who had a prevalence of 17.2%.

Approximately half of postmenopausal women report urogenital symptoms. These generally appear soon after the menopause transition and worsen with time [2].

The degree of prolapse is defined by the Pelvic Organ Prolapse Quantification System (POP-Q) as:

Stage 0 – No prolapse

Stage I – descent of the cervix but more than 1 cm above the hymen

Stage II – descent to within 1 cm of hymen, to protruding 1 cm

Stage III – descent more than 1 cm past the hymen, but no more than 2 cm

Stage IV –Complete vault eversion, also called procidentia

Managing the Menopause: 21st Century Solutions, ed. Nick Panay, Paula Briggs, and Gab Kovacs.
Published by Cambridge University Press. © Cambridge University Press 2015.

Stages III–IV POP can cause obstruction at the urethrovesical junction, with voiding dysfunction, which is more likely with older age and uterus *in situ* [1].

The female reproductive system and lower urinary tract develop from two embryological segments derived from the urogenital sinus and the Müllerian ducts. The urethra is sensitive to estrogen due to the presence of estrogen receptors in the middle and distal thirds. There is a higher concentration of estrogen receptors in the distal urethra in comparison to the proximal urethra, vault and trigone of the bladder [3]. The ligamentous structures including the endopelvic fascia and the levator ani muscles also have estrogen receptors. A proposed mechanism in the development of stress urinary incontinence is an alteration in the stimulation of the estrogen receptors in these urogenital tissues. Progesterone receptors are also found in the lower genitourinary tract, but are sparsely distributed and are less influential with regards to the development of prolapse and incontinence [2].

Both estrogen and progesterone have a significant physiologic effect on the genitourinary tract. Besides affecting the neurology of micturition on a central and peripheral level by influencing the autonomic nervous system, estrogen also affects the collagen metabolism in the lower genital tract [4]. Progesterone generally adversely affects female urinary tract function, typically decreasing the tone in the ureters, bladder and urethra [3]; this may be the reason why urinary symptoms worsen during the secretory phase of the menstrual cycle, and during pregnancy.

Risk factors for development of POP include vaginal delivery, aging and possibly pudendal nerve injury.

Age-related loss of skeletal muscle tone, volume and consequent impaired function is well recognized. This may result in excessive "load-bearing" by the ligamentous structures, fascia and other connective tissue elements of the pelvic floor. Supraphysiologic stresses may result in collagen breakdown with consequent pelvic organ prolapse, as the "new" collagen formed to "repair" the damage is often immature and does not possess the resilience of the mature collagen, resulting in a potential exacerbating factor with regards to prolapse. The dual innervation of the levator ani muscles by the pudendal nerve and by nerve roots from S3–S5 makes pudendal nerve injury a less likely cause of pelvic organ prolapse when compared with the other potential causative factors as described above.

The risk factors for development of stress urinary incontinence (SUI) are similar to those of POP. Smoking, hormone replacement therapy (HRT), diabetes and hysterectomy are positively associated with SUI. Age-related dementia and lack of mobility may also be contributing factors with regards to incontinence.

The risk factors for developing urge urinary incontinence (UUI) are also similar to that of pelvic organ prolapse. Urge urinary incontinence may be caused as a result of poor bladder compliance secondary to loss of the vesico-elastic features of the bladder leading to involuntary contractions of the detrusor muscle. Urge urinary incontinence and recurrent urinary tract infections may also result due to hypoestrogenism.

As discussed above, in the Women's Health Initiative Study, 41% of women aged 50–79 years showed some amount of pelvic organ prolapse. This included cystocele in 34%, rectocele in 19% and uterine prolapse in 14%. In a multicenter study of 1,006 women aged 18–83 years presenting for routine gynecologic care, 24% had normal support and 38% had stage I, 35% stage II and 2% stage III pelvic organ prolapse (Figure 6.1). Patients may complain of a vaginal "lump," voiding dysfunction, sexual dysfunction, vaginal flatus and sometimes defecatory dysfunction with the need to "digitate" to evacuate the bowel.

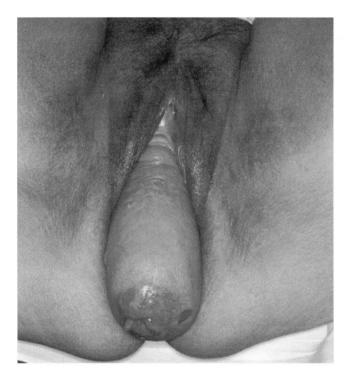

Figure 6.1. Complete procidentia.

Subtle symptoms like a dragging sensation or a strain in the lower back may indicate enterocele and lesser degrees of uterocervical descent.

Many women accept urinary incontinence as a normal part of aging, and they do not seek help for an average of 4 years [5]. Symptoms may include difficulty maintaining bladder control in association with an increase in intra-abdominal pressure (SUI) and an inability to maintain bladder control due to cortical inhibition of the sacral reflex arc during normal bladder filling, resulting in an urge to void urine when the bladder is less than full to capacity (UUI).

Management of prolapse and incontinence

Conservative management of prolapse

Conservative management of POP should be considered prior to surgical intervention. In women who are overweight, weight loss should be recommended first-line in conjunction with non-weight-bearing exercise. Kegel's exercises, to the point of muscle fatigue, are recommended several times a day. In order to do these exercises, women need to identify the appropriate muscles by stopping the flow of urine mid stream. They should then learn to contract these muscles for 10 seconds, relax for 10 seconds and repeat 10 sets at least three times daily. Directed pelvic floor physiotherapy is highly recommended. A good physiotherapist is able to coach the woman to "isolate" her puborectalis muscle and therefore provide a more directed and individualized management plan. A 4–6-month course of pelvic physiotherapy is sufficient to ascertain potential benefit. Pelvic floor muscle exercises have a positive effect on prolapse symptoms and severity, as reported in a Cochrane analysis [6]. They need to be continued lifelong.

Local estrogen (delivered directly to the vagina) is a useful treatment for women with atrophic vaginitis. It may also be helpful for women suffering from incontinence. This treatment is suitable for all women.

There are a variety of different ways of delivering this form of therapy including creams, tablets and via a vaginal ring impregnated with a low dose of estradiol with modified release over a 24-hour period.

Only one product, Vagifem®, delivering $10\,\mu g$ of estradiol daily to the vaginal epithelium has a license to be used indefinitely without the need for endometrial protection.

Pessaries can be used to manage POP and they may also be helpful in controlling SUI. There are many different types of pessary available made of either silicone or inert plastic. Ring pessaries are the first-line option as they are easy to insert and remove. The newer folding rings can be removed and re-inserted by the woman herself, which means that they can be removed for sex if preferable, and leaving them out overnight every couple of weeks reduces the risk of a discharge developing. More advanced-stage prolapse may require the use of a space-occupying pessary such as a shelf pessary or a Gellhorn pessary. These pessaries are not suitable for women who are sexually active.

Hormone replacement therapy (HRT) has been used with variable success in the management of POP. At best, it helps to improve cross-linking and maturation of collagen, which may be of benefit in postoperative outcomes. However, it has been associated with an increased incidence of all types of urinary incontinence (reported at 1 year among women who were continent at baseline) [1]. Given the possible adverse impact of HRT on urinary continence, a clinical evaluation of bladder control at the time of commencing HRT is recommended.

Surgical management of prolapse

Surgical management of prolapse usually is determined by the compartment affected, the DeLancey's [7] "levels of support" that are defective, the size of the prolapse and most importantly by informed patient choice. A variety of options are available: fascial repairs, ligamentous anchors and mesh (Figure 6.2) with or without a hysterectomy; the modality to be individualized to meet the anatomical and functional needs of the woman. The vaginal route allows for more comprehensive repairs, however, more recently laparoscopic pelvic floor repair is gaining in popularity.

Conservative management of incontinence

Lifestyle and behavioral modifications, such as weight loss, fluid management, avoidance of bladder irritants, bladder training, timed voiding, treatment of chronic cough and constipation have been shown to be of benefit in patients with urinary incontinence. Pelvic floor exercises can benefit bladder control in addition to reducing POP, but require long-term compliance. Other treatment options include biofeedback, use of vaginal cones and electrostimulation.

SUI and UUI are managed differently and therefore the history is crucial in order to offer appropriate treatment. Women with SUI will leak in association with increased intra-abdominal pressure whereas women with UUI will "toilet map" due to reduced bladder capacity.

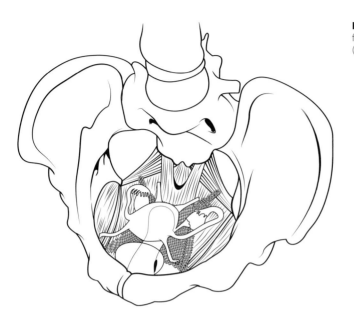

Figure 6.2. Graft (Mesh) used for vaginal prolapse repair (Cystocele).

Stress urinary incontinence does not respond to drug therapy. Use of a ring pessary with a knob, which alters the angle of the junction between the bladder and the urethra, may be helpful, but surgery is the mainstay of treatment.

Urge urinary incontinence can be managed successfully using antimuscarinic drugs, where there are no contraindications. These include having a history of acute angle closure glaucoma and cardiac arrhythmias. These drugs reduce detrusor muscle contraction and increase bladder capacity.

There are different options ranging from drugs such as oxybutynin, which is inexpensive, but often associated with intolerable side effects (most frequently dry mouth) to newer, more expensive drugs, which result in fewer side effects. These include trospium XL 60 mg (first choice for elderly women and women who are overweight), tolterodine, solifenacin and fesoterodine.

Kentera® is a patch delivering 3.9 mg of oxybutynin/24 h. Each patch contains 36 mg of oxybutynin and the patches are changed twice weekly. This is a useful option for women who have side effects with any of the oral preparations. In addition to dry mouth, women may develop gastrointestinal disturbance, blurred vision, dizziness, drowsiness, difficulty voiding, palpitations/arrhythmias and skin reactions. The most recent addition to the range of treatments available is mirabegron, a selective beta 3-adrenoceptor agonist. It has a different mode of action to the antimuscarinic agents, relaxing the smooth muscle in the bladder and enhancing urine storage, and is unlikely to interfere with the urine voiding phase as it is predominantly the activity of acetylcholine on muscarinic receptors that induces bladder contraction. This is a good drug to use for women who are unable to tolerate the side effects of any of the antimuscarinic agents.

Patients with refractory overactive bladder can be treated with sacral neuro-modulation. This can provide effective relief of overactive bladder symptoms and also neurogenic retention.

Another, non-surgical treatment is percutaneous tibial nerve stimulation.

Surgical treatment of incontinence

Where medical therapy has failed, another effective option to treat overactive bladder (OAB) is cystoscopically directed intravesicular (into the detrusor muscles) injection of botulinum toxin (100–200 IU). Patients need to be aware of the risks of urinary retention potentially requiring intermittent self-clean catheterization and the need for repeated injections every 6–9 months [8].

Repeat injections are required every 6–9 months. This seems to be a safe treatment option, but is associated with high voiding dysfunction rates [5].

Surgical intervention should be preceded by a urodynamic assessment and the women should also be assessed and deemed suitable for self-clean catheterization to manage any postsurgical voiding difficulties. For women with urodynamically proven SUI with a stable bladder, synthetic mid-urethral slings form the mainstay of treatment. This is a minimally invasive procedure, and the sling can be placed via a retropubic, trans-obturator or minimally invasive "inside-out" mini-sling approach. Success rates are comparable with all these modalities, however, for patients with "intrinsic sphincter deficiency" the retropubic approach remains the gold standard.

Women with SUI in whom mid-urethral slings have either been ineffective, or are only partly effective, may be suitable for treatment with urethral bulking injections. These act by improving urethral mucosal co-aptation and restoring the mucosal seal mechanism of continence. They are suitable for use in women with isolated intrinsic sphincter deficiency, limited urethral mobility and absence of detrusor overactivity. Urethral bulking injections are also appropriate for elderly women, women who cannot undergo surgery, those who require continued anticoagulation therapy, or have poor bladder emptying and may be at higher risk for voiding dysfunction [8].

Conclusion

Pelvic organ prolapse and urinary incontinence commonly worsen in postmenopausal women although the role of the menopause is uncertain.

In the case of Joanne, a number of treatment options are likely to be required to result in optimal symptom control.

Her systemic menopausal symptoms would be best treated with HRT. She will require additional local estrogen for her atrophic vaginitis and dyspareunia, and this may also help with her urinary problems. She understands the rationale for pelvic floor exercises and is keen to engage in those with the support of a physiotherapist. She has used a diaphragm for contraception in the past and is not fazed by the prospect of a ring pessary with a knob, which she will remove and replace herself at least once a fortnight and possibly also when she is having sex. If this is not sufficient to manage her urinary problems, she is aware that there are drugs, which might be helpful.

References

1.   Doumouchtsis SK, Chrysanthopoulou EL. Urogenital consequences in ageing women. *Best Pract Res Clin Obstet Gynaecol* 2013; 27: 699–714.

2.   Mannellaa P, Pallaa G, Bellinib M, Simoncinia T. The female pelvic floor through midlife and aging. *Maturitas* 2013; 76: 230–34.

3.   Wilson PD, Barker G, Barnard RJ, Siddle NC. Steroid hormone receptors in the female lower urinary tract. *Urol Int* 1984; 39: 5–8.

4.   Robinson D, Cardozo LD. The role of estrogens in female lower urinary tract

dysfunction. *Urology* 2003; **62 Suppl 1**: 45–51. [Epub 2003/10/11].

5. Deng DY. Urinary incontinence in women. *Med Clin North Am* 2011; **95**: 101–9.

6. Hagen S, Stark D. Conservative prevention and management of pelvic organ prolapse in women. *Cochrane Database Syst Rev* 2011; **12**: CD003882.

7. DeLancey JO. Anatomical aspects of vaginal eversion after hysterectomy. *Am J Obstet Gynecol* 1992; **166**: 1717–24.

8. Karsenty G, Denys P, Amarenco G, *et al.* Botulinum toxin A (Botox) intradetrusor injections in adults with neurogenic detrusor overactivity/neurogenic overactive bladder: a systematic literature review. *Eur Urol* 2008; **53**: 275–87.

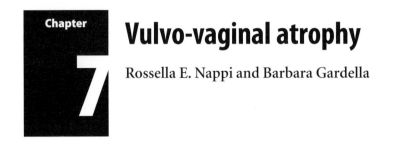

Chapter 7

Vulvo-vaginal atrophy

Rossella E. Nappi and Barbara Gardella

Gladys is 74 and comes to see you because she is sore "down below." She finds her knickers are irritating her, and sometimes she notices a pink discharge. She has been a widow for 5 years and has not been sexually active for a decade. Her "change of life" was uneventful and she has never taken hormone replacement therapy. She has also noticed that she doesn't get much warning when she needs to pass urine and this is making her life very difficult.

Introduction

The term vulvo-vaginal atrophy (VVA) defines the anatomic and physiological changes in the vulvo-vaginal tissues which are directly related to the reduced circulating estrogen levels associated with menopause and to aging. Atrophic vaginitis connotes a state of inflammation or infection that may be present in some women with VVA.

Vulvo-vaginal atrophy or atrophic vaginitis is a medical challenge because it is under-reported by women, under-recognized by health-care providers (HCPs) and, therefore, under-treated. The most common symptoms associated with VVA are dryness, itching, irritation, burning and dyspareunia that may negatively influence well-being and partnership. Even other urinary symptoms are eventually associated with VVA, such as increased frequency, urgency, dysuria and recurrent urinary tract infections (rUTIs), as well as urinary incontinence resulting mainly from pelvic floor relaxation. According to recent surveys, about 50% of postmenopausal women experience vaginal discomfort attributable to VVA. Longitudinal data showed that the prevalence of vaginal dryness, the most common symptoms associated with VVA, ranged from about 3% at premenopause to 47% at 3 years postmenopause. Epidemiologic findings are influenced by a range of factors, including age, time since menopause, frequency of sexual activity, general health, partner's availability and socio-cultural background. In addition, most of the data rely on self-reported symptoms and the severity of symptoms (from mild to severe) is rather subjective. Indeed, objective signs of VVA may be present but women may not report symptoms because they are self-treating, feel the symptoms are not important enough, abstain from sexual activity because of no partner/a partner with health/sexual problems or are embarrassed to discuss such an intimate topic.

Health-care providers should be proactive in order to help their patients to disclose the symptoms related to VVA, and to seek adequate treatment when vaginal discomfort is clinically relevant. Women are poorly aware that VVA is a chronic condition with a significant impact on sexual health and quality of life and that effective and safe treatments

Managing the Menopause: 21st Century Solutions, ed. Nick Panay, Paula Briggs, and Gab Kovacs. Published by Cambridge University Press. © Cambridge University Press 2015.

may be available. Vulvo-vaginal atrophy can lead to symptoms not only in response to sexual activity (low lubrication, pain, poor desire and arousal, impaired sexual pleasure and orgasm), but also during simple activities such as walking or exercising (itching, burning, discharge, unattractive odor, discomfort). Dyspareunia may be accompanied by postcoital bleeding and secondary vaginismus triggered by avoidance, anxiety and loss of sexual desire because of the anticipation of coital pain. A woman with VVA may also experience bleeding with minimal trauma, such as during a medical examination or practicing physical activities. That being so, it is very important to include VVA in the menopause agenda, by encouraging an open and sensible conversation on the topic of uro-genital health and performing a gynecologic pelvic examination, if indicated. According to very recent guidelines for the appropriate management of VVA in clinical practice, it is essential to overcome the vaginal "taboo" in order to optimize elderly women's health care.

Vulvo-vaginal atrophy as a chronic condition

In European countries natural menopause occurs between 51–52 years of age and the increased life expectancy means that most women will spend at least one third of their life in the postmenopausal period, a hypoestrogenic state. Menopausal syndrome is a multidimensional phenomenon in which biological variables are modulated by intrapersonal and interpersonal factors varying according to the socio-cultural environment and the health-care system.

Vulvo-vaginal atrophy is one of the many changes occurring after menopause as a consequence of the loss of estrogen production by the aging ovaries. It may occur as a consequence of other hypoestrogenic states but this is less common. Unlike hot flashes that usually may resolve over time, VVA has a chronic progressive nature throughout the menopausal transition and beyond. The areas of a woman's life most likely to be negatively impacted by VVA are sexual intimacy (64%), having a loving relationship with a partner (32%), overall quality of life (32%), feeling healthy (21%) and feeling attractive (21%). The presence and severity of symptoms are variable, from mild discomfort to great impairment, depending also on age, time and type of menopause, parity and vaginal delivery, frequency of coital activity, cigarette smoking and certain medical conditions/medications. Breast cancer survivors are a special group of women that may suffer from VVA and require an individualized care.

Estrogen stimulation is vital to maintain normal structure and function of the vagina and surrounding uro-genital tissues. Menopausal women displaying less than 50 pg/mL of estradiol suffer more from symptoms associated with VVA. The absence of estrogen stimulation contributes to the loss of mucosal elasticity by inducing fusion and hyalinization of collagen fibers and fragmentation of elastin fibers. Even mucosal hydration is reduced in the dermal layer with a reduction of intercellular acid mucopolysaccharide and hyaluronic acid. The vagina loses its rugae, the epithelial folds that allow for distensibility, and there is a shortening and narrowing of the vaginal canal. The mucosa of the vagina, introitus and labia minora becomes thin and pale, and the significant reduction of vascular support induces a decrease of the volume of vaginal transudate and of other secretions. Over time, there is a progressive dominance of parabasal cells with fewer intermediate and superficial cells as a marker of a deprived estrogen vaginal squamous epithelium which becomes friable with petechiae, ulcerations and eventually bleeding after minimal trauma. With thinning of the vaginal epithelium there is also a significant reduction of glycogen and, therefore, of the population of lactobacilli, causing an increase in vaginal pH (between 5.0 and 7.5) and a decrease of vaginal hydrogen peroxide that allow the growth of other pathogenic bacteria, including staphylococci, group B streptococci and coliforms. Similar anatomical and functional changes in the vulva, as well as in the pelvic floor and within the urinary tract, occur, resulting in an impairment of the neurovascular and neuromuscular substrates of the pelvic area. In particular, the vulvar introitus retracts, and hymeneal carunculae involute and lose elasticity, leading to significant entry dyspareunia. The urethral meatus appears prominent relative to the introitus and thinning of the urinary epithelium and weakening of the surrounding tissue may promote reduced urethral closure pressure, reduced sensory threshold in the bladder, and, in some cases, increased risk of rUTIs.

That being so, VVA is a chronic condition during the postmenopausal years and it cannot regress unless adequately treated.

How to recognize symptoms and signs of VVA

During menopausal consultation, women are often uncomfortable to report intimate symptoms spontaneously and they assume that VVA is a natural part of aging. However, postmenopausal women appreciate being asked and very simple questions may help HCPs to "break the ice" in order to discuss vaginal and sexual health. Unfortunately, HCPs tend not to take a proactive approach to uro-genital health management in the middle and later life age groups, mainly because of inadequate training, constraints of time, personal attitudes and beliefs that sex is not a priority for older patients. Whenever postmenopausal women report uro-genital symptoms in clinical practice, an accurate pelvic examination should be performed to recognize the signs of VVA (Table 7.1). Dyspareunia is generally less reported later in life mainly because older women are less likely to still have a spousal or other intimate relationship and sexually related personal distress declines with age. Tissues may be easily traumatized and irritated and a gentle approach is mandatory in the most severe cases. It has been comprehensively described that the inspection should include the tissues of the vulva, vestibule, vagina and urethra and clinical scales may be used in the attempt to quantify VVA. Organ prolapse and the muscle tone of the pelvic floor also should be noted, as well as other disorders that can cause symptoms similar to those of VVA. Although VVA is typically a clinical diagnosis, other laboratory tests may be used to

Table 7.1. Symptoms and signs associated with VVA in menopause.

Symptoms	Signs
Dryness (vaginal, vulvar, genital skin)	Decreased moisture
Decreased lubrication with sexual intercourse	Decreased elasticity
Discomfort with sexual activity	Labial resorption
Irritation/burning/itching	Pallor/erythema
Vulvo-vaginal infections	Loss of vaginal rugae
Dysuria	Tissue fragility/fissures/petechiae
Urinary frequency	Discharge
Urinary urgency	Odor/infections

Supportive findings: pH >5, increased parabasal cells on vaginal maturation index (VMI).

support the diagnosis, such as an evaluation of vaginal pH and the vaginal maturation index (VMI), which describes the relative proportion of parabasal, intermediate and superficial vaginal epithelial cells. A more alkaline pH (> 5) leads to a shift in the vaginal flora towards more coliforms and, together with the other atrophic changes, is responsible for increased susceptibility to and frequency of infections and odor, as well as traumatic bleeding associated with sexual intercourse or secondary to speculum insertion during routine gynecologic examination. A dominance of parabasal cells, calculated on specimens obtained directly from the lateral upper vaginal walls, indicates hypoestrogenism and atrophy. Thus, the shift to a higher number of superficial cells is a primary endpoint of any treatments prescribed to relieve symptoms of VVA.

The potential burden of VVA should be considered not only in sexually active post-menopausal women but also in women who abstain from sexual activity, because they may suffer even more of the long-term consequences of estrogen deprivation, especially vaginal and introital stenosis, fusion of the labia minora to the labia majora and other uro-genital conditions. Special care should be devoted to women with breast cancer and other gyneco-logic malignancies who are at very high risk of VVA and associated symptoms as a conse-quence of endocrine chemotherapy, surgery and/or radiation. Finally, severe VVA may be a barrier to adequately assess both cytological and colposcopic findings to prevent cervical cancer and it is a very common reason of urgent referral to exclude endometrial cancer and other malignancies after an episode of postmenopausal bleeding. Vaginal occlusion is uncommon but may cause vaginal synechiae and hematocolpos impeding early diagnosis of cancer.

Treatment options

The therapeutic management of VVA in the menopause is multifaceted and should include non-hormonal and hormonal preparations according to very recent guidelines. An open dialogue between women and doctor is needed in order to individualize the most suitable strategy for VVA according to the personal risk-benefit profile, women's preferences and expectations. The principles of treatment in women with clinical diagnosis of VVA are: (1) restoration of uro-genital physiology, and (2) alleviation of symptoms. Given the progression of VVA over time, it is mandatory to start an effective treatment as soon as the symptoms start bothering the woman in order to avoid severe impairment of uro-genital tissues with aging. Indeed, it has been shown that more than half of women who had experienced VVA reported having symptoms for 3 years or longer because they did not feel comfortable discussing VVA with their HCPs. By delaying the treatments, unfortunately VVA symptoms may be amplified by psychosocial factors, such as low self-esteem and poor relationships, and may become refractory to treatment.

There is a general agreement that systemic hormone replacement therapy (HRT) may be prescribed at the lowest effective dose, in the absence of contraindications. Indeed, HRT is efficacious in relieving most of the symptoms because VVA is an integral part of the climacteric syndrome. However, when VVA is the sole consequence of menopause, HRT is not indicated and local estrogen therapy (LET) is the first-line treatment for the mainte-nance of uro-gynecologic and sexual health. Moreover, around 10–25% of women using systemic HRT will still experience VVA symptoms and, therefore, a combination with LET may be useful to relieve vaginal dryness, dyspareunia and other uro-genital symptoms, after appropriate counseling. Low-dose intravaginal estrogen (conjugate equine estrogens, estradiol, estriol, promestriene) preparations in various formulations (creams, rings, tablets, suppositories, gels) are available with some differences among countries. They have been shown, when used as directed, to be safe and effective, without causing significant proliferation of the endometrium or increase in serum estrogen levels beyond the normal postmenopausal range. Local estrogen therapy provides vaginal estrogen, while minimizing systemic exposure, and results in increased blood flow, increased epithelial thickness and increased secretions, as well as reduced pH. These physiologic improvements represent a reversal of atrophy and lead to a positive clinical outcome for most postmenopausal women. In older women, LET has been shown to improve urinary urge incontinence and overactive bladder symptoms and to reduce the episodes of rUTIs. Generally, there is no need to administer progestogen because low-dose LET has not been associated with increased risk for endometrial hyperplasia. Given the comparable efficiency of the low-dose, locally administered different estrogen products, the best guide to select the type of treatment is the level of effectiveness and safety for the individual patient. In addition, it is important that patients accept and adhere to their treatment in order to fully realize the benefits, and, therefore, they have to like the treatment of choice. The intravaginal use of dehydroepiandrosterone (DHEA) is promising in the treatment of sexual symptoms associated with VVA and it has the advantage of not significantly increasing plasma levels of sex hormones. Every woman also may be helped to alleviate VVA by prescribing non-hormonal treatments, such as commercial vaginal moisturizers and lubricants with different characteristics. Lubricants are usually used on demand to relieve vaginal dryness during intercourse and therefore do not provide a long-term solution. On the other hand, women use moisturizers on a more regular basis and these local products may induce some positive modification of genital tissues according to their composition (reduction of pH, maturation of the vaginal epithelium, improvement of natural moisture). Although over-the-counter treatments may work for women with mild symptoms, they are often inadequate for women with moderate-to-severe symptoms. However, non-hormonal options are primarily indicated in women wishing to avoid hormonal therapy or in high-risk individuals with a history of hormone-sensitive malignancy such as breast or endometrial cancer. In cases of severe symptoms of VVA, it may be appropriate to discuss the relative risk of using LET with the oncology team as well as with the patient. Whereas in women taking tamoxifen following breast cancer, there is very little concern that the use of LET may compromise the effects of tamoxifen, the situation is different in women treated with aromatase inhibitors which still represent a contraindication to LET use.

In general, physical therapy including pelvic floor exercises, medical devices, laser technology and other activities with the aim to learn new sexual expertises are useful alone or in association with other treatments to improve uro-genital health. It is also important to mention that regular sexual activity, when it is possible, facilitates active blood flow to the vagina and increases vaginal lubrication. Psycho-educational programs and cognitive reconstruction have been proved highly effective in menopause, namely after gynecologic and breast cancers, and such techniques are available both for the individual woman and also for the couple. Indeed, recent data indicate that evaluation of men's attitudes regarding VVA affecting their postmenopausal partners may lead to better understanding of the impact of VVA on sexual intimacy and may help couples to address the consequences of vaginal discomfort with their HCPs.

Systemic plant-derived and herbal remedies are a very popular alternative to medical treatments, but any real effectiveness in improving VVA is not proven in well-controlled studies, even though a combination of vaginal phytoestrogens and lactobacilli has been proven effective in women with contraindication to hormone therapy.

Finally, ospemifene, a selective estrogen receptor modulator (SERM) with unique estrogen-like effects in the vaginal epithelium, is the first oral treatment approved by the US Food and Drug Administration in February 2013 for moderate-to-severe dyspareunia associated with VVA. At the dose of 60 mg, ospemifene has been shown to reduce symptoms of both dyspareunia and vaginal dryness significantly compared with placebo in a randomized, phase III study. The long-term safety of ospemifene up to 1 year has also been shown, with no significant estrogenic or clinically relevant adverse effects reported on endometrial tissue in women with an intact uterus.

Conclusion

Vulvo-vaginal atrophy is a chronic, age-dependent condition resulting from estrogen deficiency, and may worsen without appropriate treatment, leading to the vicious cycle of sexual symptoms and uro-gynecologic consequences. Early recognition and effective treatment of VVA may enhance sexual health and quality of life of women and their partners and it is part of the general strategy of HCPs to assure a successful aging long after the menopause.

Bibliography

1. Goldstein I. Recognizing and treating urogenital atrophy in postmenopausal women. *J Womens Health (Larchmt)* 2010; **19**: 425–32.

2. Mehta A, Bachmann G. Vulvovaginal complaints. *Clin Obstet Gynecol* 2008; **51**: 549–55.

3. Nappi RE, Palacios S. Impact of vulvovaginal atrophy on sexual health and quality of life at postmenopause. *Climacteric* 2014; **17**: 3–9.

4. Nappi RE, Davis SR. The use of hormone therapy for the maintenance of urogynecological and sexual health post WHI. *Climacteric* 2012; **15**: 267–74.

5. Parish SJ, Nappi RE, Krychman ML, *et al.* Impact of vulvovaginal health on postmenopausal women: a review of surveys on symptoms of vulvovaginal atrophy. *Int J Womens Health* 2013; **5**: 437–47.

6. Sturdee DW, Panay N; International Menopause Society Writing Group. Recommendations for the management of postmenopausal vaginal atrophy. *Climacteric* 2010; **13**: 509–22.

Chapter

8

Musculoskeletal system and the menopause

Jean Calleja-Agius and Mark P. Brincat

Rosemary is 57 years old. Her last menstrual period was 5 years ago. Some of her friends and work colleagues had a terrible time with hot flashes, but she did not experience anything like this. However, recently she has had problems with backache and headaches. She feels stiff and achy all the time and she no longer enjoys playing tennis. One of her friends suggested that her problems may be due to the menopause, and she comes to see you to ask whether she should try some HRT.

Introduction

In 1940, an American endocrinologist, Fuller Albright, was the first to link osteoporosis to ovarian failure when he noted that 40 out of the 42 patients admitted on the orthopedic ward with osteoporotic fractures were women and all had passed the menopause.

Postmenopausal osteoporosis is characterized by progressive loss of bone tissue occurring as a result of an imbalance between bone formation and bone resorption leading to the occurrence of fractures. The pathophysiology of osteoporosis is multifactorial, involving various cytokines, mediators and signaling pathways in combination with genetic, hormonal and environmental influences regulating the bone remodeling process.

Bone homeostasis depends on its cellular components. The development and differentiation of osteoblasts and osteoclasts is tightly controlled by growth factors and cytokines synthesized in the bone marrow microenvironment, so as to maintain a dynamic equilibrium between their formation, survival and function. The increase in osteoclastogenesis and impaired osteoblastogenesis rather than the alteration in the activity of these cells are responsible for postmenopausal osteoporosis [1].

The role of estrogen on bone turnover

Bone marrow stromal cells express two functional estrogen receptors (ER): ERα and ERβ. In human bone cells, ERα mostly predominates in cortical bone while ERβ is the predominant isoform in trabecular bone. When the ligand binds to estrogen receptors, it causes a conformational change resulting in receptor dimerization. The receptor binds to specific DNA sequences known as estrogen response elements (EREs). At the promoter, the ligand-bound receptor establishes a complex with co-activator proteins that stimulate the general transcriptional machinery and enhance the expression of target genes via chromatin remodeling. Estrogen receptors may also recruit co-repressors which down regulate estrogen receptor-dependent gene expression.

Managing the Menopause: 21st Century Solutions, ed. Nick Panay, Paula Briggs, and Gab Kovacs. Published by Cambridge University Press. © Cambridge University Press 2015.

Estrogen regulates the secretion of cytokines involved in bone homeostasis, exerting a role in bone remodeling. It inhibits the formation of locally produced pro-inflammatory cytokines and suppresses new osteoclast formation. Estrogen indirectly decreases osteoclastic activity by suppressing the formation of macrophage-colony stimulating factor (M-CSF), receptor activator of nuclear factor kappa-B ligand (RANKL), interleukins (IL)-1 and -6 and tumor necrosis factor alpha (TNF-α) by osteoblasts and stromal cells and activating the synthesis of osteoprotegerin (OPG) and transforming growth factor beta (TGF-β).

The main result of oophorectomy is a significant increase in bone resorption. This occurs because a decline in circulating estrogen results in an increase in osteoclastogenesis and prolongation of osteoclast lifespan by decreasing apoptosis. However, the unlimited rise in osteoclast number and lifespan is restrained by a compensatory increase in bone formation at each remodeling unit. Estrogen deficiency causes expansion of the pool of early mesenchymal progenitors as well as an increase in committed pluripotent precursors to the osteoblastic lineage, both enhancing the number of osteoblasts. However, lack of estrogen limits osteoblastogenesis by accelerating osteoblast apoptosis and enhancing the formation of inflammatory cytokines such as IL-7 and TNF, which inhibit the functional activity of mature osteoblasts. Thus, the overall increase in osteoblastogenesis is insufficient to compensate for osteoclastic bone resorption.

Decreased levels of bioavailable estradiol inhibit the activity of osteoblasts and stromal cells. This results in decreased OPG secretion, permitting more binding of RANKL to receptor activator of nuclear factor kappa-B (RANK), hence increasing osteoclastogenesis and bone resorption. In postmenopausal osteoporosis, the increase in bone resorption is brought about by a rise in paracrine production of bone-resorbing cytokines [1]. Decreased estradiol levels also increase the expression and secretion of IL-6, IL-11 and RANKL, which in turn directly activate more osteoclast formation and activity. The secretion of these cytokines is significantly higher in bone marrow cells isolated from postmenopausal women [2, 3].

The role of hormone replacement therapy

Hormone replacement therapy involves the administration of physiological levels of estrogen and progestin to replace and artificially boost the hormones which decline during menopause.

Hormone replacement therapy slows the rate of bone loss in osteoporotic patients. It elevates calcium absorption and as a result of a decline in the bone resorption rate, bone balance is either maintained or becomes slightly positive. This positive bone balance is mainly pronounced in trabecular bone while bone mass is maintained in areas of the skeleton rich in cortical bone.

Estrogen is known to inhibit osteoclastic activity. It causes a decline in erosion depth and osteoclast activation frequency by inducing apoptosis which is mediated by TGF-β and suppressing osteoclastogenesis. The decline in bone resorption is also mediated by a reduction in the formation and sensitivity of bone cells to IL-6, IL-1 and TNF-α, and increase in the formation of IL-4. This causes a decrease in the differentiation of precursor cells to osteoclasts. Additionally, administering HRT to postmenopausal women causes a decline in proportion of bone marrow cell to express RANKL in lymphocytes, but its concentration per cell is not altered. Hence, a decline in the formation, differentiation and survival of osteoclasts is observed. Moreover, estrogen reduces the lytic enzyme activity of osteoclasts, alters the concentration of growth factors and interferons, and affects bone collagen metabolism [4].

As estrogen receptors are present on osteoblasts, estrogen supplied through HRT acts directly on such receptors to prevent bone loss. Long-term treatment with HRT administered at high doses not only decreases bone resorption but also activates bone formation by enhancing proliferation of osteoblasts resulting in a net anabolic action. This is known to result from the non-genotropic effect of estrogen on osteoblast apoptosis.

The indirect action of estrogen involves decreasing the responsiveness of bone to parathyroid hormone (PTH) and altering its secretion. It also elevates intestinal absorption and reduces the renal excretion of calcium.

Epidemiologic studies have shown that a short-term treatment with HRT decreases the occurrence of osteoporotic fractures. It has been determined that undergoing estrogen therapy for 5 years reduces vertebral fractures by 60% whilst hip fractures may decline by 50%. Generally with estrogen treatment, bone turnover is reduced by half, decreasing postmenopausal bone loss and lowering the incidence of an osteoporotic fracture. However, once treatment with HRT is terminated, estrogen level declines and protection against osteoporosis is lost again. Most studies suggest that bone loss will progress at the same rate prior to treatment with HRT. Thus the accelerated bone loss during menopause is postponed by the duration of HRT treatment. To date, the degree of bone density and the diagnosis of osteoporosis is routinely clinically measured using a dual energy X-ray absorptiometry (DXA) bone density scan [5].

Hormone replacement therapy has been shown to be highly effective to prevent post-menopausal osteoporosis during the first 5–10 years following the onset of menopause and treatment should be continuous and lifelong. This is because the rate of bone loss is the highest during the first 2 years of menopause. However, studies suggest that when estrogen therapy is initiated beyond the age of 60 years, bone mineral density (BMD) is either maintained or increased after 2 years of use. The increase in bone mass in such patients is a result of a decline in bone resorption more than bone formation. Women who initiate HRT at an old age, gain 5–10% of bone density during the initial 2 years of therapy and then lose 0.5% of bone density each year. Studies suggest that estrogen therapy initiated in women in their early 60s is as advantageous as continuous treatment begun immediately after menopause. When HRT is discontinued, 2% of bone density is lost each year for 5 years and 1% each year thereafter.

Progestin, a chemical analog of progesterone, decreases the rate of bone resorption as it reduces urinary calcium excretion. Administration of progestin in combination with estrogen not only decreases the rate of bone loss but it has been proved to promote bone formation by enhancing osteoblast activity via suppression of glucocorticoid action. A number of studies have shown the positive effect of progesterone on bone proliferation and inhibition of bone resorption. Administration of estrogen and progestin alone may have distinct yet complementary roles in the maintenance of bone architecture.

Intervertebral discs

Each intervertebral disc is composed of high collagen content and glycosaminoglycans. Intervertebral discs are responsible for 20% of the spinal column height and allow flexion and extension of the back, and also act as "shock absorbers" of the spinal column. This may have an important role on osteoporotic compression fractures.

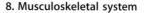

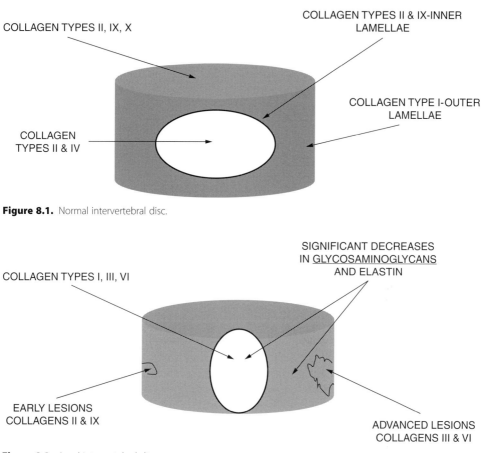

COLLAGEN TYPES II, IX, X

COLLAGEN TYPES II & IX-INNER LAMELLAE

COLLAGEN TYPE I-OUTER LAMELLAE

COLLAGEN TYPES II & IV

Figure 8.1. Normal intervertebral disc.

SIGNIFICANT DECREASES IN GLYCOSAMINOGLYCANS AND ELASTIN

COLLAGEN TYPES I, III, VI

EARLY LESIONS COLLAGENS II & IX

ADVANCED LESIONS COLLAGENS III & VI

Figure 8.2. Aged intervertebral disc.

With the aging process, there is a change in collagen type, with a more profound difference with increasing years since menopause. The collagen types I, III and VI predominate at the expense of collagen types II, IV and IX. There is also a significant decrease in glycosaminoglycans and elastin in the aged intervertebral disc. Figures 8.1 and 8.2 show the normal intervertebral disc and the changes which occur with aging respectively.

The lumbar intervertebral disc height has been shown to be significantly higher in the premenopausal group and hormone-treated group, compared with the untreated postmenopausal women. The premenopausal women and hormone-treated women had disc heights of 2.01 ± 0.09 cm and 2.15 ± 0.08 cm respectively, the latter results being significantly higher than the untreated postmenopausal group (height of three lumbar discs 1.82 ± 0.06 cm) and the osteoporotic fracture group (1.58 ± 0.1 cm) ($P < 0.0001$) [6]. Figure 8.3 shows how the intervertebral disc can be measured during a DXA bone density scan.

These results may be due to the effect that the menopause has on the connective tissue components of intervertebral discs. This may lead to loss of the shock-absorbing properties of the intervertebral disc and an altered discoid shape, influencing the occurrence of osteoporotic vertebral body fractures. After menopause, intervertebral disc space shows a progressive decrease that almost entirely occurs in the first 5–10 years since menopause,

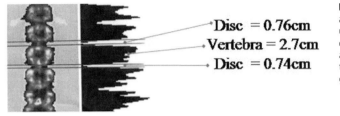

$Disc = 0.76cm$
$Vertebra = 2.7cm$
$Disc = 0.74cm$

Figure 8.3. Dual energy X-ray absorptiometry (DXA) bone scan used to measure intervertebral disc height. This is measured by applying cursors to the edges of the discs using the adjacent grayscale to increase accuracy.

suggesting that the decline in estrogen level may rapidly change connective tissue metabolism in the intervertebral discs.

Hormone-treated and premenopausal women have thicker intervertebral discs than untreated postmenopausal women. Alterations in the extracellular matrix in the intervertebral discs appear to be intimately related to the menopausal process. Loss of disc height may pre-date osteoporotic fracture.

Muscle

In menopause, there is a decline in muscle mass and strength when serum estrogen declines. Estrogen improves muscle strength. The underlying mechanism involves estrogen receptors to improve muscle quality rather than quantity. Hormone replacement therapy attenuates exercise-induced skeletal muscle damage in postmenopausal women. Postmenopausal women not using hormonal therapy experience greater muscle damage. Hormone replacement therapy modifies skeletal muscle composition and function. It gives better mobility, greater muscle power, prevents muscle weakness and thus prevents mobility limitation [7].

Thus, in order to maintain the integrity of the musculoskeletal system, the main recommendations are to do regular physical exercise, maintain protein intake, and in the postmenopause, consider estrogen replacement.

Where do we stand now?

While some studies claim that HRT is the treatment of choice for postmenopausal women, its use has become controversial following the Women's Health Initiative (WHI) Study over a decade ago. As long-term duration of therapy is needed for prevention of postmenopausal osteoporosis, HRT has been associated with various risks which limit its administration. The long-term adverse effects implicated for HRT include carcinoma mainly of the breast, endometrium and colorectal as well as cardiovascular diseases such as coronary heart disease, cerebrovascular events and pulmonary embolism. Regulatory authorities, including the European Medicines Authority, claim that HRT should not be used as a first-line treatment in prophylaxis as long-term risks may outweigh the potential benefits, and thus claim that HRT should only be considered when other treatment options have proved to be unsuccessful.

However, in view of current evidence, in particular the re-evaluation of the WHI data, the role of estrogen treatment of osteoporosis and osteoporotic fractures needs to be reassessed. The potential side effects and risks involved in taking HRT may be reduced by using lower HRT doses; minimizing or eliminating systemic progestogens; using non-oral routes in some women; and initiating HRT in symptomatic women near menopause.

Table 8.1. Current pharmacological agents indicated for the treatment of postmenopausal osteoporosis.

Conventional pharmacological treatment	
Hormone replacement therapy (HRT)	• Increases calcium absorption • Decreases the erosion depth and osteoclast activation frequency by inducing apoptosis and suppressing osteoclastogenesis • Decreases the responsiveness of bone to parathyroid hormone (PTH) and alters its secretion • Promotes calcium intestinal absorption • Decreases the renal excretion of calcium • Long-term treatment with HRT administered at high doses stimulates proliferation of osteoblasts, hence promoting bone formation
Bisphosphonates	• Decreases the activity of osteoclasts • Stimulates osteoclast apoptosis • Decreases the formation of oxygen-free radicals produced by polymorphonuclear cells which are known to promote inflammation • Decreases proinflammatory cytokines and adhesion molecules • Promotes proliferation of T-lymphocytes
Strontium ranelate	• Dual action; anti-resorptive and anabolic actions • Inhibits osteoclast recruitment and augments osteoblast proliferation and differentiation • Decreases both hip and vertebral fractures
Teriparatide	• Recombinant synthetic form of the natural human hormone • Daily subcutaneous injection enhances bone formation by activating osteoblasts and increase in bone mineral density (BMD) • Enhances calcium intestinal absorption as well as calcium reabsorption by the kidney • Decreases significantly vertebral (by 65%) and non-vertebral fractures (by 35%) excluding hip fractures • Mainly used in severely osteoporotic patients with a high fracture risk
Calcitonin	• Peptide hormone synthesized by the thyroid gland • Can be administered via subcutaneous, intramuscular or nasal routes • Nasal spray calcitonin effective in decreasing vertebral fractures in postmenopausal osteoporotic women but no effect on non-vertebral fractures • Administer calcium and vitamin D supplementation concurrently as calcitonin decreases blood calcium levels • Indicated mainly for osteoporotic women who are beyond their fifth year of menopause
Calcitriol	• Active vitamin D metabolite used to treat low calcium levels in postmenopausal women • Aids in calcium intestinal absorption • Reduces the rate of vertebral fractures, whereas it has no effect on hip fractures

Table 8.1. (*cont.*)

	Conventional pharmacological treatment

Selective estrogen receptor modulators	• Non-steroidal compounds with tissue-specific activity; estrogenic effects in certain tissues and anti-estrogenic effects in others
	• **Raloxifene**
	  • Anti-resorptive agent administered either to young postmenopausal osteoporotic women or those having low bone mass
	  • Prevents and decreases osteoporosis-related vertebral fractures by 30–50% and increases BMD at the hip and the spine by 0.5% to 1.0% respectively
	  • Decreases the risk of breast cancer in osteoporotic women and is also cardio-protective
	  • Vasomotor symptoms and thromboembolic events placed raloxifene as a second-line agent in patients who have developed intolerance to previous osteoporotic treatment
	
	• **Bazedoxifene**
	  • Elevates BMD
	  • Reduces the bone turnover markers
	  • Decreases the occurrence of vertebral fractures in postmenopausal women
	  • As opposed to other SERMs, bazedoxifene has an antagonistic activity on the uterus and the breast

Tibolone	• Synthetic steroid known as selective tissue estrogenic activity regulator (STEAR) • Exerts tissue-specific actions by enzymatic conversion of steroid into three bioactive metabolites • Suppresses bone turnover by decreasing osteoclastic activity • Bone loss is prevented at the lumbar spine and proximal femur while it can increase BMD in the phalanges and the hip • Low dose of tibolone also decreases the occurrence of vertebral and non-vertebral fractures in elderly postmenopausal women
Vitamin D/calcium	• Postmenopausal women have the highest calcium requirements • Adequate amount of dietary or supplemental calcium and vitamin D to postmenopausal women serves as a baseline treatment of postmenopausal osteoporosis • Dietary calcium intake without estrogen therapy retards but not entirely prevents postmenopausal bone loss • Concomitant intake of vitamin D with calcium enhances calcium absorption from the gastrointestinal tract • Calcium supplementation may lower the rate of bone loss following 2 years of treatment; however, during the initial 5 years of menopause, it exerts little effect on bone loss as it can be attributed to the decline in estrogen synthesis • Calcium supplementation regarded as an adjunct to other treatment regimens unless sufficient dietary intake is ensured

Table 8.1. (cont.)

Conventional pharmacological treatment
• Vitamin D may decrease the risk of hip and non-vertebral fractures in ambulatory elderly patients only if an oral supplementation of 700–800 IU is administered each day • Vitamin D/calcium supplementation increases BMD and decreases the risk of fracture. The latter is negated by some recent randomized controlled clinical trials

When HRT is initiated near menopause for symptom control, there may be additional benefits including reduced fracture and cardiovascular risk [8]. These benefits outweigh the risks, which are not significantly raised in women under age 60 years. As long as their therapy and risks are assessed on an individual basis and each patient is aware of the risks, older women with continuing symptoms should not be denied HRT. In fact, the key recommendation of most societies, including the British Menopause Society, is that all women should be able to access advice on how they can optimize their menopause transition and beyond, with particular reference to lifestyle and diet and an opportunity to discuss the pros and cons of complementary therapies and HRT [9]. A global consensus statement on menopausal HRT concludes that HRT is effective and appropriate for the prevention of osteoporosis-related fractures in at-risk women before age 60 years or within 10 years after menopause [10].

Alternatives

Selective estrogen receptor modulators (SERMs), such as raloxifene, now have a more central role in the prevention and management of postmenopausal osteoporosis. Selective estrogen receptor modulators act through estrogen receptors and are agonists for bone and antagonists for breast and uterine tissue. Bisphosphonates are also widely used. There are also newer drugs which act by interplaying with cytokines.

Table 8.1 lists the alternative treatments that can be used in the management of osteoporosis.

Conclusion

The ideal prevention of postmenopausal bone loss is to maintain premenopausal estrogen status. Estrogens have been shown to be the most effective in the prevention of osteoporosis and osteoporotic fractures. This is particularly relevant when estrogen therapy is used in the first decade after the menopause.

References

1. Calleja-Agius J, Brincat M. The effect of menopause on the skin and other connective tissues. *Gynecol Endocrinol* 2012; **28**: 273–7.

2. Rachner TD, Khosla S, Lorenz C, Hofbauer LC. Osteoporosis: now and the future. *Lancet* 2011; **377**: 1276–87.

3. Salari P, Abdollahi M. A comprehensive review of the shared roles of inflammatory cytokines in osteoporosis and cardiovascular diseases as two common old people problem – actions toward development of new drugs. *Int J Pharmacol* 2011; **7**: 552–67.

4. Clowes JA, Eghbali-Fatourechi GZ, McCready L, Oursler MJ, Khosla S, Riggs

BL. Estrogen action on bone marrow osteoclast lineage cells of postmenopausal women in vivo. *Osteoporosis Int.* 2009; **20**: 761–9.

5. Brincat M, Calleja-Agius J, Vujovic S, *et al.* EMAS position statement: bone densitometry screening for osteoporosis. *Maturitas* 2011; **68**: 98–101.

6. Muscat BY, Brincat MP, Galea R, Calleja N. Low intervertebral disc height in postmenopausal women with osteoporotic vertebral fractures compared to hormone-treated and untreated postmenopausal women and premenopausal women without fractures. *Climacteric* 2007; **10**: 314–19.

7. Dieli-Conwright CM, Spektor TM, Rice JC, Sattler FR, Schroeder ET. Hormone replacement therapy and messenger RNA expression of estrogen receptor coregulators after exercise in postmenopausal women. *Med Sci Sports Exerc* 2010; **42**: 422–9.

8. Calleja-Agius J, Brincat MP. Hormone replacement therapy post Women's Health Initiative study: where do we stand? *Curr Opin Obstet Gynecol* 2008; **20**: 513–18.

9. Panay N, Hamoda H, Arya R, Savvas M; British Menopause Society and Women's Health Concern. The 2013 British Menopause Society & Women's Health Concern recommendations on hormone replacement therapy. *Menopause Int* 2013; **19**: 59–68.

10. de Villiers TJ, Gass ML, Haines CJ, *et al.* Global consensus statement on menopausal hormone therapy. *Climacteric* 2013; **16**: 203–4.

Osteoporosis recognition and assessment

Christopher J. Yates and John D. Wark

Introduction

Postmenopausal osteoporosis (PMO) is a common disease characterized by low bone mass and micro-architectural deterioration of bone tissue leading to skeletal fragility [1]. Osteoporosis is also defined as a skeletal disorder characterized by compromised bone strength predisposing to an increased risk of fracture. Bone strength reflects the integration of two main features: bone mineral density (BMD) and bone quality [2]. Osteoporotic fractures are a major public health problem due to the associated consequences of pain, loss of independence, reduced quality of life, increased mortality and elevated health-care costs. Early recognition, assessment and treatment of PMO are necessary to reduce the significant burden of osteoporotic fractures.

Clinical assessment

Osteoporosis is known as a silent disease because no outward symptoms are noted until a fracture occurs. However, a thorough medical history from a postmenopausal woman should detect risk factors for osteoporosis, assess for underlying medical conditions that predispose to fracture and identify medications associated with bone loss and fractures. Important factors to consider include age, low body mass index, past fractures, sedentary lifestyle, calcium-deficient diet, family history of hip fracture or osteoporosis, falls history, glucocorticoid therapy, anticonvulsant medication, cigarette smoking and alcohol intake of three or more units per day. Other causes of fractures and reduced BMD such as osteomalacia, malignancy (multiple myeloma), renal osteodystrophy, liver disease, Paget's disease, hyperparathyroidism, malabsorption, inflammatory conditions, Cushing's syndrome and hyperthyroidism should also be considered. The history and physical examination may also identify abnormalities suggestive of a secondary cause of osteoporosis, or signs of vertebral fractures such as back pain, height loss of 4 cm or greater and change in appearance of the back (e.g. prominent thoracic kyphosis). While height loss is not specific to osteoporotic vertebral fracture, it is a useful guide to the possible presence of (new) fractures; hence height measurement is recommended as part of regular health monitoring in older people.

A history of low-trauma fracture is key to the clinical diagnosis of osteoporosis. A low-trauma event is defined as one occurring due to a fall from standing height or less, or an equivalent injury. It is important to elicit the level of trauma associated with fractures, particularly in older people.

Managing the Menopause: 21st Century Solutions, ed. Nick Panay, Paula Briggs, and Gab Kovacs. Published by Cambridge University Press. © Cambridge University Press 2015.

Falls risk is an important risk factor for fracture and multiple validated risk assessment tools are available, such as the QuickScreen and Falls Risk for Older People in the Community (FROP-Com) tools, which take less than 10 minutes to administer in the consultation room and identify recurrent fallers with an accuracy of over 70% in community-dwelling individuals [3, 4]. QuickScreen and FROP-Com provide a probability of falls based on the presence of risk factors such as prior falls, polypharmacy, psychotropic medication, vision impairment, peripheral sensory impairment, and deficits in strength, reaction time and balance. The assessment of multiple factors by this and other risk assessment tools could assist with guiding the implementation of multifactorial interventions to prevent falls. Other simple tools with lower predictive ability include the Timed Up and Go test and functional reach [5, 6].

Diagnosis

A clinical diagnosis of osteoporosis can be made in an individual who sustains a fragility fracture in the absence of another cause of skeletal fragility. Typical osteoporotic fragility fractures include those at the proximal femur, spine, forearm, proximal humerus, ribs, pelvis and sometimes at the tibia and fibula. Stress fractures and fractures involving the hands, feet, cervical spine and skull are not generally considered to be fragility fractures. Where there is suspicion of a vertebral fracture (a significant episode of back pain, significant height loss, kyphosis), performance of plain X-rays of the thoracic and lumbar spine should be considered. It is also important to remember that the absence of a history of back pain does not rule out osteoporotic vertebral fracture since only about one third of patients with these fractures will report a clear history of back pain.

Osteoporosis can also be diagnosed by assessing BMD at the hip, lumbar spine or distal third of the radius using dual energy X-ray absorptiometry (DXA). The World Health Organization (WHO) criteria classify BMD (in g/cm^2) according to the T-score, which is the standard deviation (SD) difference between the individual's BMD and the mean value of a young adult reference population. A normal BMD is a value greater than 1 SD below the young adult reference mean (Table 9.1). A value more than 1 SD below the young adult female reference mean but less than 2.5 SD below this value is classified as low bone mass or osteopenia, and osteoporosis is classified as a BMD 2.5 SD or more below the young adult reference mean. A diagnosis of established or severe osteoporosis is made if an individual has both a history of fragility fracture and a BMD T-score of −2.5 or lower. Although individuals with a T-score below −2.5 have the greatest fracture risk, many more fractures occur in individuals falling into the osteopenic BMD range due to the significantly larger proportion of the population within that range. A DXA Z-score is a

Table 9.1. Classification of bone mineral density by dual energy X-ray absorptiometry (DXA).

Classification	T-score
Normal	−1.0 or greater
Osteopenia (low bone mass)	−1.0 to −2.5
Osteoporosis	−2.5 or lower
Established osteoporosis	−2.5 or lower with a fragility fracture

comparison between the individual and age-matched controls and gives an indication of the severity of a bone deficit. Although it is not a criterion for the diagnosis of osteoporosis, a Z-score below −2.0 SD is considered to be a more severe reduction in BMD at any age and is generally an indication for more comprehensive investigation for underlying causes of a bone deficit.

Recommendations for the timing of DXA testing in postmenopausal women vary between countries. However, a general consensus is that testing should be performed for: all women over the age of 70 years; postmenopausal women with osteoporosis risk factors; and any women who have sustained a fracture after the age of 50 years.

A DXA scan is typically performed at the spine and hip, and radiation exposure is very low. The DXA scan is reliable with a reported precision of approximately 1–2% at the lumbar spine (though precision is less at the hip sites). There is a strong correlation between fracture risk and DXA BMD score at the proximal femur and lumbar spine. Each SD reduction in femoral neck or total hip BMD increases the age-adjusted risk of hip fracture by a factor of about 2.5, while each SD reduction in lumbar spine BMD increases the risk of spinal fracture by a factor of approximately 2.3 [7]. However, a limitation of DXA is that the image is two-dimensional and therefore provides areal rather than volumetric BMD. Quantitative computed tomography (QCT) of the spine has inadequate precision at most centres and involves higher ionizing radiation exposure, so is not a first-line investigation; QCT at the hip is primarily a research tool at this time due to limited clinical validation and availability. Peripheral QCT (pQCT) at peripheral sites (forearm and tibia) provide true volumetric BMD, but has limited clinical validation and limited availability. Quantitative ultrasound of the calcaneum is occasionally used to estimate fracture risk and has demonstrated predictive value for fractures but cannot be used to diagnose osteoporosis or to monitor therapeutic responses.

In addition to ensuring appropriate quality control for all DXA service providers, there are numerous pitfalls of bone densitometry of which clinicians should be aware. Positioning of the patient is vital as rotation of the spine or hip can result in significantly altered T-scores. Artifacts such as surgical clips or local structural changes such as osteophytes, compression fractures, scoliosis, metastases or aortic calcification can elevate T-scores (Figure 9.1). Degenerative lumbar spine disease is a very common cause of a spuriously elevated vertebral BMD, particularly in older individuals, while spina bifida or surgically excised bone (e.g. laminectomy) can cause a spuriously lower BMD.

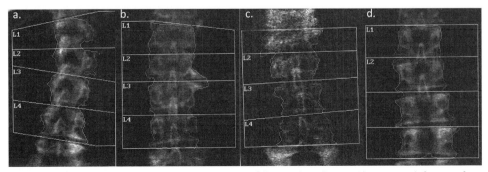

Figure 9.1. Examples of common spine DXA scanning pitfalls: a. scoliosis, b. osteophytes, c. crush fracture of first lumbar vertebra and d. laminectomy.

Vertebrae affected by local structural changes should therefore be omitted from analysis and if all vertebrae are affected then the spine BMD should be reported as invalid. In reading a DXA report from the spine it is helpful to note that BMD typically increases from the first lumbar vertebra through to the third lumbar vertebra, and T-scores for individual vertebrae are typically within 1 SD of each other. When these observations are not present, clinicians should suspect and investigate for a possible artifact or local structural change. It is usually the greatest BMD that is the spurious result in the vertebrae.

Fracture risk stratification

Fracture risk stratification is facilitated by the use of calculators such as the WHO FRAX algorithm [8] and the Garvan fracture risk calculator [9] that are applicable to postmenopausal women and predict probability of fracture better than BMD or clinical risk factors alone. FRAX is a computer-based algorithm that uses clinical risk factors, BMD and large country-specific fracture datasets to quantify an individual's 10-year probability of hip or major osteoporotic fracture (i.e. vertebral, hip, proximal humerus or distal forearm fracture). Computed parameters include femoral bone mineral density, prior fractures, parental hip fracture history, age, gender, body mass index (BMI), ethnicity, smoking, alcohol use, glucocorticoid use, rheumatoid arthritis and secondary causes of osteoporosis. FRAX can also be used without femoral neck BMD in circumstances where DXA is unavailable. Some risk factors such as falls and frailty are not included in FRAX and require further clinical judgment. FRAX also takes no account of the dose responses for several risk factors (e.g. glucocorticoid use) and may underestimate fracture risk when the lumbar spine BMD is substantially lower than the femoral neck BMD.

Laboratory investigations

Patients who have sustained a fragility fracture and those with a DXA T-score of -2.5 or below (or a Z-score of -2.0 or below) should have further laboratory investigations to screen for secondary causes of osteoporosis and bone fragility. Serum calcium, phosphate, creatinine and electrolytes should be assessed to detect primary hyperparathyroidism, secondary hyperparathyroidism and renal osteodystrophy. Serum 25-hydroxyvitamin D should be performed to assess for vitamin D deficiency and possible malabsorption. Serum alkaline phosphatase may help to identify cases of metastatic bone disease, Paget's disease and osteomalacia, and will be elevated during the healing of a major fracture; gamma GT testing is useful to discriminate hepatic and bone origin of alkaline phosphatase elevations. Other helpful investigations include ESR or CRP and full blood examination to identify inflammatory diseases and marrow infiltration, thyroid stimulating hormone (TSH) to detect thyrotoxicosis, and serum and urine protein electrophoresis to screen for multiple myeloma. Additionally, if the history is suggestive of celiac disease (e.g. gluten intolerance, relatively low body weight, other autoimmune disease, iron deficiency), celiac serology is indicated. Parathyroid hormone levels should be assessed in all patients with hypercalcemia. Bone turnover markers such as P1NP and beta CTX may also provide valuable information for predicting fracture risk. Bone turnover markers are increased after menopause, and the rate of bone loss appears to vary according to the marker value [10].

Clinical cases

Case 1

Christine is a 74-year-old white woman from England who presents for her annual health assessment. She has a history of hypertension controlled with a calcium channel blocker and of lumbar spine osteoarthritis. She does not smoke and drinks less than one unit of alcohol per day. She took HRT for 2 years after menopause. She supplements her vitamin D intake with 1,000 IU of cholecalciferol daily. Due to lactose intolerance, she consumes less than one serving of dairy products per day. She supplements her calcium intake with calcium carbonate 600 mg with her evening meal. She has no history of falls or fractures and there is no family history of osteoporosis.

On examination, she weighs 54.4 kg and is 160 cm tall, which is 4 cm less than her peak adult height. Her body mass index is 21.3. She has a mild thoracic kyphosis. Laboratory investigations including full blood count, creatinine, electrolytes, alkaline phosphatase, gamma GT, TSH and 25-hydroxyvitamin D are all within normal limits. Lumbar spine X-ray to investigate the height loss shows no significant vertebral fractures. A DXA BMD scan is performed because of her age and reveals a T-score of −1.9 at the lumbar spine and −2.0 at the femoral neck.

Discussion points: this patient has osteopenia of the lumbar spine and femoral neck. The FRAX calculator is used to evaluate her fracture risk. Her 10-year probability of major osteoporotic fracture is 10% and hip fracture is 2.8%. Based on these results she is provided with lifestyle advice and discharged to her general practitioner. A follow-up BMD is scheduled for 5 years.

Case 2

Barbara is a 60-year-old Australian woman who presents for a screening assessment for osteoporosis. She has a history of rheumatoid arthritis for 20 years for which she has been managed with prolonged glucocorticoid therapy. She has chronic low back pain and her height has reduced by 6 cm from peak height. She eats two servings of dairy food per day and her current medications include prednisolone 10 mg daily, calcium carbonate 600 mg daily and cholecalciferol 1,000 IU daily. There is no family history of osteoporosis. She is a non-smoker and does not drink alcohol.

On examination, she has mild low back pain. Her height is 160 cm and her weight is 60 kg (BMI 23.4). She has a flattened lumbar lordosis. Investigations reveal a 25-hydroxyvitamin D level of 45 nmol/L. Full blood count, creatinine, electrolytes, alkaline phosphatase, gamma GT and TSH are normal. Her DXA T-scores are −0.8 at the lumbar spine and −2.6 at the femoral neck. Lumbar spine X-ray reveals degenerative disease at L1–L3 that is confounding the lumbar spine DXA result.

Discussion points: Barbara has osteoporosis of the femoral neck with risk factors of prolonged glucocorticoid therapy and chronic inflammatory disease. The FRAX calculator is used to evaluate her fracture risk and the 10-year probability of major osteoporotic fracture is 15% and for hip fracture 6.1%. She is recommended to increase her vitamin D supplementation and commence osteoporosis-specific therapy.

Acknowledgments

We acknowledge the contributions of Professor Stephen R. Lord, Senior Principal Research Fellow of Neurosciences Research Australia and Professor Keith D. Hill, Faculty of Health

Sciences, Latrobe University, regarding the falls assessment section; and the input of Dr. Ashwini Kale, Department of Medicine, University of Melbourne, for providing the sample DXA images in Figure 1.

References

1. Peck WA, Burckhardt P, Christiansen C, et al. Consensus development conference – diagnosis, prophylaxis, and treatment of osteoporosis. Am J Med 1993; 94: 646–50.

2. Klibanski A, Adams-Campbell L, Bassford T, et al. Osteoporosis prevention, diagnosis, and therapy. JAMA 2001; 285: 785–95.

3. Tiedemann A, Lord SR, Sherrington C. The development and validation of a brief performance-based fall risk assessment tool for use in primary care. J Gerontol Ser A – Biologic Sci Med Sci 2010; 65: 893–900.

4. Russell MA, Hill KD, Day LM, et al. Development of the Falls Risk for Older People in the Community (FROP-Com) screening tool. Age Ageing 2009; 38: 40–6.

5. Russell MA, Hill KD, Blackberry I, Day LM, Dharmage SC. The reliability and predictive accuracy of the Falls Risk for Older People in the Community Assessment (FROP-Com) tool. Age Ageing 2008; 37: 634–9.

6. Scott V, Votova K, Scanlan A, Close J. Multifactorial and functional mobility assessment tools for fall risk among older adults in community, home-support, long-term and acute care settings. Age Ageing 2007; 36: 130–9.

7. Royal Australian College of General Practitioners. Clinical Guideline for the Prevention and Treatment of Osteoporosis in Postmenopausal Women and Older Men. South Melbourne: Council AGNHaMR Royal Australian College of General Practitioners; 2010.

8. Kanis JA, Johnell O, Oden A, Johansson H, McCloskey E. FRAX (TM) and the assessment of fracture probability in men and women from the UK. Osteoporos Int 2008; 19: 385–97.

9. Nguyen ND, Frost SA, Center JR, Eisman JA, Nguyen TV. Development of prognostic nomograms for individualizing 5-year and 10-year fracture risks. Osteoporos Int 2008; 19: 1431–44.

10. Delmas PD, Eastell R, Garnero P, Seibel MJ, Stepan J, Comm Sci Advisors Int O. The use of biochemical markers of bone turnover in osteoporosis. Osteoporos Int 2000; 11: 2–17.

Hormonal management of osteoporosis during the menopause

Panagiotis G. Anagnostis and John C. Stevenson

Kay is 62 and a retired radiologist. At 55 she twisted her ankle, and broke her tibia, which needed fixation with a plate. At 58 she fell and sustained a Colles' fracture. Recently she has noticed that she appears to be "shrinking." She also has back pain. A friend suggested that she may be osteoporotic, and she has come to see you for assessment and advice regarding treatment.

Bone pathophysiology

Therapies for osteoporosis have been traditionally based on our understanding of bone cell activities. Bone tissue is constantly being removed and replaced (bone turnover) by osteoclasts which resorb bone and osteoblasts which lay down new bone. Bone turnover is essential for the maintenance of a healthy skeleton by removing or repairing the microscopic damage that results from everyday physical activity. These processes of resorption and formation are linked or "coupled" so that bone turnover proceeds in an orderly fashion. When these processes become imbalanced or uncoupled, resorption can exceed formation and bone loss then occurs leading to an increased risk of fractures. Traditionally, drugs which reduce osteoclastic activity have been the mainstay of treatment. Thus agents such as estrogens and bisphosphonates have been widely used with considerable success. Agents that act directly on osteoblasts to increase bone formation are few, with parathyroid hormone being the main one. However, more recent understanding of bone biology has led to the recognition of cell signaling systems that regulate both osteoclasts and osteoblasts. New therapies are being developed which target these cell signals. Receptor activator of nuclear factor kappa-B ligand (RANKL) plays a key role in the differentiation, activation and survival of osteoclasts. RANKL, which is produced by pre-osteoblasts and osteoblasts, is a member of the tumor necrosis factor superfamily and plays a pivotal role in osteoclastogenesis. Another member of this system is osteoprotegerin (OPG), a soluble receptor for RANKL produced by osteoblasts, which acts in the opposite way by inhibiting RANKL-induced bone resorption. Antibodies to RANKL have now been developed and act as powerful inhibitors of bone resorption. A major signaling pathway to the osteoblasts is the Wnt-Low Density Lipoprotein receptor-related proteins (LRP) pathway which stimulates differentiation of pre-osteoblasts into mature bone-forming osteoblasts. This signaling pathway has two natural inhibitors, sclerostin and Dickkopf-1 (Dkk-1), and these have become targets for the development of antibodies blocking their actions and hence enhancing the stimulatory signals of Wnt-LRP. Finally, an understanding of the mechanisms by which osteoclasts resorb bone has led to the development of inhibitors of proteases secreted by osteoclasts,

Managing the Menopause: 21st Century Solutions, ed. Nick Panay, Paula Briggs, and Gab Kovacs.
Published by Cambridge University Press. © Cambridge University Press 2015.

thereby inhibiting their resorptive actions without influencing their cell activity or numbers. This potentially avoids a concomitant reduction of osteoblastic activity via the coupling mechanisms which is normally seen with agents that reduce osteoclastic cell activity.

Therapeutic options

Osteoporosis is a term used to describe a condition of bone micro-architecture deterioration and subsequent predisposition to fractures. It constitutes a major health problem, affecting millions of people worldwide, and is associated with increased morbidity and mortality. The hallmark of osteoporosis diagnosis is low bone mineral density (BMD), usually assessed by dual energy X-ray absorptiometry (DXA). Although women with the lowest BMD have the highest risk of fracture, the majority of fractures occur in women with osteopenia rather than osteoporosis, highlighting the importance of assessing fracture risk on an individual basis. The decision for treatment should thus be based both on BMD measurement and individual fracture risk profile. Medical history and clinical examination (in order to exclude causes of secondary osteoporosis and estimate fracture risk), taking into account the patient's age, lifestyle habits (exercise, smoking, alcohol) and specific medications associated with bone loss should always precede DXA assessment.

General management

Anti-fall strategies and nutritional measures, including a balanced diet with adequate calcium and vitamin D, should precede any major therapeutic intervention. Interventions which aim at modifying several risk factors associated with falls, such as decreased visual acuity, medications affecting balance, and home environment obstacles such as slippery floors, insufficient lighting and handrails, are recommended. Furthermore, avoidance of smoking, excessive alcohol and caffeine intake are also helpful in maintaining bone mass.

To gain the best available benefit with anti-osteoporosis medications, optimal calcium and vitamin D intake must be assured. Assessing 25-hydroxy-vitamin D (25(OH)D) levels prior to commencing any major anti-osteoporosis treatment may be prudent if there is suspected deficiency, because optimizing 25(OH)D concentrations may significantly increase the anti-fracture efficacy of osteoporosis treatment. In general, doses > 800 IU/day are more effective than lower doses. In patients with severe vitamin D deficiency (< 25 nmol/L) high loading doses, i.e. 300,000 IU, may be considered, which correspond to weekly doses of 50,000 IU for 6 weeks, followed by maintenance doses of 800–2,000 IU/day. Specific considerations are recommended for special patient groups, such as pregnant or lactating women, obese women, those with malabsorption disorders, or receiving corticosteroid or anticonvulsant medication. Regarding obesity, there is an inverse association between 25(OH)D concentrations and BMI or waist circumference, although the exact mechanisms have not been fully elucidated. The decreased bioavailability of vitamin D metabolites in adipose tissue and the reduced sun exposure due to a sedentary lifestyle are the most plausible explanations.

Major pharmacological interventions
Hormone replacement therapy (HRT) and tibolone

The findings from the Women's Health Initiative (WHI) trial, which was designed to assess the prevention of common chronic diseases in women, such as cardiovascular disease, cancer and osteoporosis, showed a beneficial effect of estrogen on bones. In particular, both estrogen (conjugated equine estrogens (CEE), at a daily dose of 0.625 mg) plus progestin (medroxyprogesterone acetate 2.5 mg/day) and CEE alone, were efficient in reducing the risk of vertebral and hip fractures by 33%, in comparison with placebo. Mean BMD in lumbar spine and total hip and femoral neck increased by a mean of 7.6% and 4.5%, respectively, after 3 years of treatment, compared with 1.5% and −0.3% in the placebo group. However, there was a small increased risk of venous thromboembolism (VTE). An increased risk of stroke in those initiating therapy at older ages was not seen in those initiating therapy below age 60 years. Breast cancer incidence was significantly reduced with cumulative follow-up of the estrogen-alone users. Moreover, breast cancer incidence was not significantly increased with combination therapy after adjustment for confounding variables, a finding confirmed in a more recent smaller but longer duration randomized HRT trial. For those initiating estrogen-alone HRT below the age of 60, a reduction in coronary heart disease became evident during long-term follow-up. Although not currently recommended by regulatory authorities, we believe that the use of HRT for the sole treatment of osteoporosis should be considered as first-line therapy in postmenopausal women. The risks of VTE and stroke may be minimized or even prevented by the use of appropriately low doses of estrogen on initiating therapy or by the use of non-oral administration. Hormone replacement therapy is an effective, safe and cheap therapy for osteoporosis prevention. The bone-preserving effect of estrogen is dose dependent and lower than standard doses are effective in older women. Higher doses may be necessary in young women who have premature ovarian insufficiency or have undergone a menopause induced by surgery, radiation or chemotherapy.

Tibolone is a synthetic steroid, with a mixed estrogenic, progestogenic and androgenic profile, used as an alternative to estrogen for relief of menopausal symptoms. Clinical trials have shown that tibolone 2.5 mg/day can prevent bone loss in both spine and proximal femur. In comparative studies, tibolone seems to be as effective as HRT regimens regarding its effect on BMD. Data show a significant reduction in vertebral and non-vertebral fracture risk by 45% and 26%, respectively. No adequate data exist with respect to its effect on hip fracture prevention. Tibolone has some adverse metabolic effects on lipid metabolism and insulin resistance. It may also increase the risk of stroke and its effect on breast cancer risk is unclear.

Selective estrogen receptor modulators

Selective estrogen receptor modulators (SERMS) exert estrogenic and anti-estrogenic properties, depending on the target tissue. In terms of bone, SERMS inhibit osteoclast-mediated bone resorption. Two members of this family are currently available for the treatment of postmenopausal osteoporosis, these being raloxifene and bazedoxifene. Raloxifene has estrogen agonist effects on bone and lipid metabolism and estrogen antagonist effects on uterine and breast tissue. Raloxifene administered at 60 mg daily has been associated with a significant reduction in the incidence of new vertebral fractures by 61% in women without prevalent vertebral fractures and by 37% in those with prevalent vertebral fractures. However, it has not shown any significant effect with respect to the risk of non-vertebral fractures. Raloxifene has also been approved for the prevention of invasive breast cancer. The most common side effects include increased risk of deep vein thrombosis (DVT), hot flashes, leg cramps and endometrial hyperplasia.

The other representative of this drug category, bazedoxifene, is currently available in several countries. It is effective in reducing vertebral fracture risk in postmenopausal women with osteoporosis (by 42%, compared with placebo) and that of non-vertebral fractures in high-risk populations (50% and 44% compared with placebo and raloxifene, respectively). Its effect on the endometrium is neutral. Other SERMS, which have not been approved for osteoporosis treatment, are tamoxifen and toremifene (used for prevention and treatment of breast cancer), ospemifene (approved for treatment of dyspareunia from menopausal vaginal atrophy) and lasofoxifene. A new promising formulation is the tissue selective estrogen complex (TSEC), a pairing of CEE with bazedoxifene, which allows both relief of vasomotor symptoms and prevention of bone loss without any stimulatory effect on the breast or the endometrium.

Bisphosphonates

Bisphosphonates are synthetic analogs of pyrophosphate, in which the oxygen atom has been substituted by a carbon atom. Their different action is dependent on the variable R2 side chain, bound to the carbon atom and in particular the nitrogen compound. The main representatives of this category used for the treatment of osteoporosis are alendronate, ibandronate (with their nitrogen found in the straight alkyl chain), risedronate and zoledronate (with their nitrogen being part of a cyclized aromatic ring). Their main action is inhibition of bone resorption, by inhibition of farnesyl pyrophosphate synthase, a key enzyme in the mevalonic acid pathway, which blocks specific signaling molecules (GTPases) involved in major osteoclastic functions, such as maintenance of the cytoskeleton and formation of ruffled borders. Because of the coupling of bone resorption to bone formation, the inhibition of resorption by these agents is associated with a reduction in bone formation, but the former effect is initially greater than the latter, leading to a refilling of the remodeling space and a subsequent increase in mineralization density. Consequently, they are associated with a reduction in fracture risk both due to a decrease in bone remodeling and to an increase in bone mass.

Both oral (weekly administered alendronate and risedonate or monthly ibandronate) and intravenous (i.v.) bisphosphonates (ibandronate administered every 3 months and zoledronate administered annually) have been associated with significant reductions in vertebral fractures (40–70%) and non-vertebral fractures (30–40%). Hip fracture efficacy has been shown for alendronate, risedronate and zoledronate (40–50%). Greater anti-fracture efficacy has been seen with the latter in terms of vertebral, non-vertebral and hip fractures, although direct head-to-head comparisons between bisphosphonates do not exist. It is of note that the anti-resorptive effect of zoledronate may persist for at least 5 years after a single injection, as demonstrated by a sustained reduction in bone turnover markers and increase in BMD. Extension trials show maintained benefit with 5 years of oral bisphosphonates and 6 years with zoledronate.

The overall benefits of bisphosphonate therapy generally outweigh its risks. Some concerns with oral bisphosphonates are symptoms from the upper gastrointestinal tract, such as esophagitis, esophageal ulcer and bleeding, although these have been minimized with less frequent dosing. There is conflicting evidence concerning an association with increased risk of esophageal cancer. An acute phase reaction (characterized by fever, headache, myalgia, arthralgia, malaise) may occur in 18% of patients with 24–36 hours after zoledronate infusion, lasting up to 3 days. This reaction can be significantly reduced with acetaminophen and with subsequent infusions. In the HORIZON trial, the pivotal trial of zoledronate, there was an increased risk of serious atrial fibrillation (1.3% vs. 0.5% with placebo), but the overall incidence of atrial fibrillation did not differ between the two groups. This risk has also been observed in some studies of oral bisphosphonates.

The two major concerns with bisphosphonate use are the risk of atypical subtrochanteric and diaphyseal femur fractures, and osteonecrosis of the jaw (ONJ). The absolute risk for atypical fractures is very low (around five cases per 10,000 person-years), taking also into account that these fractures constitute < 1% of all hip and femoral fractures. It is increased in cases of prolonged bisphosphonate use (> 5 years) and use of other concomitant drugs, such as glucocorticoids. With regard to ONJ, this is mostly seen in patients with underlying malignancies treated with high doses of i.v. bisphosphonates (4 mg zoledronic acid/3–4 weeks), with a reported risk of 1–10%. Osteonecrosis of the jaw is associated with prolonged suppression of bone turnover and its risk is mainly increased in patients undergoing tooth extractions, and in those with other comorbidities. The absolute risk of ONJ when bisphosphonates are administered for osteoporosis is extremely low (one case per 100,000 person-years). The prevalence of ONJ with oral bisphosphonates was found to be one case in 250,000, estimated by three identified patients in a German registry of 780,000 osteoporotic patients.

However, higher prevalence has been reported in studies by oral and maxillofacial surgeons, varying from one in 1,000 to one in 100,000.

Because of the risk of fragility fractures and ONJ, a drug holiday may be considered after perhaps 5 years of bisphosphonate therapy. Finally, it should be remembered that bisphosphonates have a prolonged skeletal retention time, perhaps around 12–15 years for alendronate and probably considerably longer for the more potent bisphosphonates. The very long-term consequences of this skeletal retention are not known, and hence caution should be taken when considering their use in younger patients. In 80-year-old osteoporotics, unknown clinical consequences some 20 years later are unlikely to be considered important, but this may not be true for those aged around 60 years.

Parathyroid hormone

Although continuous endogenous production of parathyroid hormone (PTH) (i.e. in primary hyperparathyroidism) exerts detrimental effects on bone, intermittent PTH administration leads to an increase in bone mass due to increased number and activity of osteoblasts. Recombinant PTH, consisting of the 1–34 N-terminal fragment of natural PTH molecule (which is the active one) (PTH(1–34) or teriparatide) or the intact PTH molecule (amino acids 1–84) have both been used for the treatment of osteoporosis. They stimulate bone formation and increase BMD to a greater extent than other agents, such as bisphosphonates, both in lumbar spine and femoral neck. Teriparatide appears also to improve bone micro-architecture (trabecular connectivity) at both trabecular and cortical skeletal sites, which further contributes to the reduction in fracture risk and cannot be detected by DXA. Teriparatide treatment has been associated with a significant reduction in the incidence of both vertebral and non-vertebral fractures by 70% and 38%, respectively. It is recommended for patients at high risk for fracture, such as those with T-score < −3.5, previous fragility fractures irrespective of low BMD and established glucocorticoid-induced osteoporosis. It is administered by subcutaneous injections, at a daily dose of 20 µg. Recently, a once-weekly agent has been developed, demonstrating an even greater reduction in vertebral fracture risk.

The most common adverse events are of minor concern and include hypersensitivity reactions, nausea, pain in the limbs, headache and dizziness. Hypercalcemia or hypercalciuria may occur, but are usually transient and of minor significance. Hypercortisolism has been reported. The risk of osteosarcoma reported in rats has not been confirmed in human clinical studies. Contraindications to teriparatide and PTH administration are states of abnormally increased bone turnover (such as hyperparathyroidism and Paget's disease), elevated alkaline phosphatase, prior radiation therapy of the skeleton and renal impairment. The high cost of teriparatide further limits its use.

Strontium ranelate

Strontium ranelate consists of two atoms of stable strontium combined with ranelic acid, acting as carrier. It is postulated to have a dual osteo-anabolic and anti-catabolic effect, although it has not been convincingly demonstrated in humans Although its action is not fully elucidated, strontium increases pre-osteoblast replication and osteoblast differentiation (via expression of Runx2 gene), collagen type I synthesis and bone matrix mineralization. The latter effect is mediated probably through a calcium-sensing receptor (CaR)-dependent mechanism, since strontium is a divalent cation which closely resembles calcium in its atomic and ionic properties and, thus, could act as an agonist for the CaR. Strontium also inhibits osteoclast differentiation and activity via an increase in OPG and a decrease in RANKL.

Therapy with strontium ranelate (administered daily as 2 g sachets) has been associated with a 41%, 16% and 19% reduction in the risk of vertebral, total and major non-vertebral fractures, respectively, after 3 years of treatment. In patients older than 74 years and with T-score ≤ -2.4, strontium ranelate has been also associated with a 36% reduction in the risk of hip fractures. The anti-fracture efficacy of strontium ranelate seems to be independent of the level of fracture risk. Extension studies show continuous increases in BMD for over 10 years of treatment. Renal impairment is a contraindication to treatment. Most common adverse events include nausea and diarrhea. Rare and serious adverse events are increased incidence in venous thromboembolism, eosinophilia and systemic symptoms syndrome, which may prove fatal. Recent serious concerns about a potential association with increased cardiovascular risk have severely limited its use for the treatment of osteoporosis.

Denosumab

Denosumab, a human monoclonal antibody, which acts in a similar way to OPG, exerting high affinity to RANKL, is approved for the treatment of postmenopausal osteoporosis. Given by subcutaneous injections of 60 mg every 6 months, it is a powerful anti-resorptive agent and reduces incidence of vertebral, non-vertebral and hip fractures by 68%, 20% and 40%, respectively, after 3 years of treatment. Extension trials of 8 years show that the increase in BMD is continued. In contrast to bisphosphonates, BMD declines after discontinuation of treatment (although it remains higher than baseline) and bone turnover markers increase above baseline within 3–6 months post-treatment. Denosumab is particularly indicated for the treatment of postmenopausal women with high fracture probability, defined as those with a history of osteoporotic fracture or multiple risk factors for fracture, or those who have inadequate response or are intolerant to other therapies.

It has a quite favorable safety profile. However, due to the fact that RANKL is also involved in other functions of the immune system, it has been associated with an increased risk of infections, such as cellulitis and urinary tract infections. Rare adverse effects that have been reported include increased muscle pain, increased cholesterol, hypocalcemia, ONJ and atypical femoral fractures. Renal impairment is not a contraindication to treatment.

Novel therapies under development

Further insights to bone metabolism have significantly contributed to a more targeted drug development. Novel therapies are already tested in phase III trials, such as cathepsin K inhibitors and sclerostin antibodies. The first category is a truly "anti-resorptive" agent, which inhibits a key osteoclast enzyme, cathepsin K, involved in bone matrix resorption. Because it does not affect osteoclast activity but only function, it does not influence the coupling of osteoclast and osteoblast activities and the latter does not decrease. Odanacatib, the first representative, has already been developed. Early studies have shown a significant dose-response increase in spine and hip BMD (7.9% and 5.8%, respectively, after treatment with 50 mg/weekly for 3 years), along with a significant reduction in bone resorption and a minimal effect on bone formation markers.

Sclerostin, which is produced by osteocytes, reduces bone formation and has been considered as an attractive target for treating osteoporosis. Romosozumab, the first humanized anti-sclerostin antibody, has already been developed and tested in a phase II multicenter study. The greatest gain in BMD was noticed in lumbar spine and it was shown with a 210 mg subcutaneous dose every 3 months (+11.3%), an effect that was significantly greater than the one observed with alendronate or teriparatide. Romosozumab also increased total hip and femoral neck BMD by 4.1% and 3.7%, respectively. It was associated with significant dose-dependent increases in bone formation markers and, in contrast with teriparatide, there is no compensatory increase in bone resorption. Antibodies against Dkk are also under development.

Combination therapies have also been tested recently. In patients at high risk for fracture, co-administration of teriparatide with denosumab seems to be highly effective both in lumbar spine and hip to a greater extent than either medication alone and than what has been reported with any current therapy. Thus, it may appear to be an attractive treatment option in these patients.

Conclusions and recommendations

Osteoporosis treatment should be commenced and selected on an individual basis. Optimal nutritional and lifestyle measures, and exclusion and potential treatment of secondary causes of osteoporosis, should always precede any major pharmaceutical intervention. It must be noted that although T-scores are commonly used in clinical practice for monitoring purposes, the change in BMD does not always reflect the change in fracture risk, which seems to be multifactorial. Treatment failure, after exclusion causes of secondary osteoporosis and suboptimal adherence, is considered in cases of: (a) $\geq$ two incident fragility fractures; (b) one incident fracture and elevated bone turnover markers or a significant decrease in BMD, or both; and (c) both no significant decrease in bone turnover markers and a significant decrease in BMD. Three general rules are proposed in cases of inadequate response to therapy: a weaker anti-resorptive may be replaced by a more potent drug of the same class; an oral drug may be replaced by an injectable agent; a strong anti-resorptive drug may be substituted by an anabolic agent.

The patient in the vignette has sustained two low-trauma fractures and possibly vertebral fractures. These significantly increase the risk of a new fracture. A BMD scan should be performed by DXA and treatment should be offered in the case of osteopenia. Plain radiographs of the spine, or DXA vertebral fracture risk assessment (VFA) when available, will provide further information on fracture prevalence. A low-dose HRT preparation or possibly a bisphosphonate appears to be a reasonable initial approach, depending on other menopausal risk factors and patient preference. Clinical reassessment in a year's time and BMD re-evaluation in 2 years to assess efficacy of treatment seems appropriate management.

Bibliography

1. Palacios S, Christiansen C, Sánchez Borrego R, et al. Recommendations on the management of fragility fracture risk in women younger than 70 years. *Gynecol Endocrinol* 2012; **28**: 770–86.

2. Diez-Perez A, Adachi JD, Agnusdei D, et al.; IOF CSA Inadequate Responders Working Group. Treatment failure in osteoporosis. *Osteoporos Int* 2012; **23**: 2769–74.

3. Watts NB, Bilezikian JP. Advances in target-specific therapy for osteoporosis. *J Clin Endocrinol Metab* 2014; **99**: 1149–51.

4. Gerval MO, Stevenson JC. Treatment of osteoporosis. In Studd J, Tan SL, Chervenak FA, (eds). *Current Progress in Obstetrics and Gynaecology*. Mumbai: Tree Life Media; 2014: 379–93.

5. Anagnostis P, Karras SN, Athyros VG, Annweiler C, Karagiannis A. The effect of vitamin D supplementation on skeletal, vascular, or cancer outcomes. *Lancet Diabetes Endocrinol* 2014; **2**: 362–3.

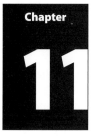

Chapter

11

Psychological aspects of the menopause

Myra S. Hunter

Introduction

Kate is 52 and always been "the life and soul of the party." However, since her periods stopped a year ago, she has been suffering from low mood. Some mornings she can hardly get herself out of bed. She sits around in her dressing gown for hours on end. She also sleeps really badly, and wakes several times a night, being unable to get back to sleep. She sometimes thinks that life is not worth living, and has thought about various ways to put herself to sleep permanently.

The menopause – the last menstrual period – takes place within a gradual process of physiologic change, but also concurrently with age and developmental changes, and within varied psychosocial and cultural contexts. Psychological perspectives on menopause include the meanings of menopause, appraisals and attributions of symptoms to menopause, as well as cognitive, affective and behavioral reactions to the menopause. Assessment and psychological interventions will be described here with particular reference to depression, anxiety, sleep and vasomotor symptoms – hot flashes and night sweats.

The relationships between menopause, hormone changes and psychological distress have troubled clinicians and researchers alike over the centuries, and women have been subject to a range of generally unhelpful and sometimes punitive treatments, including prolonged bed rest, application of leeches and gynecologic surgery. Polarized views and theories from psychoanalytic (bereavement of loss of reproductive capacity) to biomedical (estrogen deficiency) have resulted in very different treatments being offered to women depending upon where they seek help. Fortunately, today, the accumulation of anthropologic and epidemiologic research and prospective studies provide clear evidence that a biopsychosocial understanding provides the way forward in understanding these complex mind–body relationships. A biopsychosocial perspective will be described in relation to understanding Kate's depression in the following sections on assessment and treatment, but first, what does the literature tell us about the roles of psychological and social factors on women's experience during the menopause?

The psychosocial context

Anthropologic and cross-cultural studies have challenged the concept of the menopause as a universal phenomenon with wide variations in the symptom perception and reporting in women from different ethnic origins, living in different countries. Cultural explanations of these differences need to include lifestyle (diet, exercise), social factors, as well

---

Managing the Menopause: 21st Century Solutions, ed. Nick Panay, Paula Briggs, and Gab Kovacs. Published by Cambridge University Press. © Cambridge University Press 2015.

as reproductive patterns, which can affect biological processes, population differences in biology, as well as beliefs and attitudes to the menopause and the social status of mid-aged and older women. In other words this is a biopsychosociocultural process, which may vary within and between cultures and change over time.

The menopause is generally perceived as a time of poor emotional and physical health in Western societies, and attitudes to the menopause are influenced by social and cultural assumptions about older women. Nevertheless, anthropologic studies show how menopause can be a positive event, particularly when it signifies a change in social status. Much of the early research that influenced the Western view of the menopause was based on clinic samples of women who had actively sought treatment for health problems. Women attending menopause clinics have more health problems, life stresses and low mood than those who do not, as well as differing beliefs about the menopause, so it is important not to generalize these presentations to the experience of women in general. Cultural attitudes and meanings of menopause may also influence women's expectations and perceptions of symptoms. For example, menopause in many developing countries tends not to be regarded as a medical problem and thus might be accepted, with less focus on "symptoms" and more as a natural part of life. There are cultural differences in the attributions of different types of symptoms to the menopause. For example, in a study of Asian women living in the UK and in Delhi, visual changes (becoming shortsighted in middle age) were often attributed to the menopause, as well as weight gain and high blood pressure. Such attributions could result in these women not receiving the most appropriate health care.

In Western societies women tend to be valued for their physical and sexual attractiveness, reproductive capacity and youthfulness, and the menopause is often associated with emotional and physical symptoms, aging and uncertainty. In a systematic review of the evidence, Ayers et al. concluded that there is a relationship between beliefs and attitudes held before the menopause and actual experience [1]. For example, two prospective studies show that overly negative attitudes before menopause predict depressed mood and hot flashes during the menopause, suggesting that negative attitudes towards menopause can affect symptom experience – a self-fulfilling prophecy.

Menopause and mood

Determining the precise relationship between menopause and mood has been a difficult area to research because of methodological challenges (defining menopausal stages, measurement of mood and confounding factors of age and social changes). Longitudinal studies have been designed in order to address these issues. The main findings from these studies suggest that the menopause transition is not necessarily associated with psychological symptoms in healthy women. Therefore depressed mood should not be attributed automatically to the menopause transition. Past depression is the main predictor of depressive symptoms during the menopause and psychosocial factors are also highly relevant. Age is another strong predictor in that low mood is more prevalent during mid-age; psychological distress tends to rise during adulthood to middle age before declining and leveling off in old age, and after the menopause women generally report improvements in mood.

Two studies demonstrate the relationships between mood, life-stage, psychosocial factors and menopause. First the "Household Survey for England Study" of men and women (N = 94,879) investigated age bands from 16 to 84 and assessed the prevalence of psychological distress (using the 12-item General Health Questionnaire) as well as psychiatric diagnosis and use of psychiatric medications [2]. The authors examined the impact of age

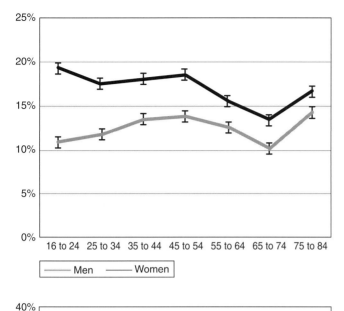

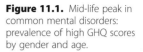

Figure 11.1. Mid-life peak in common mental disorders: prevalence of high GHQ scores by gender and age.

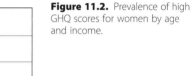

Figure 11.2. Prevalence of high GHQ scores for women by age and income.

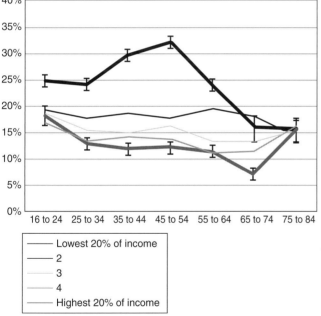

and gender on prevalence of common mental illness, and then studied these relationships by socioeconomic status (income).

The results show the increase during mid-life and also the expected gender differences – women reporting more distress and common mental illness than men (Figure 11.1); however, when the sample was divided on the basis of income, a different picture emerged. For both men and women, the mid-life increase in distress applied only to the lower income groups (bottom 20% of the income groups; the results for women are shown in Figure 11.2).

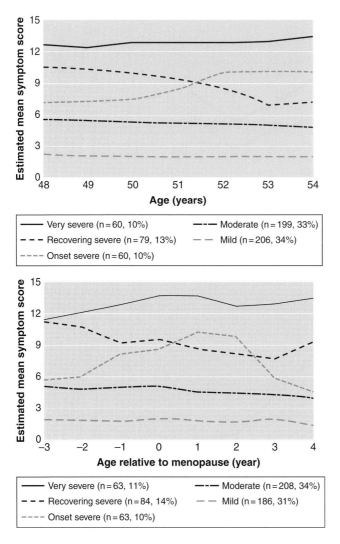

Figure 11.3. Profiles of psychological symptoms across mid-life and according to age relative to menopause (Mishra GD, Kuh D, *Br Med J* 2012; 344: bmj. e402; reproduced with kind permission from BMJ Group).

These findings are consistent with other data showing that financial and social pressures may lead to increased stress in other areas of life.

The second study by Mishra and Kuh focuses in more detail on specific changes that occur for women across the menopause transition [3]. For most women psychological symptoms generally tend to stay the same, with some increases and decreases, across the menopause transition (Figure 11.3). However, there is a proportion of women, estimated to be about 10%, who may be at a higher risk of mood changes during the transition to menopause. However, this increase in psychological symptoms tends to decrease during the postmenopause, i.e. for most, it is relatively short-lived. Factors found to be associated with psychological symptoms and depressed mood during the menopause transition include: past history of psychological problems, social factors, educational and occupational status, poor health, stressful life events, body mass index (BMI), cigarette smoking, attitudes to menopause and aging, and early life circumstances and experiences.

Psychological symptoms may also be associated with beliefs about menopause, which can affect self-esteem, vasomotor symptoms, as well as coincidental psychosocial stresses and changes. There is no clear evidence that hormonal changes predict psychological symptoms during the menopause transition, but some women present to clinics with tension and low mood, which appears to be similar to premenstrual symptomatology; premenstrual symptom reporting is also a predictor of psychological distress reported during menopause. These women are hypothesized to have a sensitivity to hormonal changes which renders them to be more at risk of psychological distress during the perimenopause. Women who have had a surgical menopause, an early menopause and those who have chronic and troublesome vasomotor symptoms also tend to report more psychological symptoms.

Vasomotor symptoms and mood

The relationship between depressed mood and hot flashes is also complex and recent evidence suggests that it is likely to be bidirectional. While depressed mood is more strongly associated with psychosocial factors than hormone changes, women who are depressed tend to report hot flashes as more problematic. There is also evidence suggesting that childhood abuse and neglect and anxiety, before the menopause, are associated with the presence and the severity of hot flashes – women with moderate or high anxiety levels being three to five times more likely to report hot flashes than women in the normal anxiety range. There is likely to be an interaction whereby vasomotor symptoms can lead to sleep problems, tiredness and low self-esteem, which can in turn result in low mood; conversely feeling depressed or overly anxious might lead to overly negative appraisals of vasomotor symptoms and unhelpful coping strategies. Hot flashes are also associated with general stress and anxiety and can themselves result in social embarrassment and discomfort, whereas night sweats tend to be associated with sleep problems and tiredness.

We also know that stress produces increases in noradrenaline and serotonin, which may affect the temperature control system in women with hot flashes and night sweats. In one study of women experiencing hot flashes, more hot flashes were reported when women were doing stressful tasks, such as mental arithmetic, than when they were involved in calm or non-stressful tasks such as reading. It is proposed that there is a narrowed thermoneutral zone in women who have hot flashes, resulting in hot flashes being triggered by small elevations in core body temperature, caused by changes in ambient temperature or other environmental triggers, such as stress. There is evidence from animal research that the thermoneutral zone is narrowed by elevated brain norepinephrine. This physiologic model provides a framework with which to understand the role of hormonal and psychological factors upon hot flashes and night sweats.

A biopsychosocial model of hot flashes and night sweats, developed by Hunter and Mann, describes how a range of psychological factors might influence the perception and appraisal of hot flashes and night sweats, as well as behavioral reactions to them [4]. Day-to-day, if we are occupied or our attention is focused on something specific, we are usually less likely to notice physical symptoms. Conversely, if we closely monitor or focus on a part of the body, we tend to notice sensations that we would normally be unaware of. Depressed mood and negative beliefs about hot flashes and night sweats (e.g. "when I have a hot flash every one will stare at me," or "if I have a night sweat I'll never get back to sleep") are the main predictors of problematic or bothersome hot flashes and night sweats. Interestingly, it is this "problem-rating," rather than frequency of hot flashes, that is strongly associated with quality of life and help-seeking, and consequently a measure of hot flash problem-rating is recommended as an important clinical outcome measure in clinical trials [4].

A biopsychosocial approach

Returning to Kate's situation, what do we need to know to understand the factors that might be important in her individual case?

Assessment

A clinical interview should include a full medical and psychosocial history, including past history of depression, psychological symptoms, help-seeking etc. However, a key aspect of a biopsychosocial assessment is to understand the patient's beliefs and understandings of the causes and influences on her symptoms. "You must have thought a lot about this – what factors do you think have influenced why you feel this way?" Explore what was happening around the time that the symptoms started – prompting for hot flashes, night sweats, menstrual changes, but also looking out for psychosocial changes. Commonly women say "nothing was happening really," but stresses accumulate during mid-life and if explored in more detail, it is not uncommon that women will describe numerous roles and stresses (family relationships, work worries, financial problems are common); if then menopausal symptoms are added to the list, they can be the last straw that tip the balance into depressed mood or anxiety. It can be useful to draw a timeline of the onset of depression, hot flashes and night sweats, and any other events in order to make sense of their possible interactions. Writing down possible influences on the biopsychosocial model (Figure 11.4) can be helpful, acknowledging that stress and biological factors often interact. Diaries can be useful to record hot flashes and night sweats and mood so that any patterns can be discussed at a subsequent appointment.

Personality factors and past depression can be explored by asking if/when she has felt this way before and how does she generally cope when she feels low. For example, Kate might respond to these questions as follows:

I was depressed about 5 years ago when I had an accident and had back pain for 2 months – I was frustrated and found it difficult not being able to do things and not being in control. I first noticed feeling low this time when the night sweats started – I couldn't sleep and it was a time

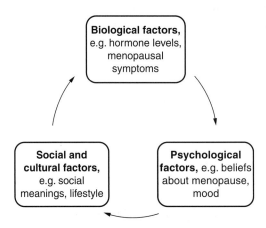

Figure 11.4. A biopsychosocial model of factors influencing experience of the menopause.

when my job was really demanding so it was hard to cope. Over time I kept trying to put on a brave face and pretended that everything was fine but I started to be irritable with my husband and work colleagues, as I just felt more out of control and tired. When I woke at night I began to have thoughts that I was useless. I've always been the life and soul of the party and people won't like me if I'm miserable. I cope now by avoiding people and staying out of the way in bed. I catch up on sleep in the day, but feel very alone and hopeless about life.

When asked about her thoughts about menopause in general, she said that she had tended to think that after the menopause women were in danger of "letting themselves go," and that anything could happen, so she was concerned about the impact of menopause upon her own well-being and ability to function.

From this interview the biopsychosocial model could be completed, by inserting:

- Night sweats into the biological section.
- Self-critical thoughts (beliefs that she should be in control and life and soul of the party or otherwise people won't like her), worries about the menopause, and unhelpful behaviors (avoidance and sleeping in the day) in the psychological section.
- Work stress in the social section.

The possible influences and the relationships between her mood, sleep and night sweats, and her thoughts and feelings would be discussed. Evidence-based treatment options for depression would include exercise (for mild-to-moderate depression), cognitive behavior therapy and antidepressants [5]. Hormone therapy could also be offered to treat trouble-some night sweats. In our example, Kate opted for non-medical treatment because she was wary of side effects and wanted to be in control. She was offered a course of cognitive behavior therapy (CBT) for her mood and to help her to manage her sleep and night sweats.

Cognitive behavioral interventions for menopausal symptoms
What is cognitive behavior therapy?

Cognitive behavior therapy, literally thinking (cognitive) and behavior therapy, is a struc-tured, collaborative and time-limited intervention. Cognitive behavior therapy was initially developed in the 1960s and 70s by Aaron Beck, who noticed that emotional distress and unhelpful behaviors in his anxious and depressed patients were preceded by specific patterns of thinking. Cognitive behavior therapy offered a pragmatic and practical approach to emotional problems, such as anxiety and depression, and over the past few decades CBT has been applied to a range of mental health and physical health problems with positive outcomes.

Cognitive behavior therapy for depression

Cognitive behavior therapy is currently one of the major treatments for depression. When people are depressed, they tend to think more negatively about themselves and the world in general – it is as if their mood state takes them into a depressive and more negative-thinking state. This can also happen to people who would normally think quite differently, when they are not depressed. Cognitive behavior therapy can help people to identify overly negative thoughts, so that they can gain a perspective on their concerns and gradually learn how to manage these thoughts. Depressive thinking and behavior can lead to a cycle of self-criticism and hopelessness, and many people often withdraw and avoid situations and feel worse as a result. To combat this tendency, early on in CBT treatment patients are encouraged to gradually re-engage in activities that they previously valued and enjoyed but which they have withdrawn from since becoming depressed. This "behavioral activation" and developing a structure to the day can help to initially lift mood. However, the overall aims of CBT are led by the patient, in order to be consistent with the individual's beliefs and values; an important part of the therapy is to enable people to value their own qualities, strengths and competencies.

Cognitive behavior therapy for anxiety

The CBT model of anxiety disorders identifies "anxious thinking," such as predicting the worst possible outcomes or viewing situations as unnecessarily threatening, as contributing to and maintaining anxiety. For people with social anxiety, this can mean assuming that others will have negative thoughts about them in social situations and as a result sufferers are likely to avoid these social occasions. People with panic disorder tend to misinterpret anxiety symptoms, such as hyperventilation and increased heart rate, as being signs of imminent disaster. They believe that they might have a heart attack or faint, and this belief leads to increased arousal. People with health anxiety (a term that replaced hypochondriasis) tend to misinterpret benign or normal physical sensations as signs of serious disease and become overly worried about their health. If health anxiety becomes chronic, people can repeatedly undergo hospital investigations or even unnecessary treatments. Cognitive behavior therapy approaches to treating anxiety examine how anxious thinking tends to "catastrophize" or overestimate the likelihood of the worst-case scenario happening. Cognitive behavior therapy includes cognitive therapy for these beliefs and encouragement to systematically approach feared situations to learn that the expected consequences do not arise. Anxiety is a normal reaction, but it becomes problematic when benign and non-dangerous situations and events are regularly perceived as threats.

Cognitive behavior therapy for sleep problems

There is consistent evidence that CBT can help people to develop better sleeping habits (behaviors) and to tackle the worries about sleep and daytime performance that can keep people lying awake at three in the morning. Essentially, worry about not sleeping increases physiological arousal and therefore wakefulness. As a result, sleep is less likely to occur. Keeping a regular sleep schedule and not sleeping in the daytime is encouraged, as is a wind-down period before bed-time. Cognitive behavior therapy delivered in groups or on a one-to-one basis has helped people to understand these patterns of thinking and behavior, and to make changes, which reduce wakening as well as increase sleep time, sleep efficiency and sleep quality [6]. Furthermore, as CBT encourages long-term changes in sleep beliefs and behaviors, improvements that have been found in trials of CBT and within clinical settings tend to be maintained over time.

Cognitive behavior therapy for vasomotor symptoms

A cognitive behavioral intervention for hot flashes and night sweats, which includes relaxation, paced breathing and CBT has been developed and evaluated in different formats (one-to-one with a psychologist, in groups of six to eight women and as a self-help booklet) by comparing these forms of CBT with no treatment or usual care respectively [7]. The CBT is based on the theoretical model [4] and has been found to be effective in randomized controlled trials for women going through the menopause transition (MENOS2). Cognitive behavior therapy is also effective for women who have hot flashes and night sweats following breast cancer treatment (MENOS1) [7], for whom few effective treatment options exist that are safe and free from side effects [8].

The main elements of the CBT for hot flashes and night sweats include:

- Psycho-education about hot flashes and menopause.
- Monitoring hot flashes and night sweats, identifying precipitants.
- Paced breathing for stress and hot flashes and night sweats.
- Cognitive therapy for stress and beliefs about hot flashes and menopause.
- Behavioral experiments and strategies.
- Cognitive behavior therapy for night sweats and sleep.

Group and self-help formats (book and CD) of the CBT were equally effective in reducing problematic hot flashes and night sweats and had additional benefits to mood and quality of life. The self-help guide, used over a 4-week period, was found to be as effective as four 2-hour weekly sessions of group CBT, and in a recent study has been found to be equally effective with minimal support, which makes the intervention widely available for women. The treatment is available as a self-help book [9], and is manualized so that trained health professionals can deliver the Group CBT [10]. The effect of CBT (MENOS1 and MENOS2 trials) was mediated mainly by changes in beliefs, and to a lesser extent by improvements in mood and sleep. Women reported improved coping (using information, paced breathing and strategies) and a restored sense of control, and experienced beneficial changes, such as increased confidence, which extended beyond their menopausal symptoms.

For Kate a course of CBT for her depression, night sweats and sleep might include:

- Behavioral activation to help her to structure her day and to start to engage in more (pleasant or neutral) activities.
- Cognitive behavior therapy for sleep and night sweats – learning to schedule sleep times, to deal with problems in the day, to have a wind-down time, take exercise and not nap in the daytime, and to manage night sweats using paced breathing, calm thoughts and an automatic routine to cool down and return to bed.
- Cognitive therapy focusing on her depressive thoughts, on her self-beliefs (I should be the life and soul of the party; I must be in control), her beliefs about others (people won't like me if I am not the life and soul of the party) and her beliefs about the menopause.

Summary

Women's experience of the menopause transition is influenced by psychosocial factors, such as past depression, past anxiety, life stresses, negative beliefs and expectations about the menopause, as well as socioeconomic factors. There are bidirectional relationships between vasomotor symptoms and mood, and some common causal pathways for these symptoms. A biopsychosocial model is advocated for assessment and is a multidisciplinary approach to treatment for women with troublesome symptoms during the menopause transition. Cognitive behavior therapy is an effective non-medical treatment for depression, anxiety, sleep problems and for hot flashes and night sweats.

References

1. Ayers B, Forshaw M, Hunter MS. The impact of attitudes towards the menopause on women's symptom experience: a systematic review. *Maturitas* 2010; **65**: 28–36.

2. Lang IA, Llewellyn DJ, Hubbard RE, *et al.* Income and midlife peak in common mental disorder prevalence. *Psychol Med* 2011; **41**: 1365–72.

3. Mishra GD, Kuh D. Health symptoms during midlife in relation to menopausal transition: British prospective cohort study. *Br Med J* 2012; **344**: e402.

4. Hunter MS, Mann E. A cognitive model of menopausal hot flushes. *J Psychosom Res* 2010; **69**: 491–501.

5. National Institute for Health and Clinical Excellence (NICE) (2009) *Depression: the Treatment and Management of Depression in Adults (Update).* www.nice.org.uk/guidance/CG90.

6. Morin CM, Bootzin RR, Buysse DJ, *et al.* Psychological and behavioral treatment of insomnia: update of the recent evidence (1998–2004). *Sleep* 2008; **29**: 1398–414.

7. Hunter MS. Cognitive behavioural interventions for the treatment of menopausal symptoms. *Expert Rev Obstet Gynaecol* 2012; **7**: 321–26.

8. Rada G, Capurro D, Pantoja T, *et al.* Non-hormonal interventions for hot flushes in women with a history of breast cancer. *The Cochrane Library* 2010; issue 9.

9. Hunter MS, Smith M. *Managing Hot Flushes and Night Sweats: A Cognitive Behavioural Self-Help Guide to the Menopause.* New York, NY: Routledge; 2014.

10. Hunter MS, Smith M. *Managing Hot Flushes with Group Cognitive Behaviour Therapy: An Evidence Based Treatment Manual for Health Professionals.* New York, NY: Routledge; 2015.

Memory and mood in the menopause

Michael C. Craig

Introduction

Previous studies have reported that the menopause is associated with deterioration in memory and mood in some women. Also, a significant body of research suggests that hormone "replacement" therapy (HRT) specifically with estrogen may act as a *prophylaxis* against the risk for developing Alzheimer's disease (AD) and a *treatment* for perimenopausal depression. The precise nature, and biological basis, of this relationship is still not fully understood. However, it probably involves a complex interaction between genes, the environment and the mode and timing of HRT prescription. Increasing our understanding of the interplay between these factors during the menopause may permit us to target more specific treatments to vulnerable individuals. Further, it offers a window of opportunity to understand the putative role of estrogen in psychiatric disorders at other times of the reproductive cycle. The current chapter will focus on the role of estrogen on Alzheimer's disease and depression during the menopause.

Alzheimer's disease

By the year 2050 it has been estimated that 30% of the population in Western Europe will be over the age of 65 and as many as 10% will have Alzheimer's disease [1]. Also, mild cognitive impairment (i.e. a preclinical stage of AD) has an estimated prevalence of 20–30% in elderly people [2]. Dementia currently costs the UK health-care system approximately £17 billion per year and is predicted to reach £35 billion within 20 years [3]. The social and economic implications of this are greatest among women because their life expectancy, and risk of developing AD, are greater than for men [4]. However it has been calculated that *if* severe cognitive impairment could be reduced by 1% per year, this would cancel out the estimated increases in the long-term health-care costs [5], as well as reducing the significant emotional costs.

Support for the protective effect of sex hormones on cognition has come both from studies into the negative effects of early surgical oophorectomy, prior to the onset of menopause, and the positive effects of HRT prescribed post menopause. In the former category it has been reported, for example, that oopherectomy before 49 years of age is associated with a significant increased relative risk of dementia, and this risk increased the earlier the age of oophorectomy [6]. Further, the risk disappeared if women were prescribed HRT until at least 50 years of age. Case-control and cohort studies have also reported a reduced relative risk of AD in postmenopausal women treated with HRT, compared with

---

Managing the Menopause: 21st Century Solutions, ed. Nick Panay, Paula Briggs, and Gab Kovacs.
Published by Cambridge University Press. © Cambridge University Press 2015.

never-users. Meta-analyses of these studies suggested that the relative risk was reduced by up to 34% [7]. Importantly, most of these studies were carried out in the USA, at a time where typical clinical practice was to prescribe HRT from the perimenopause until around 60 years old [8]. More recently this practice has been postulated to be particularly significant. For example, a prospective observational study reported that although HRT initiated early post menopause protected against AD, that hormonal treatment initiated after the age of 60 years did not [4]. Further, in a large multicentered randomized controlled study (RCT) (the Women's Health Initiative Memory Study), women over 65 years old randomized to HRT (+ medroxyprogesterone acetate) had an increased risk of "all-cause" dementia compared with the placebo group [9].

In summary, studies to date suggest that HRT prescribed to older women may have a neutral or negative effect, particularly if it is combined with MPA. However, HRT prescribed at a "critical period" around the time of menopause (particularly postsurgical menopause in younger women) may reduce the risk of dementia in later life. Larger, appropriately powered RCTs are still needed to test the "critical period" hypothesis further. The primary difficulty in designing such studies is the long delay between randomization and development of (or protection against) symptoms of dementia. A compromise to this obstacle is to study the effects of HRT on a marker for subsequent AD. One such marker is *verbal episodic memory*, as a subtle decline in this cognitive ability has been reported prior to the development of AD [10].

There currently are two large RCTs underway that have been designed to analyze differences in verbal memory performance in women following "natural" (i.e. not surgical) menopause up to 5 years post-randomization to either placebo or (a) HRT (oral conjugated equine estrogens (CEE) or transdermal estradiol) + micronized progesterone <3 years post last menstruation [11] or (b) HRT (oral estradiol) ± vaginal progesterone gel either <6 years or >10 years postmenopause [Early versus Late Intervention Trial with Estradiol, Clinical-Trials.gov identifier NCT00114517]. Results from both these studies should add to our current understanding of the putative benefits of HRT prescribed during the "critical period" on memory. However, these studies will still suffer from some of the confounding factors discussed above and a definitive study will still be needed. Further, studies are also required to facilitate our understanding into the neurobiological mechanisms underpinning the putative effects of HRT on memory and AD [12].

Depression

Major depressive disorder is the leading cause of disease-related disability among women worldwide [13]. Further, there is increasing evidence that fluctuation in reproductive hormones, such as at the time of the perimenopause, increases the risk of a major depressive episode in some women [14–23]. The biological basis of this risk is probably multifactorial. However, most of the evidence, albeit not all, suggests that it is predominantly driven by effects of estrogen on the brain. This is supported, to some degree, by studies into the effects of estrogen therapy on mood in the perimenopause. For example, a 6-week RCT of 34 women with perimenopausal depression (major and minor) reported that 17β-estradiol (50 μg) was associated with a significant improvement in mood compared with placebo [24]. These findings were replicated in a 12-week double-blind RCT of 17β-estradiol (100 μg) in 50 women with perimenopausal depression (major/minor) or dysthymic disorder [25]. Further, these results were still significant at the 4-week follow-up. Consequently, some doctors in the UK prescribe sex hormones as the first line of treatment in women with reproductive depression [26–30]. Nevertheless, the biological evidence to support this approach is limited and prescription for clinical depression (i.e. as defined by the *Diagnostic and Statistical Manual of Mental Disorders, Fifth Edition* (DSM–V) or the *International Statistical Classification of Diseases and Related Health Problems, Tenth Revision* (ICD–10)) in this patient group remains controversial. Studies are required that directly compare the effects of estradiol, preferably in the form of an implant, patch or gel (i.e. to avoid the effects of first-pass metabolism) with antidepressant medication and/or cognitive behavior therapy (CBT).

It is outside the scope of this chapter to comprehensively review earlier basic science and animal studies into these mechanisms but these can be found elsewhere [31]. Instead the remainder of the chapter will focus on some of the recent *in vivo* techniques that have been used to study the neurobiological mechanisms that underpin estrogen's effects on the brain over the menopause.

Neurobiological mechanisms

Estrogen is a steroid hormone synthesized by aromatization of androgenic precursors (i.e. androstenedione and testosterone). Naturally occurring estrogens include, in order of potency, 17β-estradiol, estrone and estriol. Estradiol is mainly produced by ovarian granulosa and theca cells and is the predominant form of estrogen found in premenopausal women. Research in ovarectomized rhesus monkeys has recently demonstrated that estradiol can also be produced *directly* by neurons [32]. This finding suggests a novel role for "neuroestrogen" as a neurotransmitter.

Estradiol mainly exerts its effects by binding to two intracellular estrogen receptors (ERs), ERα and ERβ [33]. However, subsequent modulation of brain function includes an interaction with a number of neurotransmitter systems [34, 35]. This interaction has been studied *indirectly* using neuroendocrine challenge tests and, more recently, more *directly* using *in vivo* brain imaging.

Neuroendocrine studies

This early *in vivo* technique provided an indirect method to explore the effects of estrogen on neurotransmitter systems important to memory, AD and mood in the menopause. Studies have reported modulatory effects on HRT on the cholinergic, serotonergic and dopaminergic systems.

Cholinergic system

Many different lines of research have highlighted the importance of the cholinergic system in learning and memory. Perhaps the oldest hypothesis into the cause of AD is the "cholinergic hypothesis" [36, 37], which proposed AD is caused by reduced cholinergic system activity. The role of the cholinergic system in mood is less understood. However, depressed mood has been reported to be associated with hypercholinergic neurotransmission which, paradoxically, may be mediated through excessive neuronal nicotinic receptor activation [38]. We have reported that postmenopausal women on long-term HRT (i.e. initiated at around the time of menopause) had greater responsivity to pyridostigmine challenge of the cholinergic system (measured by growth hormone response) than never-users. Further, amongst long-term HRT users there was a significant positive correlation between response and duration of estrogen exposure [39].

Dopaminergic system

Dopamine has an important role in mood [40] and memory [41]. Previous studies have reported that the response to dopaminergic challenge is increased in women taking the combined oral contraceptive pill [42], during phases of the menstrual cycle associated with high estrogen [43] and on the fourth day postpartum in women at risk of puerperal psychosis compared with controls [44]. We have also reported greater responsivity to dopaminergic challenge, with apomorphine, in postmenopausal women on long-term HRT compared with never-users [45]. Further, most women in the HRT arm had commenced treatment immediately post hysterectomy and bilateral oophorectomy during the "critical period."

Serotonergic system

The serotonergic system plays a key role in mood and memory [46]. Greater responsivity (relative to HRT never-users) to serotonergic challenge (e.g. to d-fenfluramine) has also been reported in young postmenopausal women (mean age 49 years old) following short-term HRT [47] and in older women (mean age 60 years old) following long-term HRT [39]. In the latter study, women had been prescribed HRT for a mean of 13 years (i.e. starting around the time of menopause), suggesting that in both studies women received treatment during the "critical period" immediately post menopause.

In summary, neuroendocrine challenge studies suggest that HRT prescribed around the time of menopause is associated with greater responsivity of several neurotransmitter systems that are central to memory, AD and mood. However, these studies have several shortcomings. First, they were all observational, cross-sectional studies and although groups were matched (e.g. for age and IQ), it is possible that findings were still confounded by other factors (e.g. the "healthy user bias") [48]. Second, neuroendocrine studies only provide an indirect method for analyzing the effects of HRT on receptor responsivity at the hypothalamic-pituitary axis. They are not informative about the effects of HRT on brain regions that are more critical to AD and mood (e.g. prefrontal cortex and hippocampus).

The development of *in vivo* brain imaging techniques, however, has led to a more direct approach to studying the effects of HRT on brain structure and function and contributed to significant recent advances in our understanding of the effects of HRT on the brain.

In vivo brain imaging studies

Early studies into structural integrity of neural tissue in postmenopausal women using structural magnetic resonance imaging (sMRI) reported that HRT had a neutral effect on gray and white matter volumes [49–51]. Others, including our group, have found that compared with never-users, HRT has positive effects on regional gray and white matter concentrations [52–54]. This has included modulation of brain regions that are known to be important in memory and mood. For example, studies have reported atrophy of the hippocampus, prefrontal cortex and medial temporal lobe regions (e.g. amygdala) following *chronic* depression and/or stress [55]. Further, atrophy of these same regions is also associated with memory impairment. A consistent finding reported in sMRI studies post menopause has been that HRT users had regional sparing of gray matter in prefrontal regions [52, 56] and the hippocampus [52, 54]. It has also been reported that HRT users had sparing of white matter in medial temporal lobe regions [52]. Furthermore, white matter hyperintensities (a putative marker of brain aging) have been reported to be less extensive in HRT users than non-users in cross-sectional [57] and longitudinal [58] studies. In summary, studies in postmenopausal women suggest that HRT either improves or has a neutral effect on the structural integrity of neural tissue in brain regions important to memory and mood.

The inconsistencies between findings in these studies are probably due to a variety of methodological factors. First, the effects of HRT may be limited to gray or white matter compartments within brain regions that are vulnerable to the effects of aging [59–61]. Thus studies that specifically focused on other brain regions [50] or whole brain gray and white matter volumes [49] may not detect significant between-group differences. Second, some studies failed to explicitly exclude ex-users of HRT among "non-users" [49, 50] and/or may have included women that did not receive HRT around the time of menopause with current users [49, 50, 57]. The "critical period" hypothesis, however, predicts that these factors would reduce between-group differences. Third, as described above, it is probable that factors such as the type of HRT used (e.g. CEE versus estradiol), whether HRT is opposed or unopposed by progestogens, and the mode of administration (e.g. oral or implant) may modulate the putative protective effects of HRT on brain aging [62]. Finally, the methodological technique applied to analyzing brain structure may be important. Thus although brain morphometry of bulk regions (a combined measure of both white and gray matter of whole brain or lobes) can be examined using hand-tracing methods, subtle regional differences in gray and white matter may occur that are undetectable using this approach. This difficulty has largely been overcome by studies using voxel-based morphometry (VBM), which generate statistical parametric maps of the significant between-group differences in gray matter concentration [52, 56]. In summary, studies suggest that initiation of HRT at the time of menopause may modulate age-related differences in regional gray and white matter concentration in regions that are important to memory and mood. Further studies, using functional imaging, suggest that HRT may also modulate brain activity in these regions.

Functional magnetic resonance imaging (fMRI) and positron emission tomography (PET) techniques have permitted analysis of the effects of estrogen on brain function in peri- and postmenopausal women. Several observational studies have reported a significant effect of HRT on brain function in postmenopausal women. An early PET study [49] that compared long-term HRT users to non-HRT users reported significant differences in the relative regional cerebral blood flow (rCBF) in brain regions that included the frontal and parahippocampal gyri during verbal memory, and parietal and parahippocampal cortices during visual memory. Further, these changes were associated with improved memory performance – suggesting that these functional differences had significant behavioral consequences. A subsequent PET study in postmenopausal long-term HRT+ users, HRT– non-users, and women with AD reported that HRT– women had metabolic ratios that were intermediate to HRT+ women and AD patients in brain regions characteristically hypometabolic in AD (including the dorsolateral prefrontal, middle temporal and parietal cortices) [63]. Although the behavioral performance did not differ between HRT+ and HRT– women, it was suggested that the relative hypometabolism in HRT– women might be an early indicator of future cognitive decline.

The above studies of *long*-term HRT use have been supported by research into the *short*-term effects of HRT in women closer to the "critical period." For example, a placebo-controlled, cross-over fMRI study reported that HRT+ was associated with increased activation of frontal, prefrontal and inferior parietal regions during a verbal memory task [64].

In summary, studies of brain function in older women report that long-term HRT, if prescribed since around the time of menopause, and short-term HRT, if prescribed close to the time of menopause, probably has positive modulatory effects on brain function in brain regions that are important to memory. These findings have been supported by studies in younger, premenopausal women.

Pseudo-menopause

A useful model to research the effects of reduced ovarian function on the brain is to study the consequences of acute ovarian steroid suppression (i.e. post-GnRHa) in premenopausal women. One advantage of this approach is that it avoids confounding effects of the "healthy user" bias. Studies using this approach by our group and others have reported a significant reduction in brain activity in similar regions reported postmenopause, including the dorso-lateral prefrontal and parietal cortex [65, 66]. Further, these changes have been reported to be reversed following estrogen (and progesterone) add-back [65] or the return of ovarian function [67].

In summary, studies into the effects of HRT on brain function in younger and older women suggest that it modulates brain function in regions critical to memory and mood, including the prefrontal cortex and hippocampus. However, these studies do not provide insight into putative biological mechanisms that might underpin these actions. One mechanism indirectly suggested by neuroendocrine challenge studies is that HRT might modulate specific neurotransmitter systems in these regions.

To study this we extended our earlier findings and analyzed the interaction between GnRHa and a muscarinic antagonist, scopolamine. We used a verbal memory task to probe specific brain regions important to memory, and mood. We reported that scopolamine reduced activation in the left inferior frontal gyrus (LIFG) during encoding, which was attenuated further by GnRHa [35]. Further, using a visual working memory task we also found an interaction at the parahippocampus [68]. These findings were also associated with significant behavioral effects. Following pseudo-menopause with GnRHa, cholinergic antagonism produced a more significant deficit in response accuracy and response time respectively. In summary, these findings suggest that one mechanism via which acute loss of ovarian hormones might modulate brain function is via an interaction with the cholinergic system in frontotemporal brain regions. Another putative mechanism via which sex hormones could modulate brain function in these regions is by a direct effect on the neuronal and glial function. This effect can be studied using proton magnetic resonance spectroscopy (^{1}H-MRS).

Magnetic resonance spectroscopy

In vivo ^{1}H-MRS is a magnetic resonance imaging (MRI) technique that can measure the biochemical composition within specific brain regions. Using this technique in premenopausal women we found that ovarian suppression, with GnRHa, was associated with a significant increase in Choline (Cho) concentration in the dorsolateral prefrontal cortex (DLPFC). We also found a significant trend in the increase in Cho concentration in the hippocampus. Choline is a marker of membrane metabolism and turnover [69] that has been reported to increase with age [70]. Therefore, our findings suggest that sex hormone concentration may be associated with increased neuronal/glial membrane turnover (i.e. less neuronal stability) in brain regions associated with memory and mood.

An earlier *in vivo* ^{1}H-MRS study in postmenopausal women supported these findings. In this study we reported a significant reduction in Cho concentration in the hippocampus and parietal lobe of women prescribed long-term HRT+ compared with HRT naive (HRT−) women [71]. Other groups have also reported changes in brain chemistry in specific brain regions using ^{1}H-MRS findings. For example, reduced myo-inositol concentration has been reported in basal ganglia, frontal and hippocampal regions in women prescribed HRT compared with never-users [72]. This finding is significant as myo-inositol increases with age [73] and has been reported to be particularly high in people with Alzheimer's disease [74].

In summary, studies suggest that the effects of estrogen on brain function may be biologically underpinned by direct modulation of neuronal function or via an interaction with neurotransmitter systems such as the cholinergic. A further technique that has been used to study the effects of HRT at the neurotransmitter *receptor* level is single photon emission computed tomography (SPECT).

Single photon emission computed tomography

Single photon emission computed tomography studies into *short-term* effects of HRT on postmenopausal women reported increased cortical 5-HT$_{2A}$ receptor availability in the prefrontal cortex and anterior cingulate [75, 76]. We also found that *long-term* HRT was associated with lower 5-HT$_{2A}$ receptor availability in the hippocampus, compared with never-users [77]. Further, hippocampal 5-HT$_{2A}$ receptor availability correlated negatively with verbal memory. This was consistent with previous studies, which reported total cortical 5-HT$_{2A}$ binding potential was negatively correlated with delayed verbal memory [78]. These findings suggest that upregulation of postsynaptic 5-HT$_{2A}$ receptors is associated with short-term use; but chronic use may lead to downregulation.

Previous SPECT studies in healthy postmenopausal women have also reported an increased index of cortical cholinergic nerve terminal concentrations in multiple cortical regions (e.g. anterior and posterior cingulate, prefrontal and temporal cortex) with increasing years of HRT use [79]. In another SPECT study we investigated the relationship between m1/m4 muscarinic receptor density (using a novel ligand (R,R)[123I]-I-QNB) in premenopausal and postmenopausal women who were either long-term users of HRT, following prescription around the time of menopause, or never-users. We found that premenopausal women had more m1/m4 receptors than postmenopausal women and that HRT users had a higher density of m1/m4 receptors than never-users [80]. Thus, these data add to the evidence suggesting an important relationship between estrogen and neurotransmitters, such as the serotonergic and cholinergic system, in postmenopausal women.

Summary and conclusion

Studies suggest that the prescription of estrogen around the time of the menopause may reduce the risk of longer-term memory impairment and improve mood in some women. Research to date has suggested that this may be modulated by the effects of estrogen on the structure and function of brain regions that are central to mood and memory. However, there is still a significant need for better-designed studies to determine the clinical significance of these effects. In particular, studies are required that (a) test the "critical period hypothesis," and (b) directly compare the effects of HRT with antidepressants and/or

CBT in perimenopausal women suffering from clinical depression. It is hoped that future research in this area will address these important issues.

References

1. Evans D, Ganguli M, Harris T, Kawas C, Larson EB. Women and Alzheimer disease. *Alzheimer Dis Assoc Disord* 1999; **13**: 187–9.

2. Lopez OL, Jagust WJ, DeKosky ST, *et al.* Prevalence and classification of mild cognitive impairment in the Cardiovascular Health Study Cognition Study: Part 1. *Arch Neurol* 2003; **60**: 1385–9.

3. McCrone P, Dhanasiri S, Patel A, Knapp M, Lawton-Smith S. *Paying the Price. The Cost of Mental Health Care in England to 2026.* London: Kings Fund; 2008.

4. Zandi PP, Carlson MC, Plassman BL, *et al.* Hormone replacement therapy and incidence of Alzheimer disease in older women: The Cache County Study. *JAMA* 2002; **288**: 2123–9.

5. Comas-Herrera A, Wittenberg R, Pickard L, Knapp M. Cognitive impairment in older people: future demand for long-term care services and the associated costs. *Int J Geriatr Psychiatry* 2007; **22**: 1037–45.

6. Rocca WA, Bower JH, Maraganore DM, *et al.* Increased risk of cognitive impairment or dementia in women who underwent oophorectomy before menopause. *Neurology* 2007; **69**: 1074–83.

7. LeBlanc ES, Janowsky J, Chan BKS, Nelson HD. Hormone replacement therapy and cognition: systematic review and meta-analysis. *JAMA* 2001; **285**: 1489–99.

8. Maki PM, Sundermann E. Hormone therapy and cognitive function. *Hum Reprod Update* 2009; **15**: 667–81.

9. Shumaker SA, Legault C, Rapp SR, *et al.* Estrogen plus progestin and the incidence of dementia and mild cognitive impairment in postmenopausal women: The Women's Health Initiative Memory Study: a randomized controlled trial. *JAMA* 2003; **289**: 2651–62.

10. Schmid NS, Taylor KI, Foldi NS, Berres M, Monsch AU. Neuropsychological signs of Alzheimer's disease 8 years prior to diagnosis. *J Alzheimer's Dis* 2013; **34**: 537–46.

11. Harman SM, Brinton EA, Cedars M, *et al.* KEEPS: the Kronos Early Estrogen Prevention Study. *Climacteric* 2005; **8**: 3–12.

12. Henderson VW. Alzheimer's disease: review of hormone therapy trials and implications for treatment and prevention after menopause. *J Steroid Biochem Mol Biol* 2014; **142**: 99–106.

13. World Health Organization. *World Health Report: Shaping the Future.* Geneva: WHO; 2003.

14. Stewart DE, Boydell KM. Psychologic distress during menopause: associations across the reproductive life cycle. *Int J Psychiatr Med* 1993; **23**: 157–62.

15. Gregory RJ, Masand PS, Yohai NH. Depression across the reproductive life cycle: correlations between events. *Prim Care Companion J Clin Psychiatry* 2000; **2**: 127–9.

16. Payne JL, Roy PS, Murphy-Eberenz K, *et al.* Reproductive cycle-associated mood symptoms in women with major depression and bipolar disorder. *J Affect Disord* 2007; **99**: 221–9.

17. Chuong CJ, Burgos DM. Medical history in women with premenstrual syndrome. *J Psychosom Obstet Gynaecol* 1995; **16**: 21–7.

18. Morse CA, Dudley E, Guthrie J, Dennerstein L. Relationships between premenstrual complaints and perimenopausal experiences. *J Psychosom Obstet Gynaecol* 1998; **19**: 182–91.

19. Binfa L, Castelo-Branco C, Blumel JE, *et al.* Influence of psycho-social factors on climacteric symptoms. *Maturitas* 2004; **48**: 425–31.

20. Freeman EW, Sammel MD, Liu L, *et al.* Hormones and menopausal status as predictors of depression in women in transition to menopause. *Arch Gen Psychiatry* 2004; **61**: 62–70.

21. Aydin N, Inandi T, Karabulut N. Depression and associated factors among women within their first postnatal year in Erzurum province in eastern Turkey. *Women Health* 2005; **41**: 1–12.

22. Bloch M, Rotenberg N, Koren D, Klein E. Risk factors associated with the development of postpartum mood disorders. *J Affect Disord* 2005; **88**: 9–18.

23. Bloch M, Rotenberg N, Koren D, Klein E. Risk factors for early postpartum depressive symptoms. *Gen Hosp Psychiatry* 2006; **28**: 3–8.

24. Schmidt PJ, Nieman L, Danaceau MA, *et al.* Estrogen replacement in perimenopause-related depression: a preliminary report. *Am J Obstet Gynecol* 2000; **183**: 414–20.

25. Soares CN, Almeida OP, Joffe H, Cohen LS. Efficacy of estradiol for the treatment of depressive disorders in perimenopausal women: a double-blind, randomized, placebo-controlled trial. *Arch Gen Psychiatry* 2001; **58**: 529–34.

26. Studd J, Panay N. Are oestrogens useful for the treatment of depression in women? *Best Pract Res Clin Obstet Gynaecol* 2009; **23**: 63–71.

27. Studd J. Ten reasons to be happy about hormone replacement therapy: a guide for patients. *Menopause Int* 2010; **16**: 44–6.

28. Studd J. Why are estrogens rarely used for the treatment of depression in women? *Gynecol Endocrinol* 2007; **23**: 63–4.

29. Studd J, Panay N. Hormones and depression in women. *Climacteric* 2004; 7: 338–46.

30. Studd JWW. A guide to the treatment of depression in women by estrogens. *Climacteric* 2011; **14**: 637–42.

31. McEwen B. Estrogen actions throughout the brain. *Recent Prog Horm Res* 2002; 57: 357–84.

32. Kenealy BP, Kapoor A, Guerriero KA, *et al.* Neuroestradiol in the hypothalamus contributes to the regulation of gonadotropin releasing hormone release. *J Neurosci* 2013; **33**: 19051–9.

33. Heldring N, Pike A, Andersson S, *et al.* Estrogen receptors: how do they signal and what are their targets. *Physiol Rev* 2007; **87**: 905–31.

34. Craig MC, Cutter WJ, van Amelsvoort TAMJ, Rymer J, Whitehead M, Murphy DGM. Effects of estrogen replacement therapy on dopaminergic responsivity in postmenopausal women. *Biol Psychiatry* 2003; **53**: 210S.

35. Craig MC, Fletcher PC, Daly EM, *et al.* The interactive effect of the cholinergic system and acute ovarian suppression on the brain: an fMRI study. *Horm Behav* 2009; **55**: 41–9.

36. Davies P, Maloney AJ. Selective loss of central cholinergic neurons in Alzheimer's disease. *Lancet* 1976; **2**: 1403.

37. Bowen DM, Smith CB, White P, Davison AN. Neurotransmitter-related enzymes and indices of hypoxia in senile dementia and other abiotrophies. *Brain* 1976; **99**: 459–96.

38. Shytle RD, Silver AA, Lukas RJ, *et al.* Nicotinic acetylcholine receptors as targets for antidepressants. *Mol Psychiatry* 2002; 7: 525–35.

39. van Amelsvoort TAMJ, Abel KM, Robertson DMR, *et al.* Prolactin response to *d*-fenfluramine in postmenopausal women on and off ERT: comparison with young women. *Psychoneuroendocrinology* 2001; **26**: 494–502.

40. Dunlop BW, Nemeroff CB. The role of dopamine in the pathophysiology of depression. *Arch Gen Psychiatry* 2007; **64**: 327–37.

41. Backman L, Nyberg L. Dopamine and training-related working-memory improvement. *Neurosci Biobehav Rev* 2013; **37**: 2209–19.

42. Ettigi P, Lal S, Martin JB, Friesen HC. Effects of sex, oral contraceptives, and glucose loading on apomorphine induced growth hormone secretion. *J Clin Endocrinol Metab* 1975; **40**: 1094–8.

43. Wieck A, Hirst AD, Kumar R, Checkley SA, Campbell IC. Growth hormone secretion by human females in response to apomorphine challenge is markedly affected by menstrual cycle phase. *B J Clin Pharmacol* 1989; **27**: 700–1.

44. Wieck A, Kumar R, Marks MN, Checkley SA. Increased sensitivity of dopamine receptors and recurrence of affective psychosis after childbirth. *Br Med J (Clin Res Ed)* 1991; **303**: 613–16.

45. Craig M, Cutter W, Wickhham H, van Amelsvoort T, Murphy D. Effect of long-term estrogen therapy on dopaminergic responsivity in postmenopausal women. *Psychoneuroendocrinology* 2004; **29**: 1309–16.

46. Lamar M, Craig M, Daly EM, *et al.* Acute tryptophan depletion promotes an anterior-to-posterior fMRI activation shift during task switching in older adults. *Human Brain Mapp* 2014; **35**: 712–22.

47. Halbreich U, Rojansky N, Palter S, *et al.* Estrogen augments serotonergic activity in postmenopausal women. *Biol Psychiatry* 1995; **37**: 434–41.

48. Matthews KA, Kuller LH, Wing RR, Meilahn EN, Plantinga P. Prior to use of estrogen replacement therapy, are users healthier than nonusers? *Am J Epidemiol* 1996; **143**: 971–8.

49. Resnick SM, Maki PM, Golski S, Kraut MA, Zonderman AB. Effects of estrogen replacement therapy on PET cerebral blood flow and neuropsychological performance. *Horm Behav* 1998; **34**: 171–82.

50. Raz N, Gunning-Dixon F, Head D, *et al.* Aging, sexual dimorphism, and hemispheric asymmetry of the cerebral cortex: replicability of regional differences in volume. *Neurobiol Aging* 2004; **25**: 377–96.

51. Eberling JL, Wu C, Tong-Turnbeaugh R, Jagurst J. Estrogen-and-tamoxifen-associated effects on brain structure and function. *Neuroimage* 2004; **21**: 364–71.

52. Erickson KI, Colcombe SJ, Raz N, *et al.* Selective sparing of brain tissue in postmenopausal women receiving hormone replacement therapy. *Neurobiol Aging* 2005; **26**: 1205–13.

53. Robertson DMW, Craig MC, Van Amelsvoort T, *et al.* Effects of estrogen replacement therapy on age-related differences in grey matter volume. *Climacteric* 2009; **12**: 301–9.

54. Eberling JL, Wu C, Mungas D, Buoncore M, Jagurst J. Preliminary evidence that oestrogen protects against age-related hippocampal atrophy. *Neurobiol Aging* 2003; **24**: 725–32.

55. McEwen BS. Glucocorticoids, depression, and mood disorders: structural remodeling in the brain. *Metabolism* 2005; **54 Suppl 1**: 20–3.

56. Robertson D, Craig MC, van Amelsvoort T, *et al.* Effects of estrogen therapy on age-related differences in gray matter concentration. *Climacteric* 2009; **12**: 301–9.

57. Schmidt R, Fazekas F, Reinhart B, *et al.* Estrogen replacement therapy in older women: a neuropsychological and brain MRI study. *J Am Geriatr Soc* 1996; **44**: 1307–13.

58. Cook IA, Morgan ML, Dunkin JJ, *et al.* Estrogen replacement therapy is associated with less progression of subclinical structural brain disease in normal elderly women: a pilot study. *Int J Geriatr Psychiatry* 2002; **17**: 610–18.

59. Raz E, Tighe H, Sato Y, *et al.* Preferential induction of a Th1 immune response and inhibition of specific IgE antibody formation by plasmid DNA immunization. *Proc Natl Acad Sci USA* 1996; **93**: 5141–5.

60. Jernigan TL, Archibald SL, Fennema-Notestine C, *et al.* Effects of age on tissues and regions of the cerebrum and cerebellum. *Neurobiol Aging* 2001; **22**: 581–94.

61. Sullivan EV, Marsh L, Mathalon DH, Lim KO, Pfefferbaum A. Age-related decline in MRI volumes of temporal lobe gray matter but not hippocampus. *Neurobiol Aging* 1995; **16**: 591–606.

62. Sherwin BB, Henrya JF. Brain aging modulates the neuroprotective effects of estrogen on selective aspects of cognition in women: a critical review. *Frontiers Neuroendocrinol* 2008; **29**: 88–113.

63. Eberling JL, Reed BR, Coleman JE, Jagust WJ. Effect of estrogen on cerebral glucose metabolism in postmenopausal women. *Neurology* 2000; **55**: 875–7.

64. Shaywitz SE, Shaywitz BA, Pugh KR, *et al.* Effect of estrogen on brain activation patterns in postmenopausal women during working memory tasks. *JAMA* 1999; **281**: 1197–202.

65. Berman KF, Schmidt PJ, Rubinow DR, *et al.* Modulation of cognition-specific cortical activity by gonadal steroids: a positron-emission tomography study in women. *Proc Natl Acad Sci USA* 1997; **94**: 8836–41.

66. Craig MC, Fletcher PC, Daly EM, *et al.* Gonadotropin hormone releasing hormone agonists alter prefrontal function during verbal encoding in young women. *Psychoneuroendocrinology* 2007; **32**: 1116–27.

67. Craig MC, Fletcher PC, Daly EM, *et al.* Reversibility of the effects of acute ovarian hormone suppression on verbal memory and prefrontal function in pre-menopausal women. *Psychoneuroendocrinology* 2008; **33**: 1426–31.

68. Craig MC, Brammer M, Maki PM, *et al.* The interactive effect of acute ovarian suppression and the cholinergic system on visuospatial working memory in young women. *Psychoneuroendocrinology* 2010; **35**: 987–1000.

69. Jenden DJ. The metabolism of choline. *Bull Clin Sci* 1990; **55**: 99–106.

70. Pfefferbaum A, Adalsteinsson E, Speilman D, Sullivan EV, Lim KO. *In vivo* spectroscopic quantification of the N-acetyl-moiety, creatine, and choline from large volume of brain grey and white matter: the effects of normal aging. *Magn Reson Med* 1999; **41**: 276–84.

71. Robertson DM, van Amelsvoort T, Daly E, *et al.* Effects of estrogen replacement therapy on human brain aging: an in vivo 1H MRS study. *Neurology* 2001; **57**: 2114–17.

72. Ernst T, Chang L, Cooray D, *et al.* The effects of tamoxifen and estrogen on brain metabolism in elderly women. *J Natl Cancer Inst* 2002; **94**: 592–7.

73. Chang L, Ernst T, Poland RE, Jenden DJ. In vivo proton magnetic resonance spectroscopy of the normal aging human brain. *Life Sci* 1996; **58**: 2049–56.

74. Huang W, Alexander GE, Chang L, *et al.* Brain metabolite concentration and dementia severity in Alzheimer's disease: a 1H MRS study. *Neurology* 2001; **57**: 626–32.

75. Kugaya A, Epperson CN, Zoghbi S, *et al.* Increase in prefrontal cortex serotonin 2A receptors following estrogen treatment in postmenopausal women. *Am J Psychiatry* 2003; **160**: 1522–4.

76. Moses EL, Drevets WC, Smith G, *et al.* Effects of estradiol and progesterone administration on human serotonin 2A receptor binding: a PET study. *Biol Psychiatry* 2000; **48**: 854–60.

77. Compton J, Travis MJ, Norbury R, *et al.* Long-term estrogen therapy and 5-HT2A receptor binding in postmenopausal women; a single photon emission tomography (SPET) study. *Horm Behav* 2008; **53**: 61–8.

78. Nobury R, Travis MJ, Erlandsson K, *et al.* Estrogen therapy and brain muscarinic receptor density in healthy females: a SPET study. *Horm Behav* 2007; **51**: 249–57.

79. Smith YR, Minoshima S, Kuhl DE, Zubieta JK. Effects of long-term hormone therapy on cholinergic synaptic concentrations in healthy postmenopausal women. *J Clin Endocrinol Metab* 2001; **86**: 679–84.

80. Nobury R, Travis MJ, Erlandsson K, *et al.* *In vivo* imaging of muscarinic receptors in the aging female brain with (R,R)[123I]-I-QNB and single photon emission tomography. *Exp Gerontol* 2005; **40**: 137–45.

Libido and sexual function in the menopause

Claudine Domoney

Patricia is 50 and has been happily married for 26 years. Her periods stopped at 48, and she has not had any troublesome menopausal symptoms. She has three children, who are all at university. The family have a nice house, have good holidays and to all appearances they are a "perfect family." However for the last 4 years she has found it really difficult to have sex with her husband. She does everything she can to avoid his advances, going to bed early or staying up late, so that they do not go to bed together. On the rare occasions they do have sex, she gets no enjoyment, but merely lays back and lets him "do it," hoping that its all over quickly. She comes to see you for advice.

Introduction

Loss of libido is the most common sexual complaint of women, often being a final common pathway of many sexual disorders. Estimates range from 30–45% depending on the population sampled, increasing in the postmenopausal age group [1]. However, the degree of distress associated with loss of libido may be minimal and therefore not sexually dysfunctional. Lack of arousal and orgasmic disorders are frequently correlated with loss of libido, as are sexual pain disorders. It is important for the medical doctor to help the patient decipher the chain of events and their combination, to facilitate change and improvement. Making assumptions about a particular set of expectations is likely to lead to neglect of key factors. In psychosexual medicine, listening and observing the patient's expression of feelings can help to interpret the predominant issue(s) which can be resolved using brief psychotherapeutic intervention.

The menopause

Studies of the menopause and sexual relationships have reported a reduction in sexual activity with age. However, a US study of 18–59-year-old adults has reported sexual difficulties in 43% of women and 31% of men [2]. An Australian longitudinal study, observing women from the age of 45 to 55 suggested that female sexual dysfunction increased from 42% to 88% from the early-to-late menopause [3]. However if "distress" is included in the definition of female sexual dysfunction, this is reduced significantly [4]. There is a small variation amongst European women, country by country, which indicates that the frequency of intercourse varies, but body mass index (BMI) is the only significantly varying factor.

Managing the Menopause: 21st Century Solutions, ed. Nick Panay, Paula Briggs, and Gab Kovacs. Published by Cambridge University Press. © Cambridge University Press 2015.

There are increasing sexual difficulties with age: in women these may be correlated with estrogen levels, but not androgens, although testosterone levels have not consistently been shown to reflect sexual functioning in younger women either. Predictably women who have a sexual partner are more likely to be sexually active and to have increased satisfaction within their relationship. Cessation of sexual activity is more likely to be male partner driven within a relationship. A recent lifestyle survey from the UK, published in 2013 indicated that sexual inactivity was more common with reducing health status in both men and women, and therefore with age. One in six people reported a health condition that affected their sex life in the previous year: 24% of men and 18% of women had sought help or advice from a health-care professional. Men report an increase in ejaculation and satisfaction problems, but less erectile dysfunction, although the wide availability of phosphodiesterase inhibitors may have changed the distribution of sexual problems in men. In women, sexual satisfaction rates have been increasing overall and have been linked with earlier sexual debut and more positive attitudes to female sexuality [5]. There is a greater expectation in women to continue to be sexually active and satisfied, but this is not universal. Individual preconceptions regarding aging and behavior vary hugely.

Various studies have been contradictory with respect to menopause and the cause of sexual difficulties being age-or hormone-related. Overall when dealing with individual patients, the patient will be the "expert" in her condition and the clinician needs to help her unravel the issues around cause and effect.

Sexual disorders

The *Diagnostic and Statistical Manual of Mental Disorders* (DSM) V classification now combines desire and arousal disorders as they are almost invariably linked. Isolated genital arousal disorder may however exist in postmenopausal women due to the physical changes of the menopause causing vulvo-vaginal atrophy. Over time this condition is commonly associated with reduced desire. Development of desire disorder may be protective from distress and dissatisfaction when preceded by dyspareunia or adverse changes in sexual responsivity.

Orgasmic disorders are a separate category, which may include a lack of or reduction in quality of sex, sometimes due to direct hormonal deficiencies or a culmination of other sexual issues. Dyspareunia and vaginismus are now also classified together, but are separate from non-coital pain disorders, which can also cause severe sexual dysfunction, for example vulvodynia and bladder pain syndrome.

The duration of the problem is an important factor in diagnosis of female sexual dysfunction. Short-term issues may be normal and a manifestation of the effects of life circumstances. Sexual difficulties may also reflect the overall psychological well-being of the individual. Of importance in the menopausal woman, are the organic causes of sexual problems that may impact on psychological health. The etiological routes of anatomic, hormonal, neurologic, vascular and other abnormalities affects sexual self-esteem and functioning, given that sex is a mind and body activity.

Sexual response cycle

Although the Masters and Johnson model of human sexuality [6] has been useful in explaining the sequence of phases in the human sexual response cycle, the Basson model of female sexuality [7] facilitates a clearer understanding of the drivers and difficulties specifically involved in the female sexual response cycle. A spontaneous drive to be sexually active may be less significant in a longstanding relationship than the need for emotional and physical satisfaction and emotional and physical intimacy. A sexually neutral woman is able to be receptive to sexual stimuli in the right circumstances, and desire and arousal may occur concomitantly, rather than desire being a driver for activity. A better understanding of her emotional and relationship issues can be crucial to understanding the physical responses of a woman, particularly with the major life changes occurring at the menopause. How she perceives the changes happening to her, including her role in society, at work and within her family, all reflect her self-esteem and sexual confidence.

Hormonal impact

Estrogen deficiency has a significant impact on sexual function, including changes in urogenital anatomy, nerve transmission, blood flow, sleep disorders, mood alterations and vasomotor symptoms. Within the genital tract, shortening and loss of elasticity in the vagina occurs and along with reduced secretions and thinning of the vaginal epithelial layers, increases the risk of trauma and discomfort, particularly in association with sexual activity. Atrophy of the tissues causes pain, dryness, lack of arousal, reduction in desire, reduced orgasm and sensitivity, and increasing urinary symptoms. An alteration in vaginal pH can cause recurrent infections such as bacterial vaginosis and thrush. More covert symptoms of lack of desire and arousal, decreased orgasmic potential and postcoital bleeding causing anxiety, can all lead to avoidance of sex, deterioration in a relationship and an acceptance of sexual decline. If not recognized, this becomes a repetitive cycle that is difficult to unravel or arrest. Psychologically, behavioral patterns become embedded and their initial trigger becomes less identifiable. At this point, recovery and re-engagement with a sexual partner can be troublesome.

Aging

The menopause is associated with specific features that may directly contribute to sexual decline. Symptoms of mood change and lability, night sweats and flashing, sleep problems and urogenital atrophic changes can be dealt with by the use of medication, most appropriately hormone replacement therapy (HRT). Yet the psychology of aging, particularly in the Western world, may be more pertinent. Changes in BMI and body habitus, with their impact on self-esteem, are relevant for many women. Perception of attractiveness and self-image, as a reflection of society's view of aging, may be transferred to the individual. In addition, for some, there may be an expectation that older people should be sexually passive and discrete. Problems with teenage children and their pressures, pelvic floor dysfunction, physical illness, medication use and side effects, partner dysfunction and relationship factors are all relevant and often co-exist.

Patricia has had ongoing difficulties for 4 years and much of her behavior may have become ingrained without any recognition of the initial issues. These are likely to be complex and interactive. Allegedly she has the perfect family, nice house, good holidays and successful children. She does not report any troublesome menopausal symptoms, yet she is not able to have an intimate and satisfying relationship with her husband of 26 years.

We need to know why she has come to seek help now as it may have some bearing on the possible issues involved. Has she motivated herself to attend or has she been "sent" by someone else – her husband or friends? Is she really prepared to look at the issues or does she want or expect a "quick fix" with hormones or a perceived "magic pill"?

Although it may not be the role of the health-care professional to be a relationship counselor, it is part of our remit to understand if this appears to be the most important factor. The couple can then be directed to the most appropriate therapist. We need to be able to allow revelations of fear or fantasies in an atmosphere of trust and safety in the consultation room. We should be aware of the patient's motivation for change and her defences or reluctance for this. However, this woman has presented with an overt sexual problem, indicating that she is likely to be receptive to encouragement to change her behaviors. Accept the patient as she brings her problem and although many may feel this is a relationship issue, she has chosen to present herself to the doctor without her husband. It may be appropriate to see them both together at a later appointment, if this is what she wishes or if it seems helpful to further understand Patricia's problems.

During the genital examination, revelations can be made through verbal and non-verbal communication. The process of undertaking an examination may facilitate a "moment of truth." How she approaches getting undressed, covering herself, what she says or how she covers her genitals, how they appear, whether she has any unrecognized atrophic changes is an important part of the process of examination. Has she had any other symptoms that may have caused difficulties that she had not related to the menopause? We need to understand how Patricia perceives the menopause and how aging is changing her.

We may focus on how she understands her relationship to be with her husband now, how she wishes it to be in the future, what their sexual history has been and whether there have been any other factors that have impacted on her sexuality and her ability to respond to him. Is she sad that she no longer feels sexy or wants to be sexually active, or is she accepting of the situation, or is it what she expects in middle or old age? Does she feel sexual feelings at times other than with her husband?

Any unrecognized menopausal symptoms should be elicited, particularly urogenital symptoms, and estrogen replacement therapy and/or local estrogen therapy discussed. Estrogen replacement alone has been reported to impact positively on sexual status of women, although this may be secondary to multiple modes of action. Topical estrogens alone are more useful for local symptoms than systemic estrogen, so should be promoted when there are predominant urogenital symptoms. Vaginal moisturizers are an option for those who wish to avoid hormone treatment altogether.

Testosterone replacement therapy (see Chapter 17) is controversial, although studies have confirmed a benefit for women with low sexual desire peri- and postmenopausally [8]. These studies have included women with bilateral oophorectomy who have a significant reduction in androgens, as postmenopausal ovaries produce at least 50% of circulating androgens, and with and without estrogen replacement. Androgen levels reduce by 50% in women from their 20s to their 40s, yet many women feel greater satisfaction as they mature, although this may reflect more of a change in male attentiveness with age and female confidence. Transdermal estrogen therapy may be better for libido as sex hormone binding globulin (SHBG) levels increase with oral therapy, leading to a reduction in free testosterone. Testosterone is available for women in implant, gel and patch form. For some, testosterone may help with "kick starting" sexual sensitivity and responsiveness, such that once a regular satisfying sexual life has been re-established, it may not be necessary, similar to the use of phosphodiesterase inhibitors in men with psychogenic erectile dysfunction. Once responsiveness has been confirmed to the individual, performance anxiety will reduce and sexual encounters be less stressful, therefore more reliably pleasurable.

Simple solutions such as appropriate lubricant advice can be helpful. For some, a specifically marketed sexual lubricant will be appropriate, but for others a non-medical option such as sweet almond oil will be preferable. Contraceptive concerns also need to be clarified as there is great misunderstanding of perimenopausal requirements (see Chapter 21). If there is a partner difficulty then he can be encouraged to see either his doctor or a counselor. Sometimes just prescribing relaxation time can be important. When analyzing loss of libido and sexual difficulties, approaching the two components of motivation and drive can be helpful. With respect to motivation, factors relating to previous experiences, relationship quality, relationship duration, previous disagreements and disputes may be important. Drive may be dependent on age, health, hormone status and mood, which all interact, depending on life events and circumstances. Asking a woman about her general sexual desire and feelings of sexuality can be important. Does she feel attractive or attracted to others? Does she have fantasies, daydreams or other desires? Does this induce a need and wish to behave sexually? Is she able or was she ever able to masturbate? With respect to her relationship: are there interpersonal conflicts such as a dysfunctional partner, miscommunications and any other family or financial problems. She may have mood changes, a history of trauma in the past, self-esteem issues or other inter- or intrapersonal conflicts. Are there any other comorbidities that coincided or overlap the onset of the sexual difficulties? Are they situational only? What is the effect of her problems and the impact on her quality of life?

How does she perceive that you might help her? Does she expect hormone management or a "female Viagra"? Has she read about "cures" on the Internet or been told by friends to try a product? There is clearly a strong placebo effect with medications given for sexual issues and those that are motivated to change are more likely to be thinking about sex – the lack of which may be part of the problem. Does she express feelings of pain – if she does where is that pain coming from? Pain is often expressed as physical although it can be psychological in origin. Yet this disparity is reported more commonly in younger women in comparison to older women, who often have more problems with lubrication and sexual interest.

For some women, a specific approach using the PLISSIT model may be helpful: Permission giving in the form of talking or changing behaviors, Limited Information regarding the areas suitable for the patient, Specific Suggestions detailing exercises or regimes to help the area of sexual difficulty and lastly Intensive Therapy with deeper analysis of concerns and issues. Sensate focus is a common regime of graduated increasing re-engagement with intimacy through touch, building up to sexual intimacy. This involves "homework" and the need for both partners to be involved. Often this may be cumbersome and awkward for those who have become resistant to their sexual feelings. As the "patient is the expert" in her own symptoms and sexual history, it is imperative that she feels able and comfortable to engage with the reasons for her difficulties.

Patricia therefore requires sensitive exploration of her feelings and beliefs regarding her unsatisfying sexual life. How she perceives her future sexual life and the potential sadness involved in losing it will determine how we approach managing her as an individual patient. This may be with hormonal management – topical or systemic; relationship counseling; individual therapy – this may be brief with the primary health-care professional she presented to or it might involve referral onwards. She may require management of other physical or mental health concerns – or as is frequently the case, a combination of all of the above.

References

1. Hayes RD, Bennett CM, Fairley CK, Dennerstein L. What can prevalence studies tell us about female sexual difficulty and dysfunction? *J Sex Med* 2006: **3**; 589–95.

2. Laumann E, Paik A, Rosen R. Sexual dysfunction in the United States: prevalence and predictors. *JAMA* 1999; **281**: 537–44.

3. Dennerstein L, Alexander JL, Kotz K. The menopause and sexual functioning: a review of the population-based studies. *Ann Rev Sex Res* 2003; **14**: 64–82.

4. Dennerstein L, Guthrie JR, Hayes RD, DeRogatis LR, Lehert P. Sexual function, dysfunction, and sexual distress in a prospective, population-based sample of mid-aged, Australian-born women. *J Sex Med* 2008; **5**: 2291–9.

5. Beckman N, Waern M, Gustafson D, Skoog I. Secular trends in self reported sexual activity and satisfaction in Swedish 70 year olds: cross sectional survey of four populations, 1971–2001. *Br Med J* 2008; **337**: 151–4.

6. Masters WH, Johnson VE. *Human Sexual Response*. Boston: Little, Brown; 1966.

7. Basson R, Althof S, Davis S, *et al.* Summary of the recommendations on sexual dysfunctions in women. *J Sex Med* 2004; **1**: 24.

8. Somboonporn W, Davis S, Seif MW, Bell R. Testosterone for peri- and postmenopausal women. *Cochrane Database Syst Rev* 2005; **4**: CD004509.

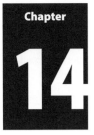
Gynecological pathology in the menopause (excluding cancers)

John Eden

Robyn is 47 years old. She has three children in their 20s. She had a sterilization after her last pregnancy 22 years ago. During the last few years her periods have become progressively heavier. Her general practitioner arranged an ultrasound, which has shown she has fibroids. She comes to see you to ask if she should have a hysterectomy [1].

Introduction

The 40s are a time of irregular and sometimes heavy menstrual loss due to fluctuating levels of sex hormones. Some months are characterized by low estrogen secretion and anovulation and others by extremely high levels of estradiol (E2). In a 20-year-old woman, E2 usually peaks at 500–1,000 pmol/L. In contrast, some perimenopausal women may have cycles where E2 levels peak at around 5,000 pmol/L. These high levels of estrogen are often not followed by ovulation and so progesterone is either not secreted at all, or levels are too low to counter these high-estrogen months. As we will see shortly, many gynecologic pathologies are driven by these unbalanced sex-hormone levels.

The perimenopause is also a time when gynecologic pathology is common. By age 40 years, around one in three women will have at least one fibroid; adenomyosis and endometriosis are also common. All three of these conditions are driven by sex hormones and are cured by menopause. Prior to the advent of the levonorgestrel-containing intrauterine system (LNG-IUS) and endoscopic surgery, as many as one in three women had an abdominal or vaginal hysterectomy for painful, heavy periods associated with fibroids, adenomyosis and/or endometriosis.

Abnormal uterine bleeding is very common at this stage of life. Apart from the conditions already mentioned, the endometrium is often the target of pathology as well. Polyps are common and can cause pain and bleeding. Potentially more sinister, endometrial hyperplasia can be a precursor to endometrial carcinoma. In contrast to younger women, where the vast majority of ovarian cysts are benign and transient, in this age group, persistent, premalignant cysts are common.

In this chapter, we will examine the pathophysiology of those gynecologic conditions that can cause significant distress for the woman who is approaching her menopause. First, the pathophysiology of these pathologies will be considered and then second, the various clinical presentations.

Managing the Menopause: 21st Century Solutions, ed. Nick Panay, Paula Briggs, and Gab Kovacs. Published by Cambridge University Press. © Cambridge University Press 2015.

Pathology

Fibroids

Fibroids are benign fibromuscular tumors arising from the myometrium. Some are very slow growing, but occasionally they can grow rapidly. Malignant transformation into a sarcoma is possible but exceedingly rare (around 1/1,000). The site of the fibroid is critically important. Those that are intramural or growing sub-serosally (under the uterine serosa) are less likely to result in menorrhagia than those inside the uterine cavity (intracavity) or under the endometrium (sub-mucus).

Beneath the endometrium is a rich plexus of blood vessels. Thus, a fibroid that is growing towards the uterine cavity will "push" these vessels ahead of it. Hysteroscopic examination of such a sub-mucus fibroid typically shows large vessels coursing over the benign tumor. When these vessels bleed, haemorrhage can be quite vigorous. Sub-mucus fibroids can become pedunculated over time and so crampy pain is common. Occasionally pain can be severe, especially if the uterus attempts to pass a pedunculated fibroid through the cervix.

Fibroids probably arise from a somatic myometrial stem cell. They usually have estrogen receptors (ERs) and progesterone receptors (PRs). After menopause, with the loss of sex-steroid drive, fibroids typically shrink and disappear, although some will become calcified.

Adenomyosis

This is a type of endometriosis and is defined by the presence of endometrial tissue within the uterine wall. It is probably due to the basalis layer of the endometrium growing into the myometrium. It usually affects the posterior wall of the uterus more than the anterior. Typically, the uterus is diffusely enlarged, although it is possible for adenomyosis to resemble a fibroid, producing a localized tumor (Figure 14.1). Adenomyosis usually hyper-expresses ER. It is often associated with fibroids, polyps and endometrial hyperplasia [2].

Endometriosis

This is an estrogen-dependent inflammatory disease that affects around 10% of reproductive-aged women. It is typified by the presence of endometrial-like tissue found outside the endometrial cavity, often associated with bleeding and inflammation (leading to scarring). The inflammation can irritate nerve fibers causing severe pain, as well as damaging adjacent structures such as the fallopian tubes (leading to blockage) or bowel (leading to pain and rectal bleeding). Infertility may result from the factors already mentioned or by adverse effects on uterine receptivity, sperm function or even the embryo itself. There may be a link with ovarian cancer.

Blood levels of CA-125 can be elevated in cases of endometriosis, but the only sure method of diagnosis is visual, usually by laparoscopy. The lesions are typically black or red but can be clear and are often seen on the pelvic peritoneum, especially the Pouch of Douglas, on the ovaries, bladder, bowel and uterine serosa. It can form (chocolate-) cysts within the ovary. There does appear to be a link between endometriosis and other autoimmune conditions [3].

The etiology of endometriosis still remains elusive. One theory speculates that endometrial cells implant on the peritoneum because of retrograde menstruation. Another theory suggests that the disease is the result of celomic metaplasia. It can be inherited in a polygenic way and it often runs in families. Endometriosis usually hyperexpresses ER;

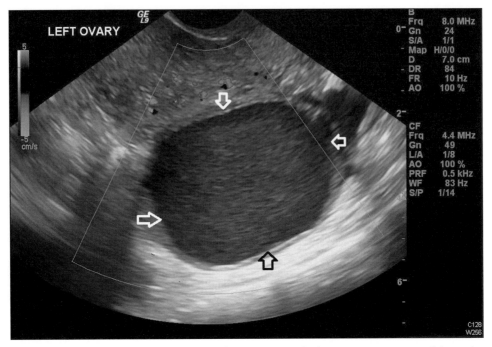

Figure 14.1. An ultrasound scan of an ovarian endometrioma. Note the homogenous appearance of the ovarian mass. Picture courtesy of Dr. Yasmin Tan, Women's Health and Research Centre of Australia.

whereas PR is usually downregulated and within the lesions, aromatase is hyperexpressed also. Prostaglandins are produced in high amounts by the endometriotic tissue and so contribute to the pain and inflammation.

Simple ovarian cysts

These are benign tumors, greater than 4–5 cm in diameter with a simple thin capsule and no internal solid features. As in younger patients, if they are ovulation-type cysts, they typically resolve in a couple of months. Cystadenomas are increasingly common as women age and are seen in this age group. Most are of a serous or mucinous type. They do not resolve spontaneously, but rather increase in size over time and can become malignant.

Most serous tumors are partly cystic and solid. Inside the cystic component are papillary structures and grossly, they can resemble ovarian cancer but without invasion or atypia. Microscopically, there are small uni- or multi-locular cysts lined by a single layer of tall, columnar, ciliated cells resembling normal tubal epithelium, or cuboidal non-ciliated cells resembling ovarian surface epithelium. In a third of cases they are bilateral. Autoimplants may occur on the ovarian surface that appear identical to non-invasive desmoplastic (serous epithelium with or without Psammoma bodies within abundant fibrous or granulation-like tissue) changes that can occur outside the ovary (e.g. on the fallopian tube).

Mucinous cystadenomas can grow very large and mimic fibroids or even pregnancy. The epithelium is usually tall and columnar with basal nuclei and abundant intracellular mucin. Stroma may be fibrous. Calcifications and microscopic cyst rupture may be present.

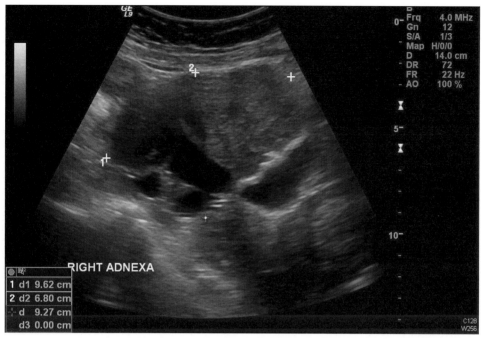

Figure 14.2. A complex ovarian mass as seen on ultrasound. Fluid shows up as "black" on ultrasound. This mass has both cystic and solid features. Picture courtesy of Dr. Yasmin Tan, Women's Health and Research Centre of Australia.

Around 5% are bilateral. If the tumor ruptures (spontaneously or at surgery), spill into the peritoneal cavity can result in pseudomyxoma peritonei (a gelatinous type of ascites).

Solid or complex ovarian cysts

Solid or complex ovarian cysts are fluid-filled structures with a diameter greater than 4–5 cm which also contain some internal solid tissue (Figure 14.2). A corpus luteum can appear as a complex ovarian cyst but will resolve over time. The differential diagnosis of a growing complex cyst includes a dermoid (teratoma; containing skin, neuronal tissue, teeth, hair etc.), ovarian cancer or an endometrioma (an ovarian cyst of endometriosis; a so-called "chocolate cyst") [4].

Endometrial hyperplasia

This condition is characterized by proliferation and thickening of the endometrium. It is typically due to a prolonged, unopposed estrogen effect, which of course commonly occurs during the perimenopausal years. It is also linked to age over 40 years, tamoxifen usage, and postmenopausal bleeding. It may progress to a variety of degrees of atypia (mild, moderate or severe). In its simplest form, endometrial hyperplasia is microscopically characterized by mild stratification of the endometrium with round glands, perhaps with some cystic dilatation; mitotic figures are occasional and vessel uniform in distribution.

As the disease progresses to complex endometrial hyperplasia (with varying degrees of atypia), the microscopic features become more intricate. This may include rounding of nuclei and nucleoli formation, epithelial stratification, an increase in mitosis rate, cytomegaly and pleomorphism. Endometrial hyperplasia (with or without atypia) may progress to

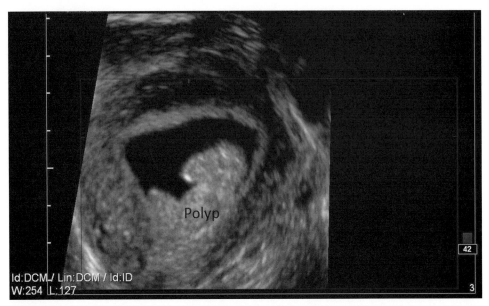

Figure 14.3. An endometrial polyp as seen on a sonohysterogram. Saline is instilled via the cervix to better define the uterine cavity. Picture courtesy of Dr. Yasmin Tan, Women's Health and Research Centre of Australia.

endometrial carcinoma and can often be reversed by moderately high doses of progestins. This usually presents with abnormal uterine bleeding, as will be discussed later.

Endometrial polyps

These are benign lesions that arise from the endometrium on a stalk fed by, often, a single blood vessel (Figure 14.3). They can range from a few millimeters to centimeters in size. They often present as abnormal uterine bleeding and are rarely premalignant (unlike bowel polyps).

Clinical scenarios and diagnostic options

Pelvic pain

Acute sudden and severe pelvic pain suggests either torsion of an ovarian cyst or perhaps rarely, in the setting of a perimenopausal woman, an ectopic pregnancy. Often the patient presents to the emergency ward and is in so much pain that she may be difficult to examine adequately.

Most of the time, pelvic pain is more chronic and often relates to the cycle. Patients with fibroids and/or adenomyosis may describe the pain as a dull ache, or feeling "bloated." Pressure symptoms from the bladder or rectum may be present. Endometriosis often produces pain that is more sharp and crampy and relates to the menses. Premenstrual spotting or staining and pain with intercourse are also often present with endometriosis. Gynecologic pain is often also referred down the legs and around to the back.

Clinical examination might reveal a large, firm irregular mass arising out of the pelvis (fibroids or ovarian cancer). The presence of ascites would make the diagnosis of ovarian cancer much more likely. If endometriosis is present, often painful nodules can be palpated vaginally (in the Pouch of Douglas, behind the uterus) and in severe cases, the uterus might be fixed in position and non-mobile. Sometimes endometriotic nodules on the rectum can be palpated too.

Blood testing may demonstrate iron deficiency and anemia. Tumor markers such as CA-125 can be elevated in cases of endometriosis as well as some ovarian cancers.

Abdominal and transvaginal ultrasound is the single most useful test. In expert hands, high-quality ultrasound can usually easily diagnose fibroids and describe their location; adenomyosis is often, but not always, picked up on ultrasound. In contrast, most patients with endometriosis have a normal scan, unless an endometrioma is present.

Abnormal uterine bleeding

The perimenopausal phase is a time when irregular menstrual loss is common and it may be challenging for the clinician to decide which patient needs investigation. A variety of types of abnormal uterine bleeding (AUB) are described [5]. Heavy menstrual bleeding (HMB) or menorrhagia is usually defined as more than 80 ml of measured blood per menses (at least for research purposes). However, in clinical practice, few clinicians will actually measure menstrual loss. Typically, menorrhagia is associated with the passage of menstrual clots and flooding. Prolonged menstruation is usually defined as bleeding for more than 8 days. Intermenstrual bleeding is also considered abnormal. The causes of AUB are typically benign but malignancy (endometrial, cervical) should always be considered. In most series of AUB around 70% will have a benign cause, 15% a malignancy and 15% a premalignant lesion.

Postmenopausal bleeding, defined as bleeding after 12 months of amenorrhea, always requires uterine assessment. The cervix should be visualized and cytology performed. Systematic reviews have shown that transvaginal (TV) ultrasound is a very good first test and if the endometrial thickness (ET) is 4 mm or less, then significant endometrial pathology is unlikely. Endometrial thickness greater than 4 mm (5 mm or more) or repeated episodes of postmenopausal bleeding (even if the ET is 4 mm or less) is an indication for a sonohysterogram (SHG) or (usually) hysteroscopy and biopsy.

A SHG involves the instillation of saline into the uterine cavity (Figure 14.4). It is an accurate test and cheaper than hysteroscopy. A SHG misses around 7% of intracavity lesions, usually a small polyp. The workup aims to document the cause of the bleeding, exclude malignancy and precisely locate any pathology such as fibroids.

Hysteroscopy can be performed under local or general anesthetic and involves inspecting the endocervical canal and uterine cavity using either CO_2 or saline (or another solution). Targeted biopsies can be performed and polypoid lesions resected.

For most episodes of AUB, the minimum workup is a TV scan, cervical smear (if due) and an endometrial biopsy. Sexually transmitted infections (STIs) such as chlamydia can present with irregular vaginal bleeding and should always be considered in the differential diagnosis. A sensitive PCR-based test is available and can be performed on a swab, urine or liquid cytology. Endometrial biopsy may be performed using a Pipelle in the consulting room, or at the time of hysteroscopy.

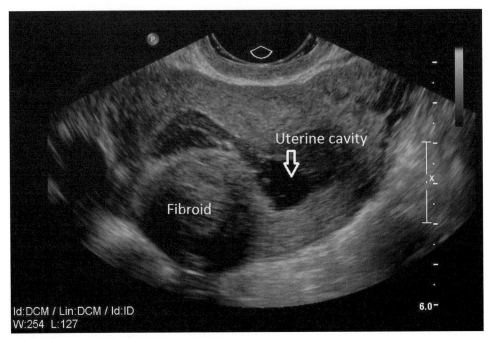

Figure 14.4. Sonohysterogram. Note a fibroid is protruding into the uterine cavity. Picture courtesy of Dr. Yasmin Tan, Women's Health and Research Centre of Australia.

Pelvic mass

Sometimes patients may present with a large mass arising out of the pelvis. Pressure symptoms on the bowel or bladder are common too. Ultrasound again is extremely helpful at clarifying the type of mass. If ovarian cancer is suspected then tumor markers should be ordered.

Management

In the recent past hysterectomy with or without removal of the ovaries was often performed to cure these gynecologic pathologies. Over the last 20 years, many more medical options have become available, along with endoscopic approaches, so that far fewer hysterectomies are now performed.

Fibroids

Depending on the patient's symptoms, fibroids can be managed expectantly, medically, radiologically or surgically. For many patients with few or no symptoms, it is reasonable to simply monitor the fibroids using ultrasound, anticipating that the menopause will cure the disease. Our patient described at the beginning of this chapter has many choices. If she is healthy, normotensive and a non-smoker then a low-estrogen contraceptive pill may be adequate to control her heavy periods. Tranexamic acid (1 g 3–4 times a day) can be taken during menses and often markedly reduce blood loss. Another approach can be to suppress menstruation completely using a moderate dose of a progestin (e.g. norethisterone 5 mg daily, medroxyprogesterone acetate [MPA] 30–50 mg or by injection 150 mg 3-monthly, Depo-Provera). If there are no intracavity fibroids, a LNG-IUS has around an 80% success rate.

A novel approach recently described is the use of ulipristal acetate (Esmya®, PreLem SA) administered orally at 5 mg/day for several weeks, thus shrinking the fibroids and enabling the insertion of a LNG-IUS [6].

Gonadotropin-releasing hormone (GnRH) agonists used for 3–6 months can effectively shrink fibroids, but are not a useful long-term option because of the risk of osteoporosis (and in some cases, severe hot flashes), and the fibroids often regrow after stopping the hormone.

Uterine artery embolization (UAE) involves an angiogram performed via the femoral artery. The uterine arteries are identified and then microspheres are injected to embolize the distal branches that supply the fibroids. Most patients will get a very good result but around 20% will still need a surgical option. Systematic reviews have shown that around 3% will develop severe pain and fever (occasionally requiring emergency hysterectomy), 1.5% will expel the fibroid, 1.5% will suffer a uterine infection, and 0.3% will have a groin complication from the angiogram [7].

Removal of the fibroids, or myomectomy, is usually performed where fertility preservation is requested. Our patient may opt for an endometrial ablation which often controls heavy menstrual loss in this setting. Any sub-mucus fibroids should be resected first. Finally, she may opt for a hysterectomy which could be performed abdominally or endoscopically (depending on the size of the uterus). A large uterus can sometimes be shrunk with a 3-month course of GnRH agonist so that a subtotal hysterectomy can be performed endoscopically. The body of the uterus can be morcellated (minced) to facilitate removal through a small port.

Adenomyosis

A minority of patients with adenomyosis have no symptoms. Most will have heavy painful bleeding. Some have continual pelvic pain and some have painful sexual intercourse. Over 90% of cases occur in multiparous women. Tamoxifen appears to be a definite risk factor for this disease. It can reactivate adenomyosis in menopausal women. In one study more than half of women on tamoxifen had evidence of adenomyosis. Also, the majority of women with adenomyosis have other uterine pathologies such as fibroids, polyps or endometrial hyperplasia.

Pain may respond to anti-inflammatories. GnRH agonists, danazol, LNG-IUS and high-dose systemic progestins have all been used to treat adenomyosis with varying success. Superficial disease may respond to endometrial ablation, but if the disease has penetrated deeply into the myometrium, then an ablation can result in severe pelvic pain. The only definitive cure for this problem is hysterectomy which may be performed endoscopically, abdominally or vaginally.

Endometriosis

Since endometriosis can only be definitively diagnosed by laparoscopy it follows that most will also be treated surgically. Lesions can be excised or vaporized using laser or diathermy. Ovarian endometriomas need to have the capsule removed, otherwise the disease will recur. However, there are also many effective medical options. Endometriotic lesions hyperexpress ER, prostaglandins and aromatase, and so treatments that suppress the menstrual cycle, ER and aromatase can be effective. As such, anti-inflammatories often relieve the pain and combined oral contraceptives (COCs), moderate doses of progestins, aromatase inhibitors and GnRH agonists can be useful. Patients who wish to delay child-bearing can have a LNG-IUS fitted at the time of endoscopic surgery.

A minority of patients with endometriosis and other painful pelvic conditions will develop neuralgias, often involving the pudendal nerve or its branches. This type of pain is often described as "burning," "tingling," like "electricity" or "sharp" and can be severe and disabling. Commonly, the pelvic floor becomes involved in this pain syndrome and goes into a state of chronic contraction (pelvic floor myalgia) causing more pain and dyspareunia. The neuralgic component sometimes responds to nerve modulators such as low-dose amitriptyline, gabapentin or pregabalin. Pelvic floor myalgia requires skilled physiotherapy (pelvic floor relaxation and/or dilators) and sometimes responds to Botox (infiltrated into the pelvic floor muscles under an anesthetic).

Ovarian cysts

Small ovarian cysts found on ultrasound (size <5 cm) are followed up with a repeat scan in 2 months or so and many will resolve. If still present, or larger on the repeat scan, then surgery will be required (usually endoscopic). Ovarian cysts with solid features are always viewed as potentially more sinister. However, a corpus luteum often has solid features, and will resolve in 2 months. A high CA-125 level does not inevitably indicate cancer, as it can be raised in the presence of endometriosis. Thus a solid ovarian lesion could be an endometrioma, a dermoid or ovarian cancer. A persistent ovarian cyst with solid features will always need to be removed.

Endometrial hyperplasia

Simple endometrial hyperplasia usually responds to progestins given orally or by the endometrial route using the LNG-IUS. The risk of progression to carcinoma is low (around 2–3%). In contrast, if atypia is present on the biopsy, then the risk of malignant progression is much higher (8–30%). In one systematic review simple hyperplasia responded equally well to oral progestin or the LNG-IUS (89% vs. 96%) [8]. However, the LNG-IUS was superior to oral progestin when the hyperplasia was complex (92% vs. 66%) or when atypia was present (90% vs. 69%). Patient compliance is also higher with the LNG-IUS over oral therapy.

Conclusions

The time leading up to the menopause is commonly associated with a number of sex hormone-responsive gynecologic pathologies. These typically present clinically with pelvic pain and/or AUB. When menopause finally occurs, these conditions such as fibroids, endometriosis and adenomyosis go into remission. Premalignant conditions such as endometrial hyperplasia with/without atypia are common after 40 years of age and usually present with AUB (including postmenopausal bleeding).

In the recent past, most of these pathologies were treated by hysterectomy (and often bilateral removal of tubes and ovaries). With the advent of improved medical options, in particular the LNG-IUS, the hysterectomy rate has fallen from around 30% to 3% now [9]. Radiologic options are now also available for those with symptomatic fibroids. Finally, the rise of endogynecology and operations such as endometrial ablation has now made many gynecologic techniques day (or overnight) procedures.

References

1. Van Voorhis B. A 41-year-old woman with menorrhagia, anemia and fibroids. *JAMA* 2009; **301**: 82–93.

2. Bergeron C, Amant F, Ferenczy A. Pathology and pathophysiology of adenomyosis. *Best Prac Res Clin Obstet Gynaecol* 2006; **20**: 511–21.

3. Bulun SE. Endometriosis. *N Eng J Med* 2009; **360**: 268–79.

4. McCluggage WG. Ovarian borderline tumours: a review with emphasis on controversial areas. *Diag Histopath* 2011; **17**: 178–91.

5. Munro MG, Critchley HOD, Fraser IS. The FIGO classification of causes of abnormal uterine bleeding in the reproductive years. *Fert Ster* 2011; **95**: 2204–8.

6. Briggs P. The management of heavy menstrual bleeding associated with uterine fibroids using Ulipristal acetate, 5 mg daily (Esmya®, Preglem) followed by the introduction of a Levonorgestrel – Intrauterine System (LNG-IUS, Mirena®, Bayer). *Giorn Ital Ostet Ginecol* 2013; **XXXV**: 150–2.

7. Martin J, Bhanot, Athreya S. Complications and reinterventions in uterine artery embolization for symptomatic uterine fibroids: a literature review and meta-analysis. *Cardiovasc Intervent Radiol* 2013; **36**: 395–402.

8. Gallos I, Shehmar M, Thangaratinam S, *et al.* Oral progestogens vs levonorgestrel-releasing intrauterine system for endometrial hyperplasia: a systematic review and meta-analysis. *Am J Obstet Gynecol* 2010; **547**: e1–10.

9. Heliövaara-Peippo S, Hurskainen R, Teperi R, *et al.* Quality of life and costs of levonorgestrel-releasing intrauterine system or hysterectomy in the treatments of menorrhagia: a 10 year randomized controlled trial. *Am J Obstet Gynecol* 2013; **209**: 535e1–e14.

Estrogens used in current menopausal therapies

David Crook

Introduction

Attempts at developing estrogen replacement therapies (expertly reviewed by Diczfalusy and Fraser [1]) can be tracked back to the French physiologist Brown-Sequard's 1890 claim of "revitalizing" benefits with injecting extracts of animal gonads. The search for an orally active estrogen therapy became a reality with Doisy's 1929 isolation of a pure crystalline estrogen – mostly estrone – from the urine of pregnant women. Butenandt in Germany, working towards the same objective, proposed a chemical structure for this molecule and the modern phase of estrogen endocrinology began.

Various estrogen therapies were marketed throughout the 1930s, often based on urine-derived estrone. Recruiting pregnant women and arranging the collection, storage and delivery of their urine was expensive and time-consuming, and so attention turned to animal sources, in particular horses. Pregnant mares produce large amounts of steroid-rich urine and can be kept indoors so that a nappy system could be used to collect the urine. A further advantage was that horses can be repeatedly impregnated, ensuring a reliable long-term source of base material.

The 1930s also saw the announcement from Inhoffen and his group in Germany that they had successfully synthesized ethinyl estradiol. This major development in the pharmacological maintenance of women's health was to some extent overshadowed by Dodds' 1938 synthesis of the potent non-steroidal estrogen diethylstilbestrol (DES). Compared with ethinyl estradiol and other estrogens, DES was inexpensive to synthesize in large amounts and had high biologic activity when administered orally. This promise slowly faded as DES side effects were found to outweigh any benefits on menopausal symptoms. The therapeutic use of DES was discontinued due to the finding of an increased risk of adenocarcinoma of the vagina and cervix in females exposed to the drug *in utero*.

In 1939 the US pharmaceutical company Ayerst (subsequently Wyeth and now Pfizer) revisited the concept of pregnant mares' urine as a source of menopausal therapies. By improving extraction methods they were able to produce a mixture of conjugated equine estrogens (CEE) such as estrone sulfate that seemed to be as potent as DES but with fewer adverse effects. Premarin® (**Pre**gnant **Mar**es Ur**in**e) was introduced in Canada in 1941, in the USA in 1942 and in the UK in 1956.

Magazine and journal articles began to report huge (often anecdotal) successes in treating menopausal women with Premarin®. In 1966 the field exploded with Robert A. Wilson's best-selling (and industry-funded) book *Feminine Forever* [2]. He described

Managing the Menopause: 21st Century Solutions, ed. Nick Panay, Paula Briggs, and Gab Kovacs.
Published by Cambridge University Press. © Cambridge University Press 2015.

the menopause as a "cruel trick" on women, setting them off on a life of "living decay." But help was at hand: a simple course of estrogen therapy could restore youth, health, good looks and marital harmony. The forceful marketing of Premarin® (both to women and to their doctors) was irresistible and this drug was soon to become one of the most prescribed medicines in the USA: one of the first drugs to reach a billion dollars in sales.

In other countries there was continued interest in like-for-like replacement of a woman's own major premenopausal estrogen (17ß-estradiol) and this became the steroid of choice when developing non-oral forms of HRT.

The estrogens currently used in UK-prescribed formulations are listed in Table 15.1. A helpful listing of formulations available in the USA has recently been published [3]. In women with an intact uterus a progestogen must be co-administered, other than in the case of the very low estrogen doses used for vaginal administration. Menopausal therapies involving drugs with estrogen-like activities (selective estrogen receptor modulators; SERMs) and tibolone will be reviewed elsewhere in this book.

Hormone replacement therapy with natural estrogens

Nomenclature is always a problem when referring to steroid hormones – think of the difficulties that came with the use of "generations" when referring to progestogens. The word "natural" is used in this chapter to describe steroids with estrogenic activity that can be found in living organisms (humans, other animals, plants). The route by which a specific steroid is produced is immaterial: a steroid may have been developed from plant (soy or yam) or animal (urine) starter material or synthesized de novo in a laboratory. To the end user (the human cell) the resulting molecules would be indistinguishable.

"Natural" does not necessarily mean "better" or "safer." We are now in a world in which "synthetic" is becoming synonymous with "dangerous," but much modern health care has benefitted from the development of "synthetic" drugs. Conversely, both arsenic and cobra venom qualify as "natural."

The Women's Health Initiative (WHI) taught us that there is no substitute for carefully planned, long-term randomized controlled trials looking at real-world endpoints (and not biomarkers). Of course there may be individual patient/prescriber preferences – ethical concerns relating to animal welfare, price, evidence base – but the branding of some formulations as "more natural" is a poor substitute for an evidence base.

Natural estrogens native to humans

The classic trio of human estrogens is formed of 17ß-estradiol (coded E2), estrone (E1), estriol (E3). The "E" shorthand refers to the number of hydroxyl groups on the molecule (Figure 15.1). In the gynecologic field, claims are being made for the potential thera-peutic benefits of estetrol (E4), a weak estrogen produced solely by the fetal liver during pregnancy [4].

Estradiol is the most potent human estrogen, with estrone about half as active and estetrol and estriol having much less activity than estrone. For HRT, both estradiol and estrone need their 17-OH group to be in the ß orientation: α-oriented isomers have little biologic activity. Some interconversions are possible, for example estradiol can be reversibly oxidized to estrone. When excreted into urine these steroids have mostly been conjugated during hepatic processing – for example, by addition of a hydrophilic side chain such as a

Table 15.1. Estrogens currently used in UK-prescribed formulations.

HRT estrogen component and route of administration	HRT estrogen dose (mg/day)	Brands
ORAL HRT		
Estrogen monotherapy		
17ß-estradiol	1.0–2.0	1.0 mg: **Elleste-Solo 1 mg**® (Meda) 2.0 mg: **Bedol**® (ReSource Medical), **Elleste-Solo 2 mg**® (Meda), **Zumenon**® (Abbott Healthcare)
Estradiol valerate	1.0	**Climaval**® (Novartis), **Progynova**® (Bayer)
Conjugated equine estrogens	0.3	**Premarin**® (Pfizer)
Estradiol, estrone, estriol mix	0.6 (E2), 1.4 (E1), 0.27 (E3)	**Hormonin**® (AMCo)
Combined therapy		
17ß-estradiol	0.5–2.0	0.5 mg: **Femoston-conti**® **0.5 mg/2.5 mg** (Abbott Healthcare) 1.0 mg: **Femoston-conti**® **1 mg/5 mg** and **Femoston**® **1 mg/10 mg** (both Abbott Healthcare), **Angeliq**® (Bayer), **Elleste-Duet** ®**1 mg** (Meda), **Kliovance**® and **Novofem**® (both Novo Nordisk) 2.0 mg: **Clinorette**® (ReSource Medical), **Elleste-Duet**® **2 mg** (Meda), **Femoston**® **2 mg/10 mg** (Abbott Healthcare), **Nuvelle**® **continuous** (Bayer), **Kliofem**® and **Trisquens**® (both Novo Nordisk)
Estradiol valerate	1.0–2.0	1.0 mg: **Climagest**® **1 mg** (Novartis), **Indivina**® **1 mg/2.5 mg** and **1 mg/5 mg** (both Orion) 2.0 mg: **Climagest**® **2 mg** or **Climesse**® (both Novartis), **Cyclo-Progynova**® (Meda), **Indivina**® **2 mg/5 mg** and **Tridestra**® (both Orion)
Conjugated equine estrogens	0.3–1.25	0.3 mg: **Premique**® **Low Dose** (Pfizer) 0.625 mg: **Premique**® and **Prempak C**® **0.625** (both Pfizer) 1.25 mg: **Prempak C**® **1.25** (Pfizer)
NON-ORAL HRT (17ß-estradiol in all cases)		
Estrogen monotherapy		
Transdermal patches	0.025–0.100	0.025 mg: **Estraderm MX 25**® and **Estradot 25**® (both Novartis), **Evorel 25**® (Janssen) 0.040 mg: **Elleste-Solo MX**® (Meda) 0.050 mg: **Estraderm MX 50**® and **Estradot 50**® (both Novartis), **Evorel 50**® (Janssen), **FemSeven 50**® (Merck Serono), **Progynova TS 50**® (Bayer)

Table 15.1. (*cont.*)

HRT estrogen component and route of administration	HRT estrogen dose (mg/day)	Brands
		0.075 mg: **Estraderm MX 75**® and **Estradot 75**® (both Novartis), **Evorel 75**® (Janssen), **FemSeven 75**® (Merck Serono)
		0.100 mg: **Estraderm MX 100**® and **Estradot 100**® (both Novartis), **Evorel 100**® (Janssen), **FemSeven 100**® (Merck Serono), **Progynova TS 100**® (Bayer)
Estradiol gel	variable	**Oestrogel**® (Besins), **Sandrena**® (Orion)
Vaginal ring	0.0075	**Estring**® (Pharmacia)
Combined therapy		
Transdermal patches	0.050	**Evorel Conti**® and **Evorel Sequi**® (both Janssen), **FemSeven Conti**® and **FemSeven Sequi**® (both Merck Serono)

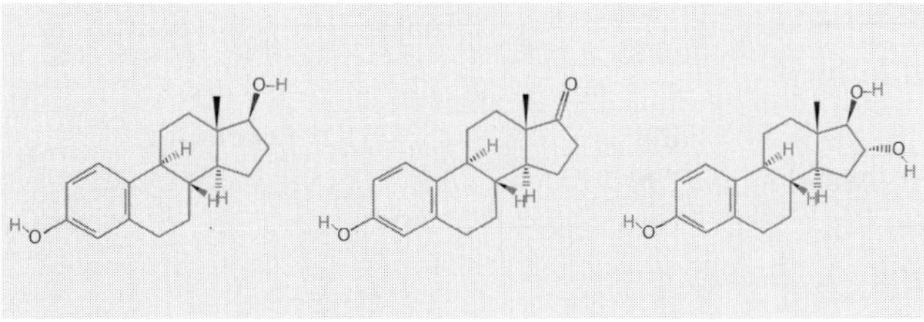

Estradiol (E2)   Estrone (E1)   Estriol (E3)

Figure 15.1. Structure of the three classic human estrogens. (*Source*: http://pubchem.ncbi.nlm.nih.gov/.)

sulfate or a glucaronide moiety. Some conjugated estrogens are biologically inactive but they also can reconvert (or be persuaded by a chemist to reconvert) back to the initial hormone. The clinical relevance of such conversions is not clearly understood.

For purposes of HRT, 17ß-estradiol is typically used at doses of 1.0–2.0 mg/day when administered orally and 50 µg/day when administered through transdermal patches. The esterified form, estradiol valerate, is also popular, quickly being converted to the estradiol valerate on oral administration and so given in similar doses. Such esterification is a pharmacologist's trick to ensure good activity following oral administration. Estradiol gels and implants have also been used for relief of menopausal symptoms. Where the concern is vaginal symptoms, a ring has been developed that delivers an even smaller dose. Estradiol pessaries, creams and tablets are also available for vaginal administration.

The major development in estrogen-based HRT over the last few decades has been the refinement of transdermal delivery systems (patches) that are replaced once or twice a week. The rationale for this delivery system has been in part a concern that some of the health hazards emerging from epidemiologic studies of HRT users, such as venous thromboembolism, were due to the initial impact of orally administered estrogens on the liver, resulting in increased protein synthesis of elements of the coagulation and fibrinolysis system. There was also an interest in demedicalizing the menopause by avoiding the ritual of pill-taking.

It can be argued, based largely on research into biomarkers, that some of the adverse health consequences of estrogen-based HRT will be avoided if the oral route is bypassed, but the RCT evidence so far is unconvincing.

Natural estrogens derived from horses

The most commonly used HRT estrogen worldwide is Premarin®, a complex mixture of CEE and other substances, extracted from the urine of pregnant horses. The precise composition of Premarin® continues to be the subject of considerable recent controversy, initiated by the desire of some pharmaceutical companies to market either (a) a generic version of this venerable medicine or (b) a simplified version, perhaps focusing on those components thought likely to improve menopausal symptoms, omitting the other components. All such applications to regulators have been and continue to be vigorously opposed by the manufacturer of Premarin®. The basis of this opposition has been that the new formulations lack (or contain suboptimal concentrations of) a key component of Premarin®, and so could not be expected to have the same protective effect on, for example, bone fracture. This claim led to the Food and Drugs Administration in the USA pointing out that Premarin® itself has not been appropriately characterized [5]. There is now an impasse in that pharmaceutical companies wishing to compete for the immense market share enjoyed by Premarin® cannot apply to the FDA for approval until the current manufacturers have completed their characterization and had this information accepted by the FDA. This is likely to be a slow process.

Traditionally, Premarin® has been considered to have 10 major estrogenic components, mostly present in their sulfated form:

- estrone
- estradiol (both 17ß and 17α forms)
- equilin
- dihydroequilin (both 17ß and 17α forms)
- equilenin
- dihydroequilenin (both 17ß and 17α forms)
- delta(8)-estrone.

In contrast, one review [6] suggests that Premarin® contains at least 230 compounds, including previously unidentified estrogens, progestogens and androgens. These complex issues have recently been reviewed in detail [7].

Premarin® is almost exclusively used as an oral therapy, although a vaginal gel is available in some countries. The original doses of 2.5 mg/day or higher have been replaced by lower doses (0.3–1.25 mg/day) in response to concerns over adverse effects. The extent to which the benefits seen in the earlier pivotal studies with 2.5 mg/day or higher doses will be seen with these lower doses is not known.

Natural estrogens derived from plants

Plants such as yams and soya represent a rich source of precursor molecules that can be chemically converted into estradiol and other hormones. However, these plants contain other molecules with estrogenic activities (phytoestrogens) that have led to them being promoted as "natural" HRT, implying that they are "safer" than conventional menopausal therapies. To make matters worse, these compounds are often promoted as nutritional supplements, an easier ride in terms of marketing.

Some phytoestrogens are being appropriately researched [8]. The evidence that iso-flavones, lignans and coumestans can reduce the intensity (and in some cases the frequency) of hot flashes is increasingly plausible, although such benefits do not appear as strong as with conventional estrogen-based HRT. There is some evidence for benefits in term of bone density, as well as some other menopausal symptoms. These claims for efficacy need to be balanced by data on safety, and that will require long-duration comparative trials with real-life clinical endpoints.

The "bioidentical" estrogen story

The WHI Study team concluded that the expected benefits in terms of osteoporotic fracture and colorectal cancer were outweighed by higher than expected risks of stroke and breast cancer in some treatment arms, plus disturbing data on an increased risk of dementia. There was an inevitable move from some HRT specialists to distance their practice by challenging the use of CEE or CEE/MPA as used in the WHI. This has ended up as strong media promotion of (a) "safer" forms of HRT and (b) recommendations for personalized prescribing of HRT.

Members of the "bioidentical" cult argue that plant-derived estradiol, estrone and estriol can be used as an effective but also safer form of HRT, with much distance being placed between these components and the "drugs" used in conventional HRT. The basic proposition is that a precise blend of these steroids can be tailored by compounding pharmacies to rectify an individual woman's perceived endocrine deficiencies on the basis of a saliva or blood test. The concept has been celebrity-endorsed and massively promoted direct to the USA public, even though the evidence for either the saliva/blood testing or the subsequent titration strategy is weak [9]. The 2013 International Menopause Society Guidelines counsel against this approach [10].

Visiting some of these "bioidentical" websites fills one with a most peculiar feeling of *déjà vu*, with unconditional guarantees of a return to a lean body, shining hair, thick skin etc. that are eerily reminiscent of Wilson's early claims for the "marriage-saving" miracle of Premarin® [2].

References

1. Diczfalusy E, Fraser I. The discovery of reproduction steroid hormone and recognition of their physiological roles. In Fraser I, Jansen R, Lobo R, Whitehead M, (eds). *Estrogens and Progestogens in Clinical Practice*. London: Churchill Livingstone; 1998: 3–11.

2. Wilson RA. *Feminine Forever*. New York, NY: M Evans and Company; 1966.

3. Sood S, Faubion SS, Kuhle CL, Thielen JM, Shuster LT. Prescribing menopausal hormone therapy: an evidence-based approach. *Int J Women's Health* 2014: **6**: 47–57.

4. Coelingh Bennink HJ, Holinka CF, Diczfalusy E. Estetrol review: profile and potential clinical applications. *Climacteric* 2008; **11 Suppl 1**: 47–58.

5. http://www.fda.gov/drugs/drugsafety/informationbydrugclass/ucm168836.htm (accessed August 1, 20/14).

6. Stanczyk FZ. Estrogens used for replacement therapy in postmenopausal women. *Gynecol Endocrinol* 2001; **15 Suppl 4**: 17–25.

7. Bhavnani BR, Stanczyk FZ. Pharmacology of conjugated equine estrogens: efficacy, safety and mechanism of action. *J Steroid Biochem Mol Biol* 2014; **142**: 16–29.

8. Bedell S, Nachtigall M, Naftolin F. The pros and cons of plant estrogens for menopause. *J Steroid Biochem Mol Biol* 2014; **139**: 225–36.

9. Huntley AL. Compounded or confused? Bioidentical hormones and menopausal health. *Menopause Int* 2011; **17**: 16–18.

10. de Villiers TJ, Gas MLS, Haines CJ, *et al.* Global Consensus Statement on menopausal hormone therapy. *Climacteric* 2013; **16**: 203–4.

Progestogens used in hormone replacement therapy

David H. Barlow

Introduction

Progestins are a fundamental component of HRT and it is important that the actions and effects of progestins are well understood by practitioners. I would argue that, as a group of molecules, the diversity of progestins and their activities is more complex than for estrogens and therefore the mechanism of progestin interactions at the cellular level is given prominence below. In HRT we use progestin for its endometrial effect but it is inevitable that the other progestin effects come into play and some of these properties may be undesirable. With a reasonable understanding of progestin action it is possible to better decide on which progestin to favor and in which circumstances.

Terminology

Recently the North American Menopause Society has provided a recommended approach to progestogen terminology which will be used in this chapter. In the NAMS terminology "progestogen" covers all molecules with significant activity at the progesterone receptor. This is consistent with the terminology for the other sex steroids, androgens and estrogens. This group of molecules includes the major endogenous progestogen, progesterone, and the diverse group of synthetic progestogens for which the term "progestin" is recommended.

Mechanism of progestogen action – the progesterone receptor and other steroid hormone receptors

The progestins are a diverse range of synthetic molecules which have sufficient structural similarity with progesterone that they have good affinity for the progesterone receptor (PR) and thus activate progesterone-receptor regulated genes. However it needs to be recognized that, like progesterone itself, the progestins may have affinity and agonist or antagonist activity at a variety of other steroid hormone receptors.

The steroid hormone receptors are members of the large superfamily of nuclear receptors. These function as transcription factors which can interact with appropriate hormone ligands to activate appropriate genes, and this is modulated by intracellular co-activators and co-repressors that will be tissue specific. Within this superfamily is a subfamily of steroid hormone receptors which have sufficient structural and functional coherence that many steroid-like molecules will have significant affinity for several of these

Managing the Menopause: 21st Century Solutions, ed. Nick Panay, Paula Briggs, and Gab Kovacs.
Published by Cambridge University Press. © Cambridge University Press 2015.

receptors. This subfamily includes the estrogen receptor and the ketosteroid receptors – the androgen (AR), progesterone (PR), glucocorticoid (GR) and mineralocorticoid (MR) receptors. Common features of these receptors are four functional domains. There is an N-terminal variable domain, a DNA binding domain, a hinge region and a C-terminal ligand binding domain. The variable domain and the ligand binding domain have segments that can bind activation and inhibitory factors that will modulate the activation of gene transcription. The key binding of the appropriately activated ligand-receptor dimer complex to the hormone response element of the DNA makes possible the transcription of the hormone-regulated genes. Depending on the ligand, the balance of co-activators and co-repressors in the receptor complex, the binding to the hormone response element might, or might not, result in expression of the hormone-regulated genes. In this way a hormone ligand may act as a full or partial agonist or an antagonist.

In the case of the PR, the progestins function as agonists. However there are now selective progesterone receptor modulators (SPRM) available and when these function as ligands at the PR, they express a mixture of tissue-specific agonist or antagonist activity that provides a new range of therapeutic options. These molecules have applications in benign gynecology, particularly fibroid shrinkage and emergency contraception. This family of molecules includes mifepristone, ulipristal and asoprisnil. Their actions include inhibition of ovulation and a direct endometrial effect with rapid induction of amenorrhea without arrest of ovarian follicular activity.

There are two PR isoforms, PRA and PRB. The PRB isoform has an additional N-terminal region that confers further binding activity. The two isoforms differ in their tissue distribution. PRA and PRB generally influence different groups of genes and in some situations their activities are in opposition. For example, in human choriocarcinoma cells the expression of the GnRH receptor gene is downregulated by PRA and upregulated by PRB.

Any understanding of the actions of progesterone and the progestins needs to encompass the likely actions of these molecules at multiple steroid hormone receptors, and the spectrum of this activity will vary between molecules. As a starting point in understanding this we need to realize that even progesterone itself does not act only at the progesterone receptor. It has significant agonist at the glucocorticoid receptor and it is a significant antagonist at the mineralocorticoid receptor. The activity of different progestins at the different steroid hormone receptors will be influenced by their parent origin. Principally there are progestins related to progesterone (17-hydroxy progesterone derivatives or 19-norprogesterone derivatives) and those related to testosterone (the 19-nortestosterone derivatives). Table 16.1 provides a useful overview of the different progestin groupings and shows the diverse activity of progesterone and the progestins at the different steroid hormone receptors. It indicates the similarity of activity of progestins in the same grouping [1].

Overall the range of progestin-specific variables that determine the clinical effects of progestins in different tissues will include: (i) differential absorption on oral administration; (ii) differential levels of protein binding and bioavailability; (iii) differential tissue distribution of the isoforms of the progesterone receptor and the other steroid hormone receptors; (iv) differential levels of binding to the range of isoforms of the steroid hormone receptors (PR, AR, MR, GR); (v) the potential for the activity at the AR, MR or GR to be partial agonist or partial antagonist depending on the circumstances.

The different progestin binding profiles introduce the possibility of tailoring the progestin to the woman's experience of side effects and her potential tolerance of these [2].

Table 16.1. Biological activities of natural progesterone and synthetic progestogens. Reproduced from Schindler *et al.* 2003 [1] with permission.

Progestin	Progesto-genic	Anti-gonado-tropic	Anti-estrogenic	Estro-genic	Andro-genic	Anti-andro-genic	Gluco-corticoid	Anti-mineralo-corticoid
Progesterone	+	+	+	–	–	±	+	+
Dydrogesterone	+	–	+	–	–	±	–	±
Medrogestone	+	+	+	–	–	±	–	–
17α-Hydroxy-derivatives								
Chlormadinone acetate	+	+	+	–	–	+	+	–
Cyproterone acetate	+	+	+	–	–	+	+	–
Megestrol acetate	+	+	+	–	±	+	+	–
Medroxyprogesterone acetate	+	+	+	–	±	–	+	–
19-Norprogesterone-derivatives								
Nomegestrol acetate	+	+	+	–	–	±	–	–
Promegestone	+	+	+	–	–	–	–	–
Trimegestone	+	+	+	–	–	±	–	±
Spirolactone-derivatives								
Drospirenone	+	+	+	–	–	+	–	+
19-Nortestosterone-derivatives								
Norethisterone	+	+	+	+	+	–	–	–
Lynestrenol	+	+	+	+	+	–	–	–
Norethinodrel	±	+	±	+	±	–	–	–
Levonorgestrel	+	+	+	–	+	–	–	–
Norgestimate	+	+	+	–	+	–	–	–
3-Keto-desogestrel	+	+	+	–	+	–	–	–
Gestoden	+	+	+	–	+	–	+	+
Dienogest	+	+	±	±	–	+	–	–

(+) effective; (±) weakly effective; (–) not effective.

Metabolic impact of progestogens

The metabolic impact of progestins will be significantly mediated via the extent of activation of the AR, GR and MR. These activities will drive the potential side effects. Androgenic activity will stimulate adverse metabolic lipid changes and androgenic symptoms such as acne; mineralocorticoid activity will affect water retention and weight; glucocorticoid activity will affect salt and water retention. The metabolic profile might influence progestin choice generally but it will be especially important when prescribing HRT to women who are already metabolically compromised, for instance in diabetes, since it is possible to select a progestin which does not appear to affect insulin sensitivity.

The metabolic impact of estrogen/progestin therapy varies and with respect to cardiovascular health, the choice of progestin will influence factors that may have an adverse influence by the effect on insulin resistance, glucose tolerance and the lipoprotein profile. The effect is more likely to be adverse for cardiovascular health if androgenic progestins are used. The most neutral effect is reported with progesterone or dydrogesterone, however even with the generally favorable lipid profile impact of dydrogesterone there is a negative feature, the rise in triglycerides. The complex topic of the metabolic impact of progestins and their effects on cardiovascular health are well reviewed by Rosano et al. [3].

Progestin action in the endometrium

Progestins are a fundamental component of HRT because of their action on the endometrium. Once an endometrium has been estrogen-primed there is induction of progesterone receptors. The endometrium will be proliferating and addition of progestogen induces secretory differentiation. Subsequent withdrawal of the hormone will usually result in endometrial shedding and menstruation. The other effect of the progestogen is the induction of an atrophic endometrial state. This is most likely with sustained progestin administration as in continuous combined HRT regimens.

There is strong evidence that unopposed estrogen HRT is associated with an increased risk of endometrial cancer whereas with combined estrogen and progestin HRT this is rare. With sequential regimens the risk is minimal but detected in observational studies after around 5 years of sequential HRT use. With continuous combined regimens the risk of endometrial cancer appears to be lower than in the background population. If an endometrium is exposed to a sustained estrogenic proliferative stimulus it is a physiological response for reversible simple hyperplasia to develop in many cases. It is with the progression to complex, and particularly, atypical hyperplasia that the reversibility becomes less sure and the risk of progression to cancer more of a concern. The risk of simple, complex and complex atypical hyperplasia progressing to endometrial cancer has been estimated to be 1%, 3% and 29% respectively. These changes may be reversed by the use of progestin, with the chance of persistence or progression of complex or atypical hyperplasia despite progestin treatment, being approximately 25–30%. Generally progestins rather than progesterone have been favored for this role in HRT because they have been developed to have more focused endometrial potency. Figure 16.1 illustrates the spectrum of endometrial histology most likely to be encountered with HRT, namely unopposed estrogen effect (Figure 16.1–A); simple hyperplasia (Figure 16.1–B); secretory transformation on sequential progestin (Figure 16.1–C); and atrophic change on continuous progestin (Figure 16.1–D). The topic has been reviewed by the Cochrane Collaboration [4].

A   B

C   D

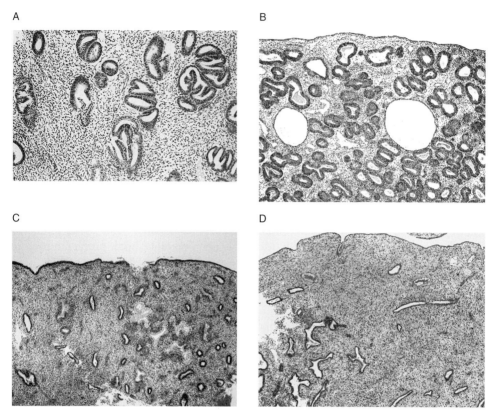

Figure 16.1. Endometrial histology with and without progestin in HRT. Images reproduced with the permission of Professor ARE Williams, University of Edinburgh. (a) Unopposed estrogen effect – disordered proliferative endometrial pattern. The endometrial glands have an irregular architectural pattern, but are distributed evenly throughout the stroma, without significant crowding, and with no increase from normal in the gland–stroma ratio. (b) Simple non-atypical endometrial hyperplasia. The endometrial glands mostly have a simple tubular architecture, some showing cystic dilatation. The epithelium is active in appearance, composed of tall columnar cells in which mitotic activity is present (not seen at this magnification). There is an increase in gland–stroma ratio. (c) Secretory differentiation in HRT effect. Glands are widely dispersed amongst endometrial stroma showing confluent decidual change. The glandular epithelium is mostly inactive, but some glands show obvious secretory differentiation with vacuolation of cytoplasm and a tortuous architecture, reminiscent of the mid-secretory phase. There is a decrease in the gland–stroma ratio. (d) Atrophic changes of continuous combined HRT. Glands show a flattened inactive appearance, and are widely dispersed in stroma showing confluent decidual change.

Estrogen/progestin regimes in HRT

The first estrogen/progestin regimens to be developed were sequential and today these are usually designed to provide 28-day cycles involving continuous estrogen and with progestin added for 12–14 days. On such regimens most women bleed for a few days from near the end of the progestin phase, but in any one cycle some women will not bleed and a small proportion of women are consistently free of bleeding. The absence of bleeding is not thought to indicate failure of endometrial protection. Such regimens are suitable for women both in the perimenopause requiring HRT and in the established menopause. The more recently introduced continuous combined estrogen/progestin regimens aim at achieving freedom from bleeding for a majority of women. On the standard regimens of this form

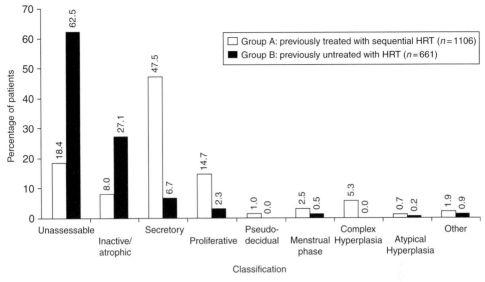

Histological results of endometrical biopsies before starting Kliofem.

Figure 16.2. Endometrial histology in women treated with sequential estrogen/progestin HRT and untreated women. Reproduced from Sturdee *et al.* 2000 [5] with permission.

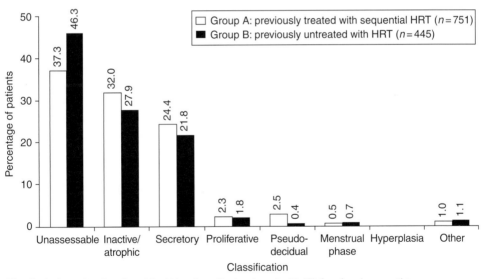

Histological results of endometrical biopsies after treatment with Kliofem for nine months.

Figure 16.3. Endometrial histology in women treated with continuous combined estrogen/progestin HRT in women previously untreated or previously treated with a sequential HRT regimen. Reproduced from Sturdee *et al.* 2000 [5] with permission.

around 80% of women become bleed-free, though a proportion will experience irregular bleeding, especially in the initial months. These regimens are not suitable before the menopause is established. It is expected that a majority of women on continuous combined regimens will have atrophic endometrium. Figures 16.2 and 16.3 illustrate the diversity of endometrial histology seen in untreated women and women using a wide range of sequential HRT preparations, all biopsied before starting on a continuous combined HRT preparation, Kliofem (Figure 16.2), or biopsied after 9 months' Kliofem (Figure 16.3) [5]. In this study the endometrial biopsies labeled as unassessable were taken to be additional cases of inactive/atrophic endometrium. The study illustrates the diversity of endometrial histology in postmenopausal women whether using HRT or not. The most consistent pattern appears to be in women using continuous combined HRT which may correlate with the evidence that this form of HRT appears to reduce endometrial cancer risk below the background rate.

Mammographic breast density

In untreated women increased breast density is important, both because increased density on mammography may mask small lesions and because there is a suggested association between increased breast density and breast cancer risk. It is known that estrogen/progestin HRT regimens increase breast density. It is not proved that this necessarily raises breast cancer risk but it may increase the difficulty in detecting lesions. Studies that compare sequential and continuous combined regimens suggest that the increase in breast density is more marked with continuous combined regimens. Currently the issue of mammographic breast density is attracting considerable attention in the USA where several states have introduced legislation concerning the responsibility of doctors to communicate information about increased breast density to women. A Swedish study of mammographic breast density reported that compared with untreated women, the risk ratio for increased density in sequential estrogen/progestin HRT was 3.6 (95% Cl 1.6–7.7) whereas with continuous combined HRT the risk ratio was 12.4 (95% CI 6.3–24.4). The rates were even higher if only women over 50 years were considered [6]. In the light of this it is of interest that the European Prospective Investigation into Cancer and Nutrition reported that overall the risk ratio for higher risk with continuous combined HRT compared with sequential HRT was 1.43 (95% CI 1.19–1.72). In their analysis, country by country, they observed the point estimate for breast cancer risk to be higher in association with continuous combined HRT regimens than with sequential HRT regimens in Denmark, France, Germany and Norway whereas the reverse was found for British women [7].

Progestins and safety – estimating the influence of progestins in HRT from trials

Progestogens have been accepted as an essential safety component of any HRT regimen where there has not been a hysterectomy. By including a progestogen in HRT the regimens facilitate more predictable scheduling of monthly bleeding, or even the possibility of freedom from bleeding for many women if the progestogen is given continuously. Unfortunately the additional actions of progestogens beyond the specific endometrial target introduces the potential for effects that might affect risk in the long term. This potential contribution to any long-term risk associated with HRT is ideally explored in appropriate clinical trials [8, 9].

In the past 20 years there has been a growing emphasis on the difficult task of studying the effects of HRT in large randomized controlled trials. The results of the small number of these major trials that have been carried out will be addressed elsewhere in this book (cancer in Chapter 22, and venous thromboembolism in Chapter 23) but an aspect directly relevant to this chapter is where these trials provide insight into the contribution of progestin in HRT. This was highlighted, in particular, by the reports from the Women's Health Initiative (WHI) trials in American women where some adverse outcomes appeared more common if a progestin was included in the HRT. It is important that the effects of adding progestin to HRT are discussed here but it must be emphasized that although there is discussion about its possible negative impact, there is no strong voice proposing that women who have a uterus would do better using HRT without progestogen. However there has undoubtedly been a trend towards exploring lower-dose estrogen and progestin HRT preparations with a view to maximizing safety.

It is a reflection of the predominance of continuous combined regimens after the menopause that the landmark WHI trial opted for a continuous combined estrogen/progestin regimen (conjugated equine estrogens + medroxyprogesterone acetate) for women who required uterine protection. These trials will have been described elsewhere in this book but here it is necessary to emphasize that the key difference between the two trials was that the larger trial compared this estrogen/progestin HRT regimen against placebo whereas the other WHI trial in women who had hysterectomy compared estrogen-only HRT (conjugated equine estrogens) against placebo. In this chapter the two trials are referred to as the E+P trial and the E-only trial respectively. Comparison of the women in the two trials revealed that the hysterectomy E-only trial population was "more racially diverse, had less favorable cardiovascular risk profiles and more commonly had oophorectomy and prior hormone use" [8].

There has been considerable interest in the differences in outcomes between these two WHI trials, and the specific therapeutic difference is involvement of progestin in the E+P study. Now more than 10 years later we have the major WHI publication that provides a "comprehensive integrated overview of findings from the two Women's Health Initiative hormone therapy trials with extended post-intervention follow-up" [8]. In focusing on this it is important to express some caveats. Firstly that a single progestin, medroxyprogesterone acetate, was used in these trials and that we do not have this weight of evidence concerning other progestins. Secondly it is important to note that because the intention of WHI was to look at health outcomes in HRT use in older women it is not straightforward to transpose the outcomes of a 50–79-year-old population to the majority of likely users of HRT who are largely under 60 years of age. On the other hand, though with less statistical power than the global studies, WHI has provided the outcomes for the 50–59-year-old subgroup. In addition to that major randomized controlled trial we now also have the data from the Danish Osteoporosis Study which focused on women below 60 years of age and which provided extended treatment and follow-up data on women randomized to use a sequential estradiol/norethisterone regimen or placebo [9].

The Women's Health Initiative trial

The 16,608-woman estrogen/progestin trial (E+P) was discontinued in 2002 at a median treatment duration of 5.6 years and the 10,739-woman estrogen-only trial (E-only) was discontinued in 2004 at a median treatment duration of 7.2 years. Extended follow-up was until 2010, which provided a median post-intervention follow-up for the two trials of 8.2 years and 6.6 years respectively. The outcomes were presented as events per 10,000 patient-years (PY) and the hazard ratio (HR) provided for the period of active treatment and for the composite of active treatment and post-treatment follow-up [8]. For many outcomes the difference between active and placebo therapy did not achieve statistical significance and these cannot be claimed to be true differences. For the purpose of exploring the long-term effect of progestin in HRT, the interest is in where the findings of the two trials differed.

The primary endpoints of the trial were coronary heart disease and invasive breast cancer. For both endpoints the active treatment phase outcomes and the outcomes which included cumulative follow-up gave similar results. For coronary heart disease, the E+P trial absolute difference in events was six additional cases per 10,000 PY on E+P than on placebo and in the E-only trial the equivalent was three fewer cases per 10,000 PY on E compared with placebo. The respective hazard ratios were 1.18 (CI 0.95–1.45) and 0.94 (CI 0.78–1.14) and in neither case was the difference significant. For invasive breast cancer, in the E+P trial there were nine additional cases per 10,000 PY on E+P (HR 1.24, CI 1.01–1.53) and in the E-only trial there were seven fewer cases on E (HR 0.79, CI 0.61–1.02) compared with placebo. These differences were numerically the same when cumulative follow-up was considered and the respective HRs were E+P (1.28, CI 1.11–1.48) and E-only (0.79, CI 0.65–0.97). Thus for invasive breast cancer an increase in risk was statistically significant in the active phase E+P trial and also when cumulated with follow-up data. In contrast in the E-only trial there was a trend to a reduction in risk in E users which failed to reach statistical significance in the active treatment phase but when cumulated with follow-up data was a significant reduction in invasive breast cancer risk.

For the primary outcomes of the trials we can conclude that neither estrogen/progestin HRT nor estrogen-only HRT affected the risk of coronary heart disease in the populations studied. We can conclude that a 24% increase in risk of invasive breast cancer was demonstrated in users of E+P in contrast to a 21% reduction in risk in E users which only became significant when the full cumulative follow-up data were included. In the two studies the placebo group rate of invasive breast cancer was 34 per 10,000 PY, so it is certainly tempting to conclude that the adverse difference in the risk of invasive breast cancer relates to the addition of the progestin.

For the three other major cardiovascular outcomes, i.e. stroke, pulmonary embolism and deep venous thrombosis, there was no major difference between the pattern seen in the E+P and E-only trials. Thus for these cardiovascular outcomes the progestin did not appear to play a significant role, though for pulmonary embolism and deep venous thrombosis the HRs were numerically higher in the E+P group in both cases.

The other cancer outcomes that are reported do not suggest a difference related to progestin, and for "all cancer types" and "cancer deaths" there was no difference between the active study arms, whether E+P or E-only, and placebo. Obviously there are two cancers where a comparison is not relevant. There can be no risk of endometrial cancer in the hysterectomy E-only trial and since many women in that category will have had oophorectomy, the E-only trial did not report on ovarian cancer. For the E+P trial the ovarian cancer HR point estimate of 1.41 was not a significant increase in risk (CI 0.75–2.66).

Since the progestin is specifically included in the HRT regimen for prevention of endometrial cancer, it is reassuring that the use of continuous combined E+P was associated with a non-significant reduction in the point estimate for endometrial cancer risk (HR 0.83, CI 0.49–1.40) and a significant reduction in the risk on the cumulative follow-up data (HR 0.67, CI 0.49–0.91).

The one cancer which showed, if anything, better performance in women receiving E+P was colorectal cancer. In the E+P trial there was a significant reduction in colorectal cancer risk on E+P (HR 0.62, CI 0.43–0.89) which was not seen in the E-only trial (HR 1.15, CI 0.81–1.64).

The expected positive outcome in HRT users was fracture reduction. This was expressed in terms of "all fractures", "hip fracture" and "vertebral fracture." For each fracture category a significant, approximately 30% reduction in fractures was achieved in the active treatment arm of both trials. The results show very similar fracture reductions whether or not the HRT included progestin.

Most women who use HRT for menopausal symptom relief are younger than 60 years so the most relevant subgroup of WHI is the 50–59-year-old subgroup. The trial was not powered to provide potentially statistically significant results in subsets so it is not surprising that very few statistically significant differences were reported for this interesting subgroup. However it is important that we do not assume that differences that fail to reach statistical significance are definitely not real differences.

For women under 60 years of age in the E+P trial, the only major outcome that significantly differed in the active treatment group compared with placebo, and only when in the cumulative data incorporating the follow-up, is invasive breast cancer (HR 1.34, CI 1.03–1.75). For the E-only trial, again it was only with incorporation of the follow-up data that some major outcomes for the active treatment group differed significantly from the placebo group. These were coronary heart disease (HR 0.65, CI 0.44–0.96), total myocardial infarction (HR 0.60, CI 0.39–0.91) and all cancer types (HR 0.80, CI 0.64–0.99). For each of these three significant positive results in favor of the E-only group there was no significant difference on the E+P trial, but in each disease the E+P point estimate was in the opposite direction from the E-only trial. What we learn from the presentation of the 50–59-year-old, subset data is that the absolute level of risk for most of the major disease outcomes studied is relatively low and that the differences in the absolute event rates are low.

In conclusion, even though it is not possible to make statistical calculations to compare the two active treatment groups, the results of the two trials suggest that the inclusion of progestin in HRT mostly does not affect the major outcomes studied in the WHI trials. What was demonstrated was an increase in the risk of invasive breast cancer only seen with E+P HRT. With respect to deep venous thrombosis risk and pulmonary embolism risk these were both significantly elevated with E+P and the extent of risk was possibly greater than in the E-only trial. On the positive side, the reduction in risk of colorectal cancer was only seen in the E+P trial and the reduction in risk of endometrial cancer, only able to be tested in the E+P trial, did show a reduction in risk associated with progestogen use.

The Danish Osteoporosis Study

This placebo-controlled randomized trial of HRT involved 1,006 recently menopausal women (45–58 years) of whom 192 had undergone hysterectomy. The hysterectomy subgroup received 2 mg estradiol valerate or placebo and the other women received a sequential preparation involving estradiol valerate and norethisterone. The HRT regime and the hormone preparations were thus distinct from the WHI regimen and preparations. Only 2% of the women had previously used HRT. It is noteworthy that across the major outcomes reported, the hazard ratio point estimates for active treatment were always lower than unity, except for deep venous thrombosis, indicating no other signal that the HRT was raising risk. The hysterectomy subgroup was too small for adequate power to explore the progestin contribution in any detail, but information is provided for some major outcomes on the event rates in those with and without hysterectomy, and for both overall mortality and the major coronary heart disease endpoint, the hysterectomy group showed hazard ratio point estimates lower than the non-hysterectomy group. On the other hand, for breast cancer the point estimates for both subgroups were below unity but similar. Thus there was no suggestion of the differential of performance seen in WHI for this outcome.

Lower doses and non-oral routes of administration

The response to the WHI trials and the emphasis on safety in HRT use is the development of lower-dose HRT regimens, particularly where progestin is also involved. Another trend is the interest in exploring non-oral approaches to the delivery of progesterone or progestins. The lower oral dose regimens have seen significant reductions in both estrogen and progestin dosage. With these regimens it is very likely that combined oral regimens will remain a prominent approach to HRT.

As alternatives, the transdermal options are probably the best explored, with transdermal matrix patches and skin gel having the longest track record. These have the advantage of avoiding first-pass liver metabolism and although the progestins used in the matrix patches are androgenic, norethisterone (140 μg/day) or levonorgestrel (10 μg/day), the metabolic impact is felt to be minimized. The other approach that is explored is direct delivery of the progestin to the key target, the endometrium, by direct intrauterine administration. Again this features levonorgestrel. The levonorgestrel-containing intrauterine system (LNG-IUS) is popular in contraceptive use and has an important role in the management of menstrual disorders. If a woman is happy to accept the insertion of an IUS, the evidence suggests that systemic absorption of levonorgestrel is limited yet very high levels are delivered to the intrauterine environment. As a result the woman is able to take estrogen by whatever route she prefers without having to add a progestin to this. As in younger women there may be irregular bleeding if the IUS is used, but many women will be bleed-free and with few side effects.

Progesterone administered to the vagina as a cream or in a vaginal ring are other potential approaches to the delivery of progesterone to the uterus. Though potentially relevant for endometrial safety in HRT these are not as yet established as HRT options, the progesterone vaginal ring, for instance, being more directly relevant to contraceptive applications.

References

1. Schindler AE, Campagnoli C, Druckmann R, et al. Classification and pharmacology of progestins. *Maturitas* 2003; **46**: S7–16.

2. Sitruk-Ware. Pharmacological profile of progestins. *Maturitas* 2004; **47**: 277–83.

3. Rosano GMC, Vitale C, Silvestri, Fini M. Metabolic and vascular effect of progestins in post-menopausal women. Implications for cardioprotection. *Maturitas* 2003; **46**: S17–29.

4. Lethaby A, Suckling J, Barlow D, et al. Hormone replacement therapy in postmenopausal women: endometrial hyperplasia and irregular bleeding. *Cochrane Database Syst Rev* 2004; **3**: CD000402.

5. Sturdee DW, Ulrich LG, Barlow DH, et al. The endometrial response to sequential and continuous oestrogen-progestogen replacement therapy. *Br J Obstetr Gynaecol* 2000; **107**: 1392–400.

6. Persson I, Thurfjell E, Holberg L. Effect of estrogen and estrogen-progestin replacement regimens on mammographic breast parenchymal density. *J Clin Oncol* 1997; **15**: 3201–7.

7. Bakken K, Fournier A, Lund E, *et al.* Menopausal hormone therapy and breast cancer risk: impact of different treatments. The European Prospective Investigation into Cancer and Nutrition. *Int J Cancer* 2011; **128**: 144–56.

8. Manson JE, Chlebowski RT, Stefanick ML, *et al.* Menopausal hormone therapy and health outcomes during the intervention and extended poststopping phases of the Women's Health Initiative randomized trials. *JAMA* 2013; **310**: 1353–68.

9. Schierbeck LL, Rejnmark L, Tofteng CL, *et al.* Effect of hormone replacement therapy on cardiovascular events in recently postmenopausal women: randomized trial. *Br Med J* 2012; **345**: e6409.

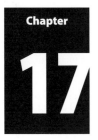

Androgen therapy for postmenopausal women

Susan R. Davis

What is androgen therapy and why is it sometimes prescribed?

Traditionally, the term "androgens" refers to a group of 19-carbon steroid hormones that are associated with maleness and the induction of male secondary sexual characteristics. This is as outdated as the concept of estrogen being only a female hormone. The major androgens circulate in concentrations greater than those of the estrogens in healthy women and androgens have a critical role in female physiology.

Testosterone is the main androgen in women, with its more potent metabolite, dihydrotestosterone (DHT), being important at a cellular level. The steroids, androstene-dione and dehydroepiandrosterone (DHEA), are classified as pre-androgens, although each exhibits very weak binding to the androgen receptor. Androstenedione and DHEA are produced by both the ovaries and the adrenals, whereas DHEA sulfate (DHEA-S) is almost exclusively a product of the adrenal glands. Dehydroepiandrosterone is a precursor for androstenedione production, which in turn can be converted to testosterone or estrone.

Androgen therapy in clinical practice refers to testosterone therapy, although DHEA is sometimes included under this heading. Androstenedione has been used as a body-building supplement, but its use as such is banned by the Food and Drug Administration of the USA and international sporting bodies because of safety concerns.

There is widespread prescription of DHEA as androgen therapy for women. Clinical trials have consistently shown that systemic DHEA therapy is not effective for the treatment of female sexual dysfunction (FSD) in women with either normal or impaired adrenal function, and should not be prescribed for this purpose [1]. Dehydroepiandrosterone does not improve mood or cognitive function in healthy women. Dehydroepiandrosterone may improve the health-related quality of life and mood in women with adrenal insufficiency, although these effects have been described as trivial [2]. There are preliminary data that daily intravaginal DHEA may alleviate vulvo-vaginal atrophy, but this requires confirmation in larger studies.

Tibolone is a synthetic compound that is used as a postmenopausal hormone therapy. It is metabolized in the gut and target tissues to isomers that exhibit estrogenic, progestogenic and androgenic actions. It therefore alleviates vasomotor symptoms and urogenital atrophy but does not activate the endometrium, and so does not cause vaginal bleeding. An active metabolite of tibolone has weak androgenic action. As a result, tibolone may improve libido and arousal [3]. As tibolone is a menopausal hormone therapy, not a specific androgen therapy, it is not discussed further in this chapter. The remainder of this chapter focuses

Managing the Menopause: 21st Century Solutions, ed. Nick Panay, Paula Briggs, and Gab Kovacs. Published by Cambridge University Press. © Cambridge University Press 2015.

on testosterone therapy for postmenopausal women as this is the androgen therapy with a sound evidence base and the most widely used.

The primary indication for the use of testosterone therapy is for the treatment of FSD, specifically, desire-arousal disorder. Initially loss of sexual desire associated with personal distress was classified as "hypoactive sexual desire disorder" in the *Diagnostic and Statistical Manual of Mental Disorders, Fourth Edition* (DSM–IV) [4]. Since it has been established that low sexual desire and low arousal are co-dependent, the two have been combined in DSM–5 as "desire-arousal disorder" [5]. Pivotal to the diagnosis of this as a disorder is that the woman must be sufficiently bothered by the problem that it causes some degree of distress. In clinical practice this usually translates to a woman presenting for treatment, although there is probably a large number of women troubled by low desire-arousal who, for a range of reasons, never raise this concern with a health-care provider. Treatment of desire-arousal disorder may involve relationship and/or sexual counseling, or it may involve a trial of testosterone therapy. Although testosterone therapy may have other favorable effects, the evidence is not strong enough for its use for any indication other than the treatment of sexual desire-arousal disorder at this time.

Basic androgen physiology

In women, androgens exert direct actions through the androgen receptor in a range of tissues. They have anabolic actions on bone and muscle, are important for normal sexual hair growth and skin sebum production, act in the cardiovascular system with positive effects on vascular endothelial function, and influence sexual function, mood and cognitive performance.

As androgens are obligatory precursors for the production of estradiol and estrone, these steroids can be considered to exert indirect actions through the estrogen receptors. For example, an adequate intra-ovarian testosterone concentration is essential for normal cyclical follicular development.

Blood levels of testosterone and androstenedione vary across the menstrual cycle, being lowest during the early follicular phase and rising to a peak by mid-cycle. The levels then fall slightly, and remain at a plateau across the luteal phase, falling to a nadir after the onset of menstruation [6]. Testosterone also appears to have a diurnal variation in young women, with levels peaking between 0400 and midday [7]. In contrast, the levels of DHEA and DHEA-S are fairly constant across the cycle.

The levels of testosterone, DHT, DHEA-S, DHEA and androstenedione decline in women from the mid 20s through to the late 40s, do not change across the natural menopause transition, but decline slowly with age thereafter [8]. The mechanism underpinning the decline in androgens during the reproductive years is not known, but may reflect ovarian aging.

An important aspect of testosterone physiology is that two thirds of circulating testosterone is bound to sex hormone binding globulin (SHBG), with the remainder bound to albumin, such that only 1–2% of testosterone circulates unbound to protein. As a consequence the concentration of SHBG determines how much testosterone circulates unbound. This is important as it is believed that the unbound fraction of testosterone exerts physiological effects. Women with higher SHBG levels have lower free testosterone and vice versa.

When are androgen levels low in women?

Most women will experience a significant age-related fall in androgen levels before they reach menopause. In addition, several spontaneous and iatrogenic conditions may cause abnormally low androgen levels.

Spontaneous causes of androgen insufficiency include:

- primary ovarian insufficiency
- hypothalamic amenorrhea
- hyperprolactinaemia (which can also be iatrogenic)
- adrenal insufficiency (due to loss of DHEA, DHEA-S and androstenedione production)
- panhypopituitism.

Iatrogenic causes of androgen insufficiency include:

- surgical menopause at any age
- chemotherapy
- radiotherapy to the pelvis
- systemic glucocorticosteroid therapy (suppression of adrenal pre-androgen production)
- oral estrogen, as the contraceptive pill or as menopausal hormone therapy, and exogenous thyroxine increase SHBG and lower a woman's free testosterone level.

Testosterone therapy

How is testosterone administered and is it effective for the treatment of FSD?

The early studies of testosterone for the treatment of FSD used oral methyltestosterone with oral estrogen. These trials showed efficacy at the expense of lowering HDL cholesterol, apolipoprotein A1, apolipoprotein B, LDL particle size, and increasing total body LDL catabolism. Other early studies involved the use of subcutaneously implanted testosterone pellets. Similarly these are highly effective, but they require a minor surgical procedure, the dissolution rate varies substantially between women, careful monitoring is required and their availability is limited.

The most extensively studied testosterone therapy for women has been a transdermal testosterone patch, which is changed twice a week, and releases approximately 300 µg of testosterone per day. The studies of this therapy have involved over 3,000 women who have received active treatment.

The transdermal testosterone patch significantly improves desire, arousal, orgasm frequency, sexual satisfaction and pleasure compared with placebo in postmenopausal women using oral or transdermal estrogen, or not on any estrogen therapy. Most recently it has also been shown to increase the number of self-reported satisfactory sexual events in women with antidepressant–associated FSD. The transdermal testosterone patch was approved for use in Europe, but approval was limited to surgically menopausal women with persistently low libido despite adequate estrogen therapy. As the uptake in Europe was low, and the European regulators refused to broaden the indication for use, the patch was withdrawn from the market. Other transdermal testosterone formulations for women, including a transdermal gel and a skin spray, with demonstrated efficacy, have not progressed through the approval process. A transdermal 1% testosterone cream for women is available in Australia. It has been shown to be effective and to have consistent pharmacokinetic properties in small studies.

Testosterone undecanoate, in a dose of 40 mg either daily or on alternate days, is used in many countries. Unfortunately this compound has highly variable absorption and can result in levels in the normal male range. Oral testosterone undecanoate also adversely affects lipoproteins and increases insulin resistance.

Fundamentally, the lack of an approved testosterone formulation for women in most countries leaves many physicians with no choice but to prescribe male formulations off-label, or recommended compounded testosterone creams or lozenges. None of these approaches can be considered safe.

Is testosterone therapy safe?

Approval of transdermal testosterone for use in postmenopausal women has been impeded by concerns about cardiovascular and cancer safety. No serious safety concerns were identified in studies of the transdermal testosterone patch, with use by women for up to 4 years.

Transdermal testosterone therapy, in a dose appropriate for women, does not alter lipoprotein levels, hemoglobin concentration, coagulation markers, inflammatory markers, fasting insulin, glucose or insulin sensitivity.

Testosterone has favorable effects on endothelial function and is a vasodilator. In women with congestive cardiac failure, transdermal testosterone was associated with significant functional improvements in exercise capacity, muscle strength and insulin sensitivity compared with placebo [9]. Transdermal testosterone has no adverse endometrial effects and has not been associated with an increase in risk of non-gynecologic cancer. The main issue of contention is whether testosterone increases the risk of breast cancer. As summarized elsewhere, oral methyltestosterone has been associated with a small increase in breast cancer risk in the Nurses Health Study, but not in other studies [9]. Two Australian studies reported no increase in breast cancer risk with testosterone implants and a 1% transdermal testosterone cream [9].

However these studies are all observational and there has been no single randomized placebo-controlled trial of sufficient size or duration to provide conclusive data. It is noteworthy that women with polycystic ovarian syndrome, who are estrogen replete and have decades of androgen excess, are not at increased risk of breast cancer.

Excessive treatment with testosterone will result in androgenic effects such as oily skin, excessive hair growth, voice change and cliteromegaly. The frequency of these effects observed with two doses of the transdermal testosterone patch, compared with placebo, in a large randomized controlled trial are shown in Figure 17.1. The use of the 300 µg/day dose patch resulted in increased hair growth, but it is of interest that withdrawals due to

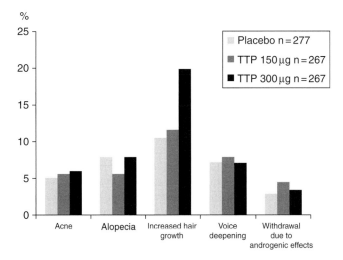

Figure 17.1. Androgenic adverse events over 52 weeks reported in a randomized controlled trial of the transdermal testosterone patch (TTP) releasing 300 µg/day or 150 µg/day. Derived from Davis *et al.* NEJM 2008 [10].

androgenic effects did not differ between the treatment groups [10]. These effects are not seen when a "female-appropriate" dose is administered. The exact "female-appropriate" dose will depend on the formulation used.

The greatest risk for women with regards to testosterone therapy is the unregulated prescribing of male formulations and compounded testosterone, often described as "bio-identical hormone therapy." Both treatment approaches put women at serious risk of excessive exposure. The International Menopause Society and the US Endocrine Society specifically recommend against the use of male testosterone products and compounded testosterone therapy for women.

Can I treat my patient with testosterone?

Testosterone should only be prescribed if there is confidence in the formulation to be used. This leaves few options presently for clinicians. There is an urgent need for a formulation for women to be approved by the regulators.

In the interim, the only options include the 1% testosterone cream available in Australia, and where available, pharmaceutically manufactured, not compounded, testosterone pellets.

Before testosterone therapy is initiated, a full medical history, including sexual history, and examination should be performed. It is important to identify the duration of the problem and whether or not it is partner-specific or generalized. The patient should be asked about ability to achieve orgasm and if not, whether this has been lifelong or of new onset. If lifelong, sexual counseling is indicated.

Prior to treating a woman with FSD with testosterone, consider and treat as indicated:

- Current circumstances.

  Relationship issues.
  Sexual health knowledge.

- Individual psychological factors.

  Body image and self-esteem.
  Experience of sexual abuse/trauma.
  Negative attitudes, inhibitions and anxieties.

- Health related factors.

  Mental health.
  Physical health.
  Medication side effects, particularly antidepressants and antipsychotics.

Although fatigue is a common complaint amongst women, if present, this may be the cause of low desire-arousal and warrants investigation. Basic investigations should include thyroid function, iron stores and fasting blood glucose.

Absolute contraindications to testosterone therapy include evidence of androgen excess, pregnancy and lactation, and a history of breast cancer.

If a woman is to be treated for desire-arousal disorder with testosterone, a baseline total testosterone level, as well as SHBG, should be measured. This is to avoid treating women with a normal testosterone level inappropriately and to guide therapy. Women with very high SHBG levels are unlikely to respond to treatment, and in the first instance an effort should be made to reduce their SHBG. For example, switching the woman from oral to transdermal estrogen therapy. If a woman has a very low SHBG level then the dose of testosterone should be lowered, as any exogenous testosterone is likely to be cleared rapidly from the circulation, increasing the risk of androgenic side effects.

Treated women should be monitored carefully as it is always possible for a woman to over-treat herself. Optimally, testosterone should be measured after a few weeks of initiating treatment, and if treatment is ongoing, then 6-monthly. A testosterone implant should never be re-inserted without checking that the testosterone levels have fallen back into the low female range. A consistent finding in studies of transdermal testosterone has been that efficacy is not observed until after 4–6 weeks of treatment. Patients need to be made aware of this. If a woman has not experienced improvements in her sexual well-being after 6 months of therapy, then treatment should cease, as an improvement after that time is not likely. Women need to be aware that treatment is a trial, as not all women will experience a benefit.

References

1. Davis SR, Panjari M, Stanczyk FZ. DHEA replacement for postmenopausal women. *J Clin Endocrinol Metab* 2011; **96**: 1642–53.

2. Alkatib AA, Cosma M, Elamin MB, *et al.* A systematic review and meta-analysis of randomized placebo-controlled trials of DHEA treatment effects on quality of life in women with adrenal insufficiency. *J Clin Endocrinol Metab* 2009; **94**: 3676–81.

3. Nijland EA, Nathorst-Boos J, Palacios S, *et al.* Tibolone and transdermal E2/NETA for the treatment of female sexual dysfunction in naturally menopausal women: results of a randomized active-controlled trial. *J Sex Med* 2008; **5**: 646–56.

4. American Psychiatric Association. *Diagnostic and Statistical Manual of Mental Disorders, Fourth Edition.* Washington, DC: American Psychiatric Press; 1994.

5. American Psychiatric Association. *Diagnostic and Statistical Manual of Mental Disorders, Fifth Edition.* Washington, DC: American Psychiatric Press; 2013.

6. Sinha-Hikim I, Arver S, Beall G, *et al.* The use of a sensitive equilibrium dialysis method for the measurement of free testosterone levels in healthy, cycling women and in human immunodeficiency virus-infected women. *J Clin Endocrinol Metab* 1998; **83**: 1312–18.

7. Vierhapper H. Nowotny P, Waldhausl W. Determination of testosterone production rates in men and women using stable isotope'dilution and mass spectrometry. *J Clin Endocrinol Metab* 1997; **82**: 1492–6.

8. Davison SL, Bell R, Donath S, Montalto JG, Davis SR. Androgen levels in adult females: changes with age, menopause, and oophorectomy. *J Clin Endocrinol Metab* 2005; **90**: 3847–53.

9. Davis SR. Cardiovascular and cancer safety of testosterone in women. *Curr Opin Endocrinol Diabetes Obes* 2011; **18**: 198–203.

10. Davis SR, Moreau M, Kroll R, *et al.* Testosterone for low libido in menopausal women not taking estrogen therapy. *N Eng J Med* 2008; **359**: 2005–17.

Selective estrogen receptor modulators used for postmenopausal women

JoAnn V. Pinkerton

Katherine is 53 with her last period about a year ago. She is complaining of severe hot flashes, night sweats and vaginal dryness. She wants to take hormonal therapy but is concerned about the increased risk of breast cancer seen in the Womens Health Initiative (WHI) Study with combination estrogen and progestin therapy. Her last periods before finally quitting were very heavy with cyclic breast tenderness. She wants relief from her hot flashes but doesn't want to develop bleeding or breast tenderness.

Background

Selective estrogen receptor modulators, commonly referred to as SERMs or estrogen agonists/antagonists, are estrogen-like compounds that may act as weak estrogen agonists and as estrogen antagonists, depending on the particular SERM and the target tissue. Selective estrogen receptor modulators have many clinical uses for postmenopausal women because of their ability to target and prevent or treat different diseases, including breast cancer and osteoporosis, and recently postmenopausal dyspareunia.

Selective estrogen receptor modulators available for postmenopausal women in the USA include tamoxifen and toremifene approved for prevention and treatment of breast cancer, raloxifene approved for prevention and treatment of osteoporosis and prevention of invasive breast cancer, and ospemifene approved for treatment of dyspareunia associated with post-menopausal vaginal atrophy. Tibolone, widely used around the world for relief of menopausal symptoms and prevention of bone loss, is not approved in the USA or Canada. Lasofoxifene prevents bone loss and improves vaginal atrophy but development has been placed on hold due to gynecologic concerns. Bazedoxefine is approved for prevention of osteoporosis in Europe. The first tissue selective estrogen complex (TSEC) approved in the USA is a pairing of conjugated equine estrogens with the SERM bazedoxefine for relief of hot flashes and prevention of bone loss. Many SERMs have been discontinued following phase III multicenter clinical trials due to adverse findings, including droloxifene, idoxifene, ormeloxifene and levormeloxifene.

An ideal SERM for postmenopausal women would be estrogenic on bone to prevent bone loss, relieve hot flashes with a neutral or estrogen antagonistic effect on the breast and endometrium to reduce cancer risks. To date, such a SERM has not been identified.

Description

Selective estrogen receptor modulators are synthetic, non-steroidal hormones that show variable or mixed estrogen agonist or antagonist properties depending on specifics found at target tissue when they bind to the estrogen receptor.

Managing the Menopause: 21st Century Solutions, ed. Nick Panay, Paula Briggs, and Gab Kovacs. Published by Cambridge University Press. © Cambridge University Press 2015.

Mechanism of action of SERMS

Mechanism of action occurs through a conformational structure change at the receptor when the SERMS bind, with effects on transcription depending on different coactivators (CoA) or corepressors (CoR) which are involved in the regulation of target gene transcription. The shape of the ligands that bind to the estrogen receptors (ERs, ERα or ERβ) allows the complex to submit variable signals, which leads to the variable tissue activity [1]. Although preclinical testing can suggest how a given SERM will behave in a given tissue, large clinical trials are needed to identify each SERM's unique tissue-selective effects in postmenopausal women. Although SERMS in general are felt to be preventive of bone loss and antagonistic at the breast, each SERM must be tested for its effects on each tissue (targeted and non-targeted) for efficacy and safety.

The hope of SERMS for postmenopausal women is to allow individual care depending on specific estrogen agonist or estrogen antagonist effects desired in a given woman.

Specific SERMS available for use for postmenopausal women

Tamoxifen

Tamoxifen is approved for prevention and treatment after breast cancer, and there is now good evidence from several prospective trials and a meta-analysis that it does decrease the incidence of recurrence, if used up to 10 years, of ER-positive breast cancer. Consequently, the American Society of Clinical Oncology (ASCO) [2, 3] has updated its guidelines for postmenopausal women with breast cancer who are hormone receptor-positive:

1. Take tamoxifen for 10 years.
2. Use an aromatase inhibitor for 5 years followed by tamoxifen for 5 years, then go back to aromatase inhibitor for up to another 5 years.
3. Take tamoxifen for 2–3 years followed by 5 years of an aromatase inhibitor.

Tamoxifen is not approved to prevent bone loss, but has been shown to be a partial agonist in bone with prevention of bone loss in postmenopausal (but not premenopausal) women at the lumbar spine and hip, although with less improvement in bone density than seen with hormone therapy.

Concerns about tamoxifen use include an increased risk of endometrial polyps, endometrial cancer (both adenocarcinoma of the endometrium and rare reports of mixed mesodermal sarcoma), venous thromboembolic events, pulmonary embolism and stroke in women over 50. The risk of endometrial cancer in postmenopausal tamoxifen users in the STAR trial was increased (RR 2.54), with an increase for women over 50 (RR 5.4), with higher risk seen with longer duration of use or prior endometrial thickening. The effect of tamoxifen on the vagina is mixed with some estrogenic effects but also adverse reports of dyspareunia, leukorrhea or vaginal dryness. Hot flashes have been reported as adverse events but reported bothersome enough to seek treatment only in 16%.

Toremifene

Toremifene is used for postmenopausal women as an adjunct in the treatment of advanced estrogen receptor-positive breast cancer and appears similar in effectiveness to tamoxifen in comparative trials [4]. Although slightly less, endometrial cancer was seen (39% compared with 44.3%), this was not significantly less [4]. Toremifene has an estrogen agonist effect on bone and lipid profiles.

Raloxifene

Raloxifene is approved for prevention and treatment of osteoporosis and for the prevention of invasive breast cancer.

Effect on breast

Several studies have shown a protective effect of raloxifene with respect to recurrence of breast cancer, with an incidence of about 50% less cases of invasive estrogen-positive breast cancer. When compared with tamoxifen, raloxifene reduced invasive breast cancers as well but with fewer endometrial cancers, venous thromboembolism (VTE), pulmonary embolism and cataracts seen in STAR trial of women at high risk [5].

Effect on bone

Raloxifene at 60 mg/day improved bone density at 3 years by 2.6% at lumbar spine and 2.1% at femoral neck ($P < 0.001$) with a significant reduction in new clinical vertebral fractures of 68% (absolute risk reduction of 1.3/1,000). At 3 years, the risk of vertebral fracture was reduced by 55% in women at high risk with T-scores of −2.5 SD or less at lumbar spine or hip, compared with a 30% reduction in women who had low T-scores and prior vertebral fracture [6]. Raloxifene has thus shown beneficial effects on prevention of bone loss and in reducing vertebral fractures associated with postmenopausal osteoporosis although it did not show prevention of hip or non-vertebral fractures [6].

Effect on endometrium

Raloxifene has been tested up to 6 months with vaginal estrogen without proliferative effects on endometrium based on transvaginal ultrasound and endometrial biopsy, but in one study combined with oral estradiol, an increase in endometrial hyperplasia was seen. Studies combining raloxifene with systemic estrogen showed a benefit on quality of life, treatment satisfaction and vaginal dryness but in some, an increase in endometrial thickness was seen as soon as 3 months with endometrial proliferation and two cases of endometrial hyperplasia both after 24 weeks. Thus combining raloxifene with vaginal estrogen appears safe, but not combining it with systemic estrogen.

Effect on vasomotor symptoms

Commonly reported side effects include hot flashes, leg cramps, VTE, along with peripheral edema, arthralgia and flu syndrome. The most significant adverse event has been hot flashes, although they were not a major cause of discontinuation in clinical trials.

Ospemifene

Ospemifene is a SERM that has been approved in the USA for treatment of dyspareunia due to postmenopausal atrophy. Several studies have shown beneficial effects on dyspareunia and positive changes on the vagina, with improvements in vaginal maturation index (increases of superficial and intermediate cells) compared with placebo, as well as improvements in vaginal pH [7].

Effect on bone and breast are largely unknown

Preclinical effect on ovariectomized rats and bone marker data in humans suggest an effect of ospemifene on prevention of bone density, but, unfortunately to date, ospemifene has not been evaluated in a large RCT for its effects on prevention of bone loss or whether it is neutral or antagonistic on the breast.

Effect on endometrium

In open-label clinical extension trial to 52 weeks [7], ospemifene was not shown to have an increased risk of endometrial proliferation on endometrial biopsy. The endometrial biopsies were atrophic or inactive, although weakly proliferative endometrium was found in two ospemifene participants at baseline and at week 52. No cases of endometrial hyperplasia or carcinoma were found in the 52-week open-label extension study, which is reassuring.

No increased risk of stroke or VTE has been seen over placebo but concern remains about potential VTE risk. No exacerbation of hot flashes was reported in the RCT.

Tissue selective estrogen complex: conjugated estrogens paired with bazedoxefine

The first TSEC tested in a large RCT and approved in the USA is conjugated estrogens (0.45 mg) combined with the SERM bazedoxifene (BZA) (20 mg) for relief of menopausal vasomotor symptoms and prevention of bone loss [8]. Bazedoxifene has been shown to prevent bone loss in osteoporosis treatment trials compared with placebo, without increase in endometrial thickness on ultrasound and without adverse effect on the breast. Preclinically and again in clinical trials, bazedoxifene has been found to be highly antiproliferative on the uterus, which means that even when combined with estrogen, there is no need for concomitant progestogen use. Both components of the TSEC (conjugated estrogens and bazedoxifene) compete for the same ligand binding on the ER.

Effect on vasomotor symptoms

Within the Selective Estrogen Menopause and Response to Therapy (SMART) trials, VMS were evaluated in highly symptomatic women in the SMART-1 trial subset of women with moderate-severe VMS of more than 7 per day or 50 per week, and SMART-2 trial (N = 332; aged 40–65 years), CE 0.45 mg/BZX 20 mg was found to have clinically meaningful decreases in the mean daily number and severity of hot flashes compared with placebo at 12 weeks ($P < 0.05$) [9, 10]. Compared with baseline in the 12-week trial of highly symptomatic menopausal women with seven or more hot flashes per day, CE 0.45 mg/BZA 20 mg reduced hot flash frequency by 74% vs. 51% for placebo [9]. An early onset of action between 2–3 weeks was found with persistence at 12 weeks and up to 2 years in the SMART-1 trial [9].

Effect on bone loss prevention

In the SMART trials, there was a consistent mildly positive effect on bone density when CE and BZA were administered together [10, 11]. This applied to bone density at the hip and lumbar spine in women at risk of osteoporosis. Bone turnover markers were reduced compared with PBO ($P < 0.01$ for all). Consistent effects were seen for prevention of bone loss in women < 5 or ≥ 5 years from menopause.

Effect on vagina

In the SMART-3 trial of postmenopausal women with VVA defined as $\leq 5\%$ superficial cells on vaginal smear, vaginal pH > 5, and ≥ 1 moderate-to-severe VVA symptoms, CE 0.45 and 0.625 mg /BZA 20 mg improved vaginal maturation index over placebo at 12 weeks [12]. The higher-dose CE 0.625 mg /BZA 20 mg reduced vaginal pH and improved severity scores over placebo for the most bothersome symptom, but this was not found with the lower-dose CE 0.45 mg /BZA 20 mg, suggesting an estrogen antagonist effect of bazedoxifene on the vagina.

Effect on breast

In the SMART trials, similar incidences of breast pain and tenderness were found for both doses of CE (0.45 mg and 0.625 mg)/BZA 20 mg and placebo, and less than with CE and MPA [13]. The breast density prospective substudy, CE 0.45 and 0.625 mg/BZA 20 mg demonstrated non-inferiority compared with PBO for change from baseline in breast density at 1 year, whereas MPA 1.5 mg/CE 0.45 mg showed a significantly greater increase compared with PBO ($P < 0.001$) [13].

Similar rates of breast cancer to placebo have been found in the SMART trials although trial durations are 2 years or less.

Effect on endometrium

High rates of amenorrhea of 84% were found, similar to placebo, unlike the higher rates of bleeding and spotting seen with CE/MPA [3, 4]. Minimal increases from baseline (<1mm) in endometrial thickness after 2 years was seen. No signal of increasing endometrial concern was seen in the SMART trials with low rates of endometrial hyperplasia $< 1\%$ similar to placebo and the active comparator CE/MPA, but longer-term studies are needed to provide evidence of safety beyond 2 years [2, 4]. Higher rates of vaginal bleeding and spotting were found with the active hormone comparator CE 0.45 mg/MPA 1.5 mg in the Smart-5 RCT [12].

Adverse events

Overall incidences of adverse events in SMART trials were similar to placebo and there were no increased risks of VTE events with CE/BZA compared with placebo [8, 11]. In SMART-1, an improvement in total cholesterol was seen with the expected increase in triglycerides from CE [8]. Cardiovascular, cerebrovascular events were similar to placebo in SMART trials up to 2 years. Compared with placebo, CE/BZA demonstrated non-inferiority for change from baseline in mammographic breast density with similar rates of breast pain/tenderness to placebo, both significantly lower than with CE/MPA [11]. The vaginal bleeding profile with CE/BZA was not significantly different from placebo and significantly better than that observed with CE/MPA [8, 11, 15]. No increase in endometrial or breast cancers were observed in trials up to 2 years. The incidence of endometrial hyperplasia with CE 0.45 and 0.625/BZA was very low ($<1\%$), similar to placebo. Limitations of the SMART trial data includes enrollment of generally healthy postmenopausal women with BMI < 30–34. Both doses were comparable to placebo in cancers or mortality [9, 12, 16].

Conclusion

Selective estrogen receptor modulators have been developed for use in postmenopausal women with targeted tissue effects which can be used to individualize therapy. Tamoxifen and toremifene are used in the prevention and treatment of breast cancer. Raloxifene is approved for both prevention of bone loss and the prevention of invasive breast cancer. Ospemifene relieves dyspareunia associated with postmenopausal vulvo-vaginal atrophy. The first TSEC is now available, offering an alternative to traditional estrogen combined with progestogen by combining estrogen and a SERM (conjugated estrogens and bazedoxefine) to relieve menopausal hot flashes and night sweats and prevent osteoporosis for symptomatic non-hysterectomized, postmenopausal women. Rates of breast tenderness, breast density, breast cancer, bleeding and endometrial cancer have been found to be similar to placebo in trials up to 2 years in duration. Continued development of novel SERMS is needed, with improved selectivity, before an ideal SERM will be available for postmenopausal women.

References

1. Maximov PY, Lee TM, Jordan VC. The discovery and development of selective estrogen receptor modulators (SERMs) for clinical practice. *Curr Clin Pharmacol* 2013; **8**: 135–55.

2. Burstein HJ, Temin S, Anderson H, *et al.* Adjuvant endocrine therapy for women with hormone receptor-positive breast cancer: American Society of Clinical Oncology Clinical Practice Guideline Focused Update. Published online before print May 27, 2014.

3. Davies C, Pan H, Godwin J, *et al.* Long-term effects of continuing adjuvant tamoxifen to 10 years versus stopping at 5 years after diagnosis of oestrogen receptor-positive breast cancer: ATLAS, a randomised trial. *Lancet* 2013; **381**: 805–16.

4. Harvey HA, Kimura M, Hajba A. Toremifene: an evaluation of its safety profile. *Breast* 2006; **15**: 142–57.

5. Vogel VG, Costantino JP, Wickerham DL, *et al.* Effects of tamoxifen vs raloxifene on the risk of developing invasive breast cancer and other disease outcomes: the NSABP Study of Tamoxifen and Raloxifene (STAR) P-2 trial. *JAMA* 2006; **295**: 2727–41.

6. Ettinger B, Black DM, Mitlak BH, *et al.* Reduction of vertebral fracture risk in postmenopausal women with osteoporosis treated with raloxifene: results from a 3-year randomized clinical trial. Multiple Outcomes of Raloxifene Evaluation (MORE) Investigators. *JAMA* 1999; **282**: 637–45.

7. Portman DJ, Bachmann GA, Simon JA. Ospemifene, a novel selective estrogen receptor modulator for treating dyspareunia associated with postmenopausal vulvar and vaginal atrophy. *Menopause* 2013; **20**: 623–30.

8. Simon JA, Lin VH, Radovich C, Bachmann GA, Ospemifene study group. One-year long-term safety extension study of ospemifene for the treatment of valvar and vaginal atrophy in postmenopausal women with a uterus. *Menopause* 2012; **20**: 418–27.

9. Lobo RA, Pinkerton JV, Gass MLS, *et al.* Evaluation of bazedoxifene/conjugated estrogens for the treatment of menopausal symptoms and effects on metabolic bone parameters and overall safety profile. *Fertil Steril* 2009; **92**: 1025–38.

10. Pinkerton JV, Utian WH, Constantine GD, Olivier S, Pickar JH. Relief of vasomotor symptoms with the tissue-selective estrogen complex containing bazedoxifene/conjugated estrogens: a randomized, controlled trial. *Menopause* 2009; **16**: 1116–24.

11. Lindsay R, Gallagher JC, Kagan R, Pickar JH, Constantine G. Efficacy of tissue-selective estrogen complex (TSEC) of bazedoxifene/conjugated estrogens (BZX/CE) for osteoporosis prevention in at-risk postmenopausal women. *Fertil Steril* 2009; **92**: 1045–52.

12. Pinkerton JV, Harvey JA, Lindsay R, *et al.*; SMART-5 Investigators. Effects of bazedoxifene/conjugated estrogens on the endometrium and bone: a randomized trial. *J Clin Endocrinol Metab* 2014; **99**: E189–98 [Epub Jan 17, 2014].

13. Kagan R, Williams RS, Pan K, Mirkin S, Pickar JH. A randomized, placebo- and active-controlled trial of bazedoxifene/conjugated estrogens (BZA/CE) for treatment of moderate to severe vulvar/vaginal atrophy in postmenopausal women. *Menopause* 2010; **17**: 281–9.

14. Pinkerton JV, Harvey JA, Pan K, *et al.* Breast effects of bazedoxifene-conjugated estrogens: a randomized controlled trial. *Obstet Gynecol* 2013; **121**: 959–68.

15. Archer DF, Lewis V, Carr BR, Olivier S, Pickar JH. Bazedoxifene/conjugated estrogens (BZA/CE): incidence of uterine bleeding in postmenopausal women. *Fertil Steril* 2009; **92**: 1039–44.

16. Pickar JH, Yeh I-T, Bachmann G, Speroff L. Endometrial effects of a tissue selective estrogen complex (TSEC) containing bazedoxifene/conjugated estrogens as a menopausal therapy. *Fertil Steril* 2009; **92**: 1018–24.

Non-hormonal treatments for menopausal symptoms

Jenifer Sassarini

Nicole is 49 and has been experiencing symptoms of the menopause for several months – hot flashes, insomnia, joint pains, headaches, vaginal dryness associated with difficulty having sex, and urinary frequency. She has a family history of breast cancer, and under no circumstances is she prepared to take HRT. She comes to see you to ask about non-hormonal solutions for her symptoms.

Introduction

There are a number of symptoms associated with perimenopause and decreasing estrogen levels, although some women will experience none of these. They include hot flashes and night sweats (vasomotor symptoms), vaginal symptoms, depression, anxiety, irritability and mood swings (psychological effects), joint pains, migraines or headaches, sleeping problems and urinary incontinence.

With improved health care and increased life expectancy, women spend a considerable proportion of their lives (30 years on average) after the menopause. At present 36% of women in the UK are over 50 years of age, and it is estimated that approximately 75% of women will experience some symptoms related to estrogen deficiency during the menopausal transition.

The most commonly reported symptoms are vasomotor symptoms. If left untreated, flashes commonly resolve within 1 year, or less, with only a third reporting symptoms 5 years after menopause; however some 20% of women will have persisting symptoms for up to 15 years.

The British Menopause Society has long held the belief that HRT is safe and effective, and has recently published the affirmation of this in the light of new data from the Danish and KEEPS trials; however there is still concern amongst general practitioners and women that the risks of HRT far outweigh the benefits and for this reason there is an interest in non-hormonal alternatives.

Care must be taken though when recommending non-hormonal alternatives as first-line therapy with the belief that they are more effective than HRT, as selective interpretation of data and personal sentiments can cloud objective evaluation of the literature. There are of course a group of women for whom hormonal therapy is not suitable and, for this reason, increasing our understanding of alternative treatments is vital.

Pathophysiology of a hot flash

The exact pathophysiology of flashing is not known, although it is generally accepted that falling estrogens play a main role; flashes generally occur at times of relative estrogen

Managing the Menopause: 21st Century Solutions, ed. Nick Panay, Paula Briggs, and Gab Kovacs. Published by Cambridge University Press. © Cambridge University Press 2015.

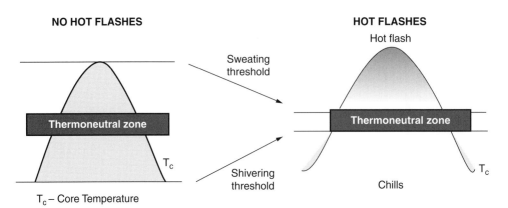

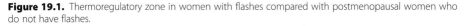

T$_c$ – Core Temperature

Figure 19.1. Thermoregulatory zone in women with flashes compared with postmenopausal women who do not have flashes.

withdrawal and replacing it will result in improvement in most women. However, whilst estrogen concentrations remain low after the menopause, most vasomotor symptoms will diminish with time, and therefore a fall in estrogen concentration does not seem to provide the complete answer. It has also been found that circulating levels of estrogen do not differ significantly between symptomatic and asymptomatic postmenopausal women.

Furthermore, it is thought that withdrawal of estrogen, rather than low circulating estrogen levels, is the central change that leads to hot flashes and there are several observations to support this theory. The abrupt estrogen withdrawal due to bilateral oophorectomy in premenopausal women is associated with a higher prevalence of flashes than in those women who experience a gradual physiological menopause, and young women with gonadal dysgenesis, who have low levels of endogenous estrogen, do not experience hot flashes unless they receive several months of estrogen therapy and then abruptly discontinue its use.

Hot flashes are characterized by a feeling of intense warmth, often accompanied by profuse sweating, anxiety, skin reddening and palpitations, and sometimes followed by chills. In this respect, flashes resemble a systemic heat dissipation response, which is controlled, in humans, by the medial preoptic area of the hypothalamus.

Studies using an ultrasensitive temperature probe suggest that hot flashes are triggered by small elevations in core body temperature acting within a narrowed thermoneutral zone in symptomatic postmenopausal women [1, 2]. Those studies found that small but significant elevations in T$_c$ precede most hot flash episodes and that postmenopausal women with hot flashes had a narrower thermoregulatory zone compared with postmenopausal women who do not flash (see Figure 19.1). This narrowing was mainly due to a lowering of the sweating threshold in symptomatic women, and estrogen replacement has been shown to elevate this threshold, with reduced hot flash occurrence.

Changes in core temperature may also be associated with alterations in neuroendocrine pathways involving steroid hormones, noradrenaline (NA), the endorphins and serotonin (Figure 19.2). Noradrenaline and serotonin, particularly, are thought to play a key role.

Non-hormonal pharmacological preparations
Clonidine
Clonidine is an α2-adrenergic agonist licensed for the treatment of hypertension, migraines and postmenopausal vasomotor symptoms.

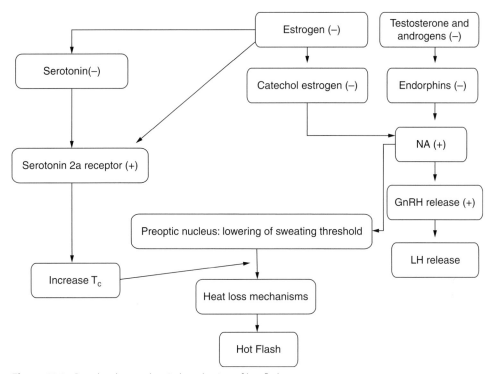

Figure 19.2. Postulated neurochemical mechanism of hot flashes.

Monoamines have been shown to play an important role in the control of thermoregulation, and animal studies have shown that noradrenaline (NA) acts to narrow the thermoregulatory zone. Noradrenergic stimulation of the medial preoptic area of the hypothalamus in monkeys and baboons causes peripheral vasodilatation, heat loss and a drop in core temperature, similar to changes which occur in women during hot flashes.

It has also been shown that plasma levels of a noradrenaline metabolite are significantly increased both before and during hot flash episodes in postmenopausal women.

The hypotensive effect of clonidine is thought to be mediated mainly through selective stimulation of presynaptic α-adrenergic receptors in the region of the vasomotor center in the medulla, however it has a dual action. When first administered, clonidine stimulates peripheral α1-adrenoceptors (ARs) resulting in vasoconstriction, but subsequently acts on the central ARs to inhibit sympathetic drive resulting in vasodilatation.

It has also been shown to widen the thermoregulatory zone in humans. Clonidine is used for postoperative shivering because it is thought that, like general anesthetic agents and sedatives, it decreases shivering thresholds by a generalized impairment of central thermoregulatory control. It has also been demonstrated to increase the sweating threshold.

A meta-analysis [3] has examined 10, poor-to-fair quality, trials in which clonidine (0.1 mg/day) demonstrated a moderate, but statistically significant, reduction in hot flash frequency and severity at 4 and 8 weeks. This suggests that clonidine is an effective alternative to hormonal therapy; however adverse effects, including dry mouth, insomnia and drowsiness, were noted in 8 out of 10 trials.

Selective serotonin (and noradrenaline) reuptake inhibitors

Serotonin is involved in many bodily functions including mood, anxiety, sleep, sexual behavior and thermoregulation. Estrogen withdrawal is associated with decreased blood serotonin levels, and short-term estrogen therapy has been shown to increase these levels.

Selective serotonin reuptake inhibitors (SSRIs) are a group of drugs typically used as antidepressants, which are thought to function by blocking the reuptake of serotonin to the presynaptic cell. This increases the amount of serotonin in the synaptic cleft available to bind to the postsynaptic cell. Selective serotonin reuptake inhibitors were commonly prescribed for the treatment of depression in women undergoing treatment for breast cancer. Anecdotally, these same women were noted to have an improvement in their vasomotor symptoms, which occurred as a side effect of treatment. Studies were then carried out to determine the efficacy of these as an effective treatment for flashing.

A meta-analysis [3] assessed two double-blind randomized placebo-controlled trials (fair and good quality) comparing paroxetine to placebo and concluded that paroxetine was more effective than placebo in reducing the frequency and severity of hot flashes. One study included predominantly women with breast cancer using tamoxifen. Doses used varied from 10 mg/day to 25 mg/day, and although efficacy did not vary with dose, those on higher doses experienced more side effects, including nausea, headaches, drowsiness or insomnia.

This same meta-analysis assessed a further two randomized controlled trials comparing venlafaxine and placebo. In one fair-quality trial, an improvement in quality of life (51% with venlafaxine compared with 15% placebo users) was demonstrated despite no reduction in frequency of flashes. In the second, a good-quality trial, venlafaxine at doses of 37.5, 75, 150 mg/day decreased hot flash frequency compared with placebo. Improvement appeared to be greater with the two higher doses, although adverse effects included dry mouth, constipation, decreased appetite, nausea and sleeplessness. Nausea typically improves in 2–3 days, and can be improved by titrating the dose slowly. Venlafaxine was also found to be superior to clonidine, decreasing flashes by 57% compared with 37% in clonidine users.

Fluoxetine (20–30 mg/day) and citalopram (30 mg/day) were no better than placebo for flash frequency or score improvement.

Two further studies, published following the meta-analysis by Nelson, and included in a Cochrane systematic review examining non-hormonal treatments in women with breast cancer [4], demonstrated a reduction in the number and severity of flashes with venlafaxine at low dose and at 75 mg/day when compared with placebo.

Desvenlafaxine is a novel serotonin-norepinephrine reuptake inhibitor, highly selective for serotonin and norepinephrine transporters, with weak or no affinity for dopamine receptors and transporters. Desvenlafaxine restored thermoregulatory function more rapidly than estrogen replacement in two rodent models of vasomotor symptoms and in two double-blind randomized placebo-controlled trials [5, 6]; 100 and 150 mg were found to decrease number of hot flashes after 12 weeks compared with placebo.

Use of these drugs in women with breast cancer using tamoxifen is common; therefore consideration must be given to potential interactions. Tamoxifen must be metabolized by the cytochrome P450 enzyme system, predominantly cytochrome P450 isoenzyme 2D6 (CYP2D6), to become active, and CYP2D6 is inhibited to varying degrees by SSRIs. Paroxetine is an exceptionally potent inhibitor, whereas sertraline inhibits to a lesser degree and citalopram and escitalopram are only weak inhibitors. Evidence is conflicting on the success rates of tamoxifen in preventing recurrence of breast cancer when using a concurrent SSRI. For those women who need to begin treatment with an SSRI for depression, citalopram or escitalopram may be the safest choice, however improvements in flashing are better with venlafaxine and desvenlafaxine, and these appear to be safe choices.

Gabapentin

The mechanism of action of gabapentin in the amelioration of vasomotor symptoms is unknown, but it is thought to involve a direct effect on the hypothalamic thermoregulatory centre.

Two double-blind randomized placebo-controlled trials, examined in a meta-analysis [3], both conducted in women with breast cancer, showed a significant reduction in frequency and severity of hot flashes when taking gabapentin 900 mg per day, but not when taking 300 mg per day. Titrated to 2,400 mg per day continued to be superior to placebo but was not significantly different to estrogen 0.625 mg/day. However, dizziness, unsteadiness and fatigue were reported in the gabapentin-treated group and resulted in a higher dropout rate than in the control group.

Non-pharmacological therapies
Phytoestrogens

Phytoestrogens are chemicals that resemble estrogen and are present in most plants, vegetables and fruits. There are three main types of phytoestrogens; soy isoflavones (the most potent), coumestans and lignans. Soyabean and red clover are also rich in phyto-estrogens. These compounds are converted into weak estrogenic substances in the gastrointestinal tract.

Isoflavones are the most researched, and Nelson's meta-analysis included 17 RCTs. From six trials comparing Promensil (red clover isoflavone) with placebo, only one fair-quality trial found a reduction in flash frequency with Promensil, although there was no overall reduction in the meta-analysis, and no improvement in flash severity was demonstrated in any of the included trials.

Soy isoflavones were compared with placebo in the remaining 11 trials. The meta-analysis revealed an improvement in hot flashes after 12–16 weeks (four trials) and after 6 months (two trials), but were not significantly decreased in studies examining 4–6 weeks' use.

A systematic review [7] was also carried out by the Cochrane Collaboration. They included five trials in a meta-analysis, which demonstrated no significant decrease in the frequency of hot flashes with phytoestrogens.

Thirty trials were also studied comparing phytoestrogens with control. Some of the trials found that phytoestrogens alleviated the frequency and severity of hot flashes and night sweats when compared with placebo but many of the trials were of low quality or were underpowered. The great variability in the results of these trials may result in part from the difference in efficacy of the various types of phytoestrogens used, the exact treatment protocol and the fraction of equol producers in the cohort. It is claimed that only 30–40% of the US population possess the gut microflora responsible for converting isoflavones to the active estrogenic equol. It should be noted that there was also a strong placebo response in most trials, ranging from 1% to 59%.

Black cohosh

Black cohosh is a native American herb that is thought to behave as a selective estrogen receptor modulator (SERM) with mild central estrogenic effects.

A meta-analysis of several short-term and relatively small RCTs comparing black cohosh use with placebo "revealed a trend towards reducing vasomotor symptoms," but only in cases of mild-to-moderate symptoms [8]. This was particularly notable when hot flashes were associated with sleep and mood disturbances. This was confirmed in another 12-week study of 304 women in addition to improvements in mood, sleep disorders, sexual disorders and sweating. In contrast, however, the recent Herbal Alternatives for Menopause Trial (HALT) [9] which compared black cohosh to both placebo and estrogen replacement over 12 months, suggested that black cohosh was ineffective in relieving vasomotor symptoms.

Whilst there has been no confirmation of its efficacy, many women, both cancer-free as well as breast cancer patients and survivors, will use black cohosh to relieve vasomotor symptoms. Nevertheless, it is important to exercise caution as there is limited information on its potential to influence breast cancer development or progression. No effect has been seen on mammary tumor development, which would suggest that black cohosh would not influence breast cancer risk if given to women before tumor formation, but there has been an increase in the incidence of lung metastases in tumor-bearing animals when compared with mice fed with an isoflavone-free control diet. Additional studies will be needed to correlate these findings to women taking different black cohosh products at various times during breast cancer development; however, these results suggest caution for women using black cohosh, especially for extended periods of time.

Hepatotoxicity has also been associated with black cohosh, however a recent critical analysis and structured causality assessment has shown no causal relationship between treatment by black cohosh and liver disease.

Vitamin E

Only one randomized placebo-controlled trial involving vitamin E is available, in which 105 women with a history of breast cancer received placebo and vitamin E 800 IU daily for 4 weeks in a cross-over design [10]. There was no improvement in frequency or severity of hot flashes with vitamin E when compared with placebo, and care must be taken when a toxic vitamin is ingested in excessive amounts.

Evening primrose oil

This is a widely used product for the treatment of menopausal symptoms, although the exact mechanism of action is not fully understood. Its effectiveness has been analyzed in a double-blind randomized placebo-controlled trial. This trial used a combination of evening primrose oil (2,000 mg/day) with vitamin E (10 mg/day) versus placebo and showed a significantly greater reduction in daytime flashes in the placebo group than in the treatment group. Unsurprisingly, there was a high dropout rate due to unrelieved symptoms, and this precluded reliable conclusions.

Lifestyle modifications

There is evidence that body mass index (BMI), smoking, alcohol consumption and sedentary lifestyle are associated with reports of vasomotor symptoms, however there are few papers reporting the direct effect that modifications have on flashes.

It may be safe to assume, though, that there will be an improvement in symptoms if a risk factor for exacerbation of those symptoms is removed. Smoking cessation and weight loss has numerous other health benefits, not exclusively alterations of endothelial function, which may be involved in the hot flash mechanism.

Exercise

As well as having significant physiologic benefits (for example cardiovascular and bone health), exercise may be one of the promising alternatives to HRT and if demonstrated to be effective in the treatment of vasomotor symptoms, is an inexpensive intervention that typically has few known side effects.

The Cochrane Collaboration carried out a systematic review [11] to examine the effectiveness of any type of exercise intervention in the management of vasomotor symptoms in symptomatic perimenopausal and postmenopausal women. Only one very small trial was considered suitable for inclusion, which found, not unexpectedly, that HRT was more effective than exercise. There is no available evidence examining whether exercise is an effective treatment relative to other interventions or no intervention.

An alternative treatment
Stellate ganglion blockade

Stellate ganglion blocks have been carried out safely for more than 60 years, for pain syndromes and vascular insufficiency; 0.5% bupivicaine is injected on the right side of the anterolateral aspect of the C6 vertebra under fluoroscopy and an effective block confirmed by the presence of Horner's syndrome.

A case report was published in 1985 of a 77-year-old man with flashing after orchiectomy. He was treated with a stellate ganglion blockade, based on the belief that the flashing centre has a sympathetic outflow to the stellate ganglion, and his attacks of flashing ceased.

A pilot study of 13 women (age range 38–71 years), with a history of breast cancer, who suffered with severe hot flashes, demonstrated reductions in flash episodes and an improvement in sleep quality following stellate ganglion blockade. A more recent study revealed a benefit in only half of the 20 women in the study [12].

Conclusion

Clonidine, SSRIs and gabapentin have all shown a significant improvement in flashing, whilst vitamin E and evening primrose oil have been shown to be of no benefit. Adverse effects may limit the use of clonidine and gabapentin, but SSRIs and SNRIs have a well-established safety profile and appear to have only minor adverse effects.

The evidence surrounding the efficacy of phytoestrogens and black cohosh is contradictory. Soy isoflavones may be more effective with longer-term use than other phytoestrogens, but black cohosh, or any compound with estrogenic properties, should be used with extreme caution in women with a history of breast cancer or any other estrogen-dependent disease.

The effectiveness of stellate ganglion blockade for vasomotor symptoms is unconfirmed, therefore further studies are required. It is also worth considering that the uptake of this treatment may be limited as it is costly, invasive and the short-term side effects of Horner's syndrome may be unacceptable to some.

References

1. Freedman RR. Biochemical: metabolic, and vascular mechanisms in menopausal hot flashes. *Fertil Steril* 1998; **70**: 332–7.

2. Freedman RR, Krell W. Reduced thermoregulatory null zone in postmenopausal women with hot flashes. *Am J Obstet Gynecol* 1999; **181**: 66–70.

3. Nelson HD, Vesco KK, Haney E, *et al.* Nonhormonal therapies for menopausal hot flashes: systematic review and meta-analysis. *JAMA* 2006; **295**: 2057–71.

4. Rada G, Capurro D, Pantoja T, *et al.* Non-hormonal interventions for hot flushes in women with a history of breast cancer. *Cochrane Database of Systematic Reviews* 2010; **9**: CD004923.

5. Speroff L, Gass M, Constantine GD, Olivier S, Study 315 Investigators. Efficacy and tolerability of desvenlafaxine succinate treatment for menopausal vasomotor symptoms: a randomized controlled trial. *Obstet Gynecol* 2008; **111**: 77–87.

6. Archer DF, Dupont CM, Constantine GD, Pickar JH, Olivier S, Study 319 Investigators. Desvenlafaxine for the treatment of vasomotor symptoms associated with menopause: a double-blind, randomized, placebo-controlled trial of efficacy and safety. *Am J Obstet Gynecol* 2009; **200**: 238e1–e10.

7. Lethaby A, Marjoribanks J, Kronenberg F, *et al.* Phytoestrogens for vasomotor menopausal symptoms. *Cochrane Database Syst Rev* 2007; **4**: CD001395.

8. Wong VC, Lim CE, Luo X, Wong WS. Current alternative and complementary therapies used in menopause. *Gynecol Endocrinol* 2009; **25**: 166–74.

9. Newton KM, Reed SD, LaCroix AZ, *et al.* Treatment of vasomotor symptoms of menopause with black cohosh, multibotanicals, soy, hormone therapy, or placebo: a randomized trial. *Ann Intern Med* 2005; **145**: 869–79.

10. Barton DL, Loprinzi CL, Quella SK, *et al.* Prospective evaluation of vitamin E for hot flashes in breast cancer survivors. *J Clin Oncol* 1998; **16**: 495–500.

11. Daley A, Stokes-Lampard H, Mutrie N, MacArthur C. Exercise for vasomotor menopausal symptoms. *Cochrane Database Syst Rev* 2007; **4**: CD006108.

12. van Gastel P, Kallewaard J-W, van der Zanden M, de Boer H. Stellate-ganglion block as a treatment for severe postmenopausal flushing. *Climacteric* 2013; **16**: 41–7.

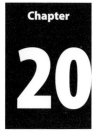

Chapter 20

Alternative therapies for the management of menopausal symptoms

Edzard Ernst and Paul Posadzki

Prevalence of alternative therapies-use by menopausal women

For the purpose of this chapter, we operationally define alternative therapies (ATs) as medical interventions which are not usually used in conventional medicine. Other terms frequently employed to describe this sector include complementary, holistic, folk, traditional, natural or integrative therapies/medicine.

The question of how many menopausal women use ATs is perhaps best answered by considering the existing evidence in this area. Our systematic review (SR) of 26 surveys including 32,465 menopausal women found that on average 50.5% of them reported using ATs specifically for their menopausal symptoms [1]. The 12-month prevalence of use was on average 47.7% (range: 33.1–56.2). Nearly one third of the surveyed women declared themselves to be current/regular AT users. Fifty-five percent did not disclose their use of ATs to their conventional health-care team. The majority of women sought information about ATs from the Internet, i.e. doctors or other health-care professionals were not considered as a source of information about ATs. The most popular AT was herbal medicine, followed by relaxation therapies and yoga. Alternative therapies were perceived as effective by 60.5% of all women using them (range: 42–98.8).

Expectations of patients using alternative therapies

For many health-care professionals, this popularity of ATs is somewhat puzzling. They point out that conventional medicine is today more effective than it ever has been, and that turning to uncertain alternatives is therefore less than rational. The reasons for the present boom in ATs are certainly not easy to define, and numerous factors are likely to play a role:

- Incessant media hype.
- Disappointment with conventional medicine.
- Fear of side effects.
- Hope for a cure without risks.
- Desperation.
- Affluence.

In this context, it is relevant to ask what patients expect from ATs. We have attempted to answer this question by conducting a SR of all 73 surveys that addressed this issue [2]. A wide range of expectations emerged. In order of prevalence, they included:

Managing the Menopause: 21st Century Solutions, ed. Nick Panay, Paula Briggs, and Gab Kovacs. Published by Cambridge University Press. © Cambridge University Press 2015.

- Hope to influence the natural history of the disease.
- Disease prevention and health/general well-being promotion.
- Fewer side effects.
- Being in control over one's health.
- Symptom relief; boosting the immune system.
- Emotional support.
- Holistic care.
- Improving quality of life.
- Relief of side effects of conventional medicine.
- Good therapeutic relationship.
- Obtaining information.
- Coping better with illness.
- Supporting the natural healing process.
- Availability of treatment.

Claims made by proponents of alternative therapies

Many patients with menopausal symptoms search the Internet in the hope of finding a safe and effective treatment for their condition. A woman using the Google search engine for "alternative treatments for menopause" would currently be inundated by more than 11 million websites. Disappointingly, very few of these sources offer reliable information. Many seem to promote unproven or disproven treatments and some even discourage the use of proven conventional therapies.

Further evidence seems to confirm the assumption that women are frequently misled: after identifying the seven best-selling lay books on ATs, we assessed which treatments their authors recommended for a range of specific conditions. For menopausal symptoms, they advised 68 different ATs. There was very little consensus amongst the seven authors as to which treatments were recommendable, and the vast majority of the recommended therapies were not supported by sound evidence [3].

The evidence for alternative therapies
Effectiveness

In an overview of the evidence from SRs, randomized controlled trials (RCTs) and epidemiologic studies of ATs for the management of menopausal symptoms, we attempted to assess the existing data critically [4]. We found that some promising evidence was available for phytosterols and phytostanols for reducing increased low-density lipoprotein (LDL) and total cholesterol levels in postmenopausal women. Similarly, regular fiber intake seemed to be effective in reducing serum total cholesterol in hypercholesterolemic post-menopausal women. Black cohosh seemed to be effective therapy for relieving menopausal symptoms, primarily hot flashes, in early menopause. Phytoestrogens, including isoflavones and lignans, appeared to have only minimal effect on hot flashes but may have other positive health effects, e.g. on plasma lipid levels and bone loss [5]. Promising evidence also existed for the effectiveness of vitamin K, a combination of calcium and vitamin D as well as for a combination of walking combined with other weight-bearing exercise in reducing bone mineral density loss and the incidence of osteoporosis/fractures in postmenopausal women [6, 7]. In premenopausal women, encouraging evidence for the effectiveness of vitamin B6 supplementation has been found [8].

Relaxation therapies seem to have positive effects on menopausal symptoms [3]. For other commonly used ATs including probiotics, prebiotics, acupuncture, homeopathy and dehydroepiandrosterone sulfate (DHEA-S), placebo-controlled RCTs are scarce and the evidence was thus unconvincing [3]. Similarly, there is insufficient evidence for the effectiveness of other popular modalities such as yoga [4] or ginseng [9].

Safety
Direct risks

Consumers often assume that ATs are inherently safe, not least because the media incessantly promote this notion. However, the assumption is clearly not correct. As there are no (or very few) systems to monitor adverse effects of ATs, it is plausible that the documented risks merely represent the tip of a much bigger iceberg. In particular, oral supplements can cause adverse effects through:

- The toxicity of an ingredient.
- Interactions with prescribed medications.
- Contamination.
- Adulteration.

Alternative therapies and therapists are usually not tightly regulated which can increase their risks considerably. Table 20.1 summarizes the known risks of the types of ATs mentioned above.

Indirect risks

Even if an AT is entirely safe, such as a highly diluted homeopathic remedy, there are indirect risks to consider [10]. The most obvious of those is that a curable condition might get treated for prolonged periods of time with a therapy that is ineffective. In fact, even the most harmless but ineffective AT can become life-threatening, if it is used as an alternative for treating a serious condition.

The risk-benefit balance

It is often argued by proponents of ATs that the risks of their treatments are far less than those of conventional therapies. This may well be true, but it is irrelevant for judging the value of any given intervention. Therapeutic decisions should never be guided by their effectiveness or their safety in isolation but by balancing the two factors. If a treatment has no or little demonstrable benefit, as seems to be the case for many ATs, then even relatively small risks would tilt this balance into the negative, and the treatment in question cannot be recommended for routine use.

Methodological problems in evaluating the effectiveness of alternative therapies

Advocates of ATs often argue that it is unfair to insist on rigorous evidence for their treatments; not only are there no funds to carry out such necessary research, but there are also significant methodological problems in testing ATs for effectiveness. These arguments

Table 20.1. Risks of particular alternative treatments for menopause.

Type of alternative treatment	Examples of adverse effects reported in the medical literature
Acupuncture	Bleeding, infections, pneumothorax, nerve injury and death
Black cohosh	Gastrointestinal upset, rash, acute hepatitis, multiorgan failure
Dietary supplements (general)	Overdosing, toxicity, interactions with prescribed drugs
Ginseng	Anxiety, burning sensation, flu, headache, insomnia, pain, skin problem, gastrointestinal upset
Herbal remedies (general)	Adulteration, contamination, toxicity, herb/drug interactions
Homeopathy	Delay of effective therapy
Prebiotics	Bloating, abdominal pain, diarrhea, increase in gastroesophageal reflux
Probiotics	Sepsis, altered metabolism, or immune system functioning, increased sensitivity to allergens
Phytoestrogens	Disruption of endogenous hormone levels and the ovulatory cycle, changes in behavior
Phytostanols	Lowered absorption of liposoluble vitamins and antioxidants
Phytosterols	Diarrhea, constipation, skin problems
Relaxation	Worsening of psychological problems
Yoga	Bone fractures, ligament tears
Vitamin B6	Arrhythmia, acne, allergic reactions, drowsiness or sedation, headache, heartburn, loss of appetite, nausea, rash, recurrence of ulcerative colitis, vomiting
Vitamin D	Nausea, vomiting, weakness, kidney problems
Vitamin K	Difficulties in breathing or swallowing, enlarged liver, skin rashes, dizziness, irritability, muscle stiffness

are, however, only partly correct. It seems high time to channel some of this money into the much-needed biomedical research.

As to the methodological problems, they mostly exist in some areas of ATs. Oral supplements, including herbal remedies, for instance, can and should be tested much like conventional medicines, i.e. by conducting placebo-controlled RCTs. When it comes to other treatments such as yoga, hypnotherapy, acupuncture etc., things can get more complex. What, for example, might be a reasonable placebo control for a trial of hypnotherapy? In some instances, this might mean that placebo controls and patient-blinding are simply impossible. However, this does not mean that RCTs comparing such ATs with standard care cannot be done.

In our experience, the biggest problem by far lies in the mind-set of alternative therapists who often are reluctant to conduct rigorous tests of their interventions. Whether this sentiment originates from the fear that such tests might be negative or from a wider anti-scientific attitude seems irrelevant; the fact is that it represents an important obstacle to progress in this area.

Common misunderstandings about alternative therapies

Because of the current popularity of ATs, it is tempting to assume that thousands of people cannot be mistaken in assuming that these treatments are effective. However, the appeal to belief, practice or popularity is a classic fallacy. Belief can be wrong, practice can be misguided and popularity is certainly not a reliable indicator for effectiveness. The history of medicine is littered with examples which demonstrate how misleading these fallacies can be.

If a menopausal woman enjoys an AT and subsequently feels better, what could be more logical than to assume that the treatment was the cause of her improvement? This conclusion seems obvious to patients and therapists alike – yet it is fallacious. Apart from the treatment *per se*, a whole range of factors can cause or at least contribute to a clinical improvement in that patient: the placebo effect, the natural history of menopause, the regression towards the mean, to mention just three. In other words, the patient can get better after administering ineffective or even mildly harmful remedies; and the word "subsequently" has not the same meaning as "consequently." Causal inferences based on anecdotes are highly problematic and rarely a sound basis for robust conclusions about the effectiveness of ATs.

Enthusiasts of ATs claim that their treatments have stood the "test of time" and that this test is more relevant than that of a clinical trial. A long tradition of use can, of course, be an *indicator* for the safety and efficacy of a treatment, but it can never be a *proof*. On the contrary, a long history might also mean that the origins of that therapy reach back to a time when our understanding of anatomy, physiology etc. was in its infancy. This in turn, might lessen the chances for any such intervention to be plausible or effective.

An entire industry has developed around the notion that ATs are natural and therefore safe. The implication is that conventional treatments are unnatural, heavily based on chemicals which are potentially harmful. Nature, by contrast, is seen as benign and "natural remedies" are therefore to be preferred. This argument is as effective for marketing purposes as it is wrong. Firstly, by no means are all ATs natural. For instance, there is nothing natural in sticking needles into a patient's body (as in acupuncture) or endlessly diluting and shaking a remedy (as in homeopathy). Secondly, nature is not necessarily benign. Even "natural" herbal extracts are not necessarily safe – just think of hemlock!

Conclusions

Many women suffering from menopausal symptoms use ATs regularly. These women deserve reliable information about the effectiveness and the risks of ATs. Despite much advertising to the contrary, very few ATs have been shown to be effective and none are entirely free of risks. Researchers need to re-double their efforts in critically evaluating ATs for a whole range of climacteric symptoms with the aim of improving health and quality of life in this population.

References

1. Posadzki P, Lee MS, Moon TW, *et al.* Prevalence of complementary and alternative medicine (CAM) use by menopausal women: a systematic review of surveys. *Maturitas* 2013; 75: 34–43.

2. Ernst E, Hung SK. Great expectations: what do patients using complementary and alternative medicine hope for? *Patient* 2011; **4**: 89–101.

3. Ernst E, Pittler MH, Wider B. *The Desktop Guide to Complementary and Alternative Medicine: An Evidence-Based Approach.* Edinburgh: Mosby Elsevier; 2006.

4. Borrelli F, Ernst E. Alternative and complementary therapies for the menopause. *Maturitas* 2010; **66**: 333–43.

5. Clement YN, Onakpoya I, Hung SK, Ernst E. Effects of herbal and dietary supplements on cognition in menopause: a systematic review. *Maturitas* 2011; **68**: 256–63.

6. Whelan AM, Jurgens TM, Bowles SK. Natural health products in the prevention and treatment of osteoporosis: systematic review of randomized controlled trials. *Ann Pharmacother* 2006; **40**: 836–49.

7. Zehnacker CH, Bemis-Dougherty A. Effect of weighted exercises on bone mineral density in post menopausal women. A systematic review. *J Geriatr Phys Ther* 2007; **30**: 79–88.

8. Williams AL, Cotter A, Sabina A, *et al.* The role for vitamin B-6 as treatment for depression: a systematic review. *Family Practice* 2005; **22**: 532–7.

9. Kim MS, Lim HJ, Yang HJ, *et al.* Ginseng for managing menopause symptoms: a systematic review of randomized clinical trials. *J Ginseng Res* 2013; **37**: 30–6.

10. Posadzki P, Alotaibi A, Ernst E. Adverse effects of homeopathy: a systematic review of published case reports and case series. *Int J Clin Pract* 2012; **66**: 1178–88.

Contraception for the perimenopausal woman

Lee P. Shulman and Jessica W. Kiley

Introduction

The North American Menopause Society (NAMS) defines perimenopause as the time from the onset of menstrual changes and menopause-related symptoms until 1 year after cessation of menses [1]. This time is typically characterized by an increasing frequency of menstrual irregularity along with menopausal-related symptoms such as hot flashes, night sweats, sleep disruption, mood fluctuations and reduced libido. There is no set time for the onset or conclusion of the perimenopause, although it usually begins when a woman is in her 40s. As the time for this transition differs from woman to woman, so does its clinical presentation. What is common among all women during the perimenopause is a gradual reduction in, but not a complete loss of, the ability to conceive. Of interest is that the unintended pregnancy rate hovers around 40% in the USA for women over the age of 40 [2]. This is an unfortunate result of a convergence of erroneous beliefs. These include:

Pregnancy is nearly biologically impossible in sexually active women during the perimenopause.

The canard that women engage in little to no sexual activity during their 40s or 50s that would place them at risk of becoming pregnant.

Highly effective contraceptive methods are not needed and should not be used by perimenopausal women because of this as well as safety concerns.

What is accurate is that, by definition, perimenopausal women who are sexually active are exposed to the risk of becoming pregnant and there are no hormonal methods of contraception, regardless of their composition or mode of delivery, that are contraindicated solely on the basis of a woman's age. In addition, such methods of contraception provide not only effective pregnancy prevention, but can also provide important non-contraceptive benefits for women during the perimenopause. To this end, we will present an overview of contraceptive methods amenable for use by women during the perimenopause and into the early years of menopause.

Contraceptive needs of the perimenopausal woman

As the perimenopause characterizes a transitional time in a woman's reproductive life, her risk of pregnancy during this time is likewise characterized by that transition, which is directly related to reduced frequency and increased irregularity of ovulation. From ages

Managing the Menopause: 21st Century Solutions, ed. Nick Panay, Paula Briggs, and Gab Kovacs.
Published by Cambridge University Press. © Cambridge University Press 2015.

40–44, the chance of pregnancy in a sexually active woman not using contraception is estimated to be approximately 30% per year while that is further reduced to 10% per year in women aged 45–49 [3]. Increasing menstrual irregularity and menopausal symptoms reflect the reduced ovulatory frequency associated with the perimenopausal transition. The likelihood of pregnancy during this time is directly related to decreased ovulatory frequency, as well as coital frequency, male partner fertility and effectiveness of contraception used.

As frequency of ovulation diminishes, menstrual cycle length increases, although increasing length of the menstrual cycle does not necessarily indicate an anovulatory cycle; 25% of cycles greater than 50 days in length are ovulatory in nature, thus making increasing menstrual irregularity a poor predictor of fertility [4]. As there are no reliable predictors of fecundity in perimenopausal women, any woman who is sexually active with menstrual activity, but using no contraception, is exposed to a risk of pregnancy and contraception is advised if pregnancy is to be avoided. As a woman ages, her aging oocytes result in an increased likelihood of fetal aneuploidy (e.g., trisomy 21) and there is a consequent increase in spontaneous fetal loss and chromosomally abnormal offspring. In addition, increasing maternal age is also associated with an increased risk of adverse maternal obstetric outcomes. These may be exacerbated by a concomitant increase in comorbidities such as obesity, hypertension and diabetes. Accordingly, contraception in sexually active women during the perimenopause is important, not only to prevent pregnancy, but also to prevent the profound morbidity and mortality associated with pregnancy during the later stages of a woman's reproductive life.

Contraceptive options during the perimenopause

When discussing contraceptive options for women during the perimenopause, it is again important to acknowledge that there are no age barriers to the use of any reversible method of contraception. Women who have decided that they no longer wish to become pregnant can choose from permanent methods of pregnancy prevention such as tubal sterilization, or a hysteroscopic tubal occlusion procedure such as the Essure™ system. For those women who may wish to conceive in the future or do not wish to undergo permanent sterilization, or may wish to avail themselves of the non-contraceptive benefits of certain reversible methods of contraception, the full array of contraceptive choices are potentially amenable for use (Table 21.1). However, while age itself does not rule out the use of any method of contraception, the onset of certain age-related conditions such as hypertension, diabetes, cancer and other cardiovascular conditions may preclude the use of certain methods of contraception, particularly those containing estrogen, because of concerns regarding safety. The effectiveness (typical use) of all methods of contraception are likely greater for women during the perimenopause because of the inherent decrease in fecundity associated with this stage in a woman's reproductive life. This is best characterized by the current practice of assessing the effectiveness of a contraceptive regimen in women in clinical trials aged 18 through 35 years, but evaluating the safety of the regimen in women aged up to 45 years.

Benefits of contraception

Aside from the prevention of pregnancy and its associated morbidities, certain hormonal contraceptive regimens can alleviate the increasing frequency and severity of the symptoms of menopause that are commonly experienced by women. In particular, regimens containing estrogen, regardless of the mode of delivery, can be effective in reducing symptoms of vasomotor instability including hot flashes and night sweats [5]. As these methods work by

Table 21.1. Non-hormonal contraceptives.

Method	Failure rate (%:perfect/typical)	Drug delivery	Dosing regimen (label)
Male condom	2/18	None	Condom placed on penis *prior* to vaginal insertion and left on until ejaculation *and* removal from vagina. May be used concomitantly with vaginal spermicidal agent
Female condom	5/21	None	Vaginal placement of condom and left *in situ* until ejaculation and removal of penis. May be used concomitantly with vaginal spermicidal agent
Cervical cap	6/12	None	Device inserted *prior* to vaginal insertion and left *in situ* until ejaculation *and* removal from vagina. May be used concomitantly with vaginal spermicidal agent
Diaphragm	6/12	None	Device inserted *prior* to vaginal insertion and left *in situ* until ejaculation *and* removal from vagina. May be used concomitantly with vaginal spermicidal agent
Vaginal spermicide	18/28	None	Gel inserted *prior* to vaginal insertion of penis
IUD	0.6/0.8	Copper	Inserted at a time when pregnancy is not likely (e.g., menses). Left *in situ* for prescribed period of effectiveness. Removed and replaced if further contraception is desired

Source: Trussell J. Contraceptive efficacy. In Hatcher RA, Trussell J, Nelson AL, Cates Jr W, Kowal D, Policar MS (eds). *Contraceptive Technology, Twentieth Revised Edition*. Valley Stream, NY: Ardent Media; 2013, pp. 69–76.

inhibiting ovulation, they can also be effective in regulating the menstrual irregularities characteristic of the perimenopause.

While progestin-only contraceptives do not contain estrogen and thus are unlikely to provide relief from the estrogen-dependent symptoms of vasomotor instability, they can be effective in managing irregular menstrual bleeding (Table 21.2). In particular, the levonorgestrel-containing intrauterine system (LNG-IUS: Mirena™) and the progestin-only pill (POP) containing 75 µg desogestrel (Cerazette™) may be effective in regulating menstrual bleeding, albeit by different mechanisms. The LNG-IUS exerts a mostly suppressive effect on the endometrium resulting in a relatively high frequency of amenorrhea after the first year of use. In addition, the LNG-IUS is effective for endometrial protection (off-label in the USA, but approved for 4 years in the UK) in women transitioning to menopausal hormone therapy. Conversely, the POP containing 75 mcg desogestrel (not available in the USA) effectively inhibits ovulation and exerts an inhibitory effect on the endometrium and

Table 21.2. Progestin-only hormonal contraceptives[1].

Method	Failure rate (%:perfect/typical)	Drug delivery	Dosing regimen (label)
Oral contraceptives	0.3/9	Oral	Daily ingestion of pill; most regimens are continuous use in nature
Injectables	0.2/6	IM/SC	Intramuscular or subcutaneous initiation for prescribed time period. Reinjection at end of the time period if continued contraception is desired
Subdermal implant	0.05/0.05	Subdermal	Subdermal placement of implant system and left *in situ* for prescribed period of effectiveness. Removed at end of time period and replaced if continued contraception is desired
Intrauterine contraceptive LNG-IUS[2]	0.2/0.2	LNG[3]	Inserted at a time when pregnancy is not likely (e.g., menses). Left *in situ* for prescribed period of effectiveness. Removed and replaced if further contraception is desired

[1] All methods are typically started at the start of or during a normal menstrual bleed, a time at which a woman is most likely to not be pregnant, and allows for best temporal management of contraception. Discontinuation of all methods should be done at the conclusion of a usage cycle, except in cases of medical emergencies (e.g., cardiovascular event such as myocardial infarction). *Source*: Trussell J. Contraceptive efficacy. In Hatcher RA, Trussell J, Nelson AL, Cates Jr W, Kowal D, Policar MS (eds). *Contraceptive Technology, Twentieth Revised Edition*. Valley Stream, NY: Ardent Media; 2013, pp. 69–76.
[2] LNG-IUS: Levonorgestrel Intrauterine System (Mirena™).
[3] LNG: Levonorgestrel.

a thickening of the cervical mucus, which is different from most POPs (those available in the USA) that contain a subinhibitory dose of progestin which fails to consistently inhibit ovulation, but exert their contraceptive effect mostly by local mechanisms of endometrial suppression and cervical mucus thickening. While these POPs would clearly provide effective contraception to a perimenopausal woman, they would likely not provide relief for the menstrual irregularity experienced by these women.

Risks of contraception

There has been much controversy concerning the risks for thromboembolic events associated with methods containing estrogen, regardless of the mode of delivery. What is not controversial is that estrogen-containing contraceptive regimens do increase the risk for thrombogenesis. They are typically associated with a 2- to 3-fold increased risk for venous thromboembolic events and ischemic stroke. What has been controversial has been whether newer contraceptive regimens that contain newer progestins, regardless of the delivery system, further increase that risk. A more detailed assessment of this literature is not in the purview of this chapter; however, it is important to recognize that the baseline risks for thromboembolic events increase with advancing age and other factors such as obesity, immobility, congenital predisposition to thromboembolic events, use of estrogen-containing regimens and pregnancy. Accordingly, women during the perimenopause are at an increased risk for thromboembolic events based solely on their age and health status, regardless of the use of any exogenous hormones. As such, only those women who do not have additional cardiovascular or thromboembolic risks should be considered candidates for combination hormonal contraception for pregnancy prevention and symptom relief. Importantly, the risk of VTE associated with the use of estrogen-containing products should be considered in the context of the risk of VTE during pregnancy. Rates of VTE in normal pregnancy are 3- to 4-fold higher than rates associated with use of low-dose combined oral contraceptive pills. Methods that do not contain estrogen do not increase the risks for thromboembolic events and thus may be used by women at increased risk for such adverse outcomes. However, such methods will likely not provide relief for the symptoms of vasomotor instability increasingly experienced by perimenopausal women.

The incidence of breast cancer is low among young women but begins to rise considerably as women begin their fifth decade, with women aged 40–49 years having an approximately 1 in 60 risk for developing breast cancer [6]. As with the risk of thromboembolic events with newer combination methods, there is much controversy in the literature concerning the impact of hormonal contraceptives on the risk for developing breast cancer, with some studies showing a small increase in risk among COC users while others show no such increase. However, as with the use of hormonal contraceptives in younger women, there is no supporting evidence that family history or age at initiation, duration of use or type of hormonal contraceptive used have a substantial impact in the risk of breast cancer [7]. Accordingly, except for those women with a contraindication to the use of hormonal contraception (i.e., women with breast cancer), the use of hormonal contraceptives during the perimenopausal years should not further increase the already increasing risk of breast cancer based on their age and other risk factors. Therefore combined hormonal contraception can be considered for pregnancy prevention and symptom relief in appropriately counseled women.

Reversible contraceptive methods

Except for those with specific contraindications to a particular method(s) of contraception, women seeking pregnancy prevention and symptom relief may choose permanent sterilization or from a variety of reversible contraceptive methods containing a progestin alone, a combination of estrogen and progestin or a non-hormonal method. The methods below are currently available reversible contraceptives amenable for use by appropriately counseled women during the perimenopause.

Barrier methods/non-hormonal methods

Barrier contraceptive methods include male and female condoms, diaphragms and the cervical cap (Table 21.1). These methods are coital-dependent and may be used with a vaginal spermicide, or the vaginal spermicide may be used by itself. As these methods are used at the time of coitus and require correct use for optimal contraception, their use is typically associated with a failure rate (pregnancy rate) of 10–15% (higher than that observed with hormonal and intrauterine methods). In addition, penile withdrawal and natural family planning options can be grouped with these methods and are also associated with comparable failure rates. For women seeking highly effective contraception for personal or medical reasons, the use of these methods alone would not be acceptable, even in a perimenopausal woman. In addition, these methods would not provide menopausal symptom relief.

All barrier methods provide non-hormonal contraception; however, there is a non-hormonal method that provides highly effective and reversible contraception. The intra-uterine device (IUD), most commonly containing copper but potentially composed of other inert materials, is a highly effective method of contraception with pregnancy (failure) rates approximating 1%. While non-hormonal IUDs do not provide symptom relief, they are one of the long-acting reversible contraceptive (LARC) methods that provide lasting and reliable contraception after insertion (by an appropriately trained clinician). Copper IUDs can also be used as a very effective emergency contraceptive option and some women will choose to continue to use the IUD for ongoing contraception (Table 21.1).

The potential for development or exacerbation of heavy menstrual bleeding (HMB), may make this a less attractive option for women in the perimenopause – a time when bleeding can become problematic in association with menstrual irregularity.

Progestin-only methods

Progestin-only methods are available in a variety of delivery systems, from pills (POPs) to subdermal implants to injectables to intrauterine delivery systems (Table 21.2). As these methods do not contain estrogen, they are not expected to provide vasomotor symptom relief, but will provide highly effective contraception without the additional risks associated with estrogen use. In addition, some progestin-only methods may provide relief for the menstrual irregularity characteristic of the perimenopause.

Progestin-only pills are generally considered to be slightly less effective than combination oral contraceptives (COCs) with a perfect-use failure rate of approximately 5–6%, though the higher-dose 75 µg desogestrel pill (see above) likely has a contraceptive effectiveness comparable to COCs. As opposed to most (but not all) COCs, POP regimens have no pill-free days in their dosing schedule.

The subdermal implant is provided in a variety of progestin-only regimens with various progestins, durations of use and number of inserted implants. There are also some combination subdermal regimens, though such combination regimens are only available in select regions, are not manufactured by major pharmaceutical companies and will not be reviewed in this chapter. All progestin-only implant regimens are considered to be LARC methods and require insertion and removal by trained clinicians, as do intrauterine contraceptive methods. Implants provide highly effective contraception (failure rates less than 1%) by ovulation suppression as well as local contraceptive effects (e.g., thickened cervical mucus, endometrial suppression). However, along with a lack of symptom relief is the frequent side effect of irregular and unscheduled bleeding patterns that may actually exacerbate a perimenopausal woman's bleeding pattern. A widely available subdermal implant is the etonogestrel implant (Implanon™; Nexplanon™; Implanon NXT™), which is a 3-year, single rod implant system that has biological plausibility as an endometrial suppressor for exogenous estrogen therapy, though with no corroborating clinical studies to demonstrate its effectiveness and side effect profile if used in this manner for peri- and postmenopausal women.

Injectable progestin-only contraceptives have been available for more than 50 years and are still widely used worldwide. The most commonly used injectable is depot-medroxyprogesterone acetate (DMPA) that contains 150 mg of MPA in a depot (crystalline) form that is injected intramuscularly and provides highly effective contraception (failure rates of approximately 1%) by ovulation inhibition and local effects for up to 3 months. While this method is associated with a high rate of amenorrhea (no vaginal bleeding) (up to 70% at 1 year of use), return to fertility may be delayed after discontinuation, which may be a problem for women seeking pregnancy during the later stages of their reproductive lives.

Progestin-only intrauterine systems are LARC methods that provide highly effective contraception (failure rates of approximately 1%) and require insertion and removal by trained clinicians. Up until recently, the LNG-IUS (Mirena™, see above), a contraceptive that lasts for up to 5 years, was the only such method that was universally available and associated with an increased likelihood (approximately 30%) of no vaginal bleeding at 1 year of use. A LNG-IUS provides endometrial protection in association with estrogen making it amenable for transition to menopausal hormone therapy. A lower-dosed LNG-IUS (Jadelle™, also known as Skyla™) has recently been introduced and is licensed to provide contraception only for up to 3 years, though without the same reduced bleeding frequency characteristic of the higher-dosed LNG-IUS.

Emergency hormonal contraception (EHC) can also be used in the perimenopause.

The most frequently used emergency contraceptive regimen is levonorgestrel 1.5 mg, taken orally as a single dose up to 5 days after unprotected intercourse (licensed to be used up to 72 hours, but commonly used up to 120 hours outside the product license). The effectiveness of this method is dependent on several factors, including baseline fertility and the day in the menstrual cycle when the unprotected sex occurs. Effectiveness estimates range from 80–90%, and it is reasonable to hypothesize that perimenopausal women would see higher effectiveness, again as a result of reduced fecundity. The World Health Organization and the Centers for Disease Control do not restrict use of levonorgestrel emergency contraception in older women – in fact, there is no medical condition in which emergency contraception is contraindicated.

The use of ulipristal acetate, in stat dose of 30 mg (available in some countries for EHC) is not contraindicated in perimenopausal women.

Combination hormonal methods

All combined hormonal contraceptive methods currently contain an estrogen and progestin and are widely available in a variety of delivery systems including pills, transdermal patches and vaginal rings (Table 21.3). All such methods provide highly effective contraception when used consistently and correctly, as well as potential relief from vasomotor symptoms associated with the perimenopause, though all are associated with the aforementioned safety issues (i.e., thrombogenesis) associated with estrogen use. Almost all such methods include a hormone-free interval in the dosing regimen. This dates back to the introduction of higher-dosed COC regimens in the early 1960s that included a respite from hormone ingestion (most commonly 7 days) in order to provide a consistently timed menstrual-like withdrawal bleed. However, as the doses in combined methods have decreased considerably over the decades and more women have become interested in reducing or eliminating the withdrawal bleed, that interval can be reduced from the original 7-day interval after a 3-week dosing regimen to 4 days or less. It has been completely eliminated in some regimens ("trimonthly pills") or by off-label use.

Over the years, the progestin component has seen the most variation with new progestins being developed to ostensibly improve the tolerability of the regimen; until recently, the estrogen component has mostly been ethinyl estradiol (EE), which has been progressively reduced in daily dose from 100 µg to as low as 10 µg. In addition, several new COC pills

Table 21.3. Combination hormonal contraceptives[1].

Method	Failure rate (%:perfect/typical)	Drug delivery	Dosing regimen (label)
Oral contraceptives	0.3/9	Oral	Daily ingestion of pill; most regimens still 21/7, though more with 24/4 and 26/2 and some continuous use regimens
Vaginal ring	0.3/9	Vaginal	Vaginal placement of ring and left *in situ* for 3 weeks; removed for a 1 week ring-free interval before replacing a new ring
Transdermal patch	0.3/9	Skin	Transdermal patch placement and left *in situ* for 1 week. Patch is then removed and replaced with new patch. Repeated for 3 weeks and then followed by a patch-free week before reinitiation

[1] All methods are typically begun at the start of or during a normal menstrual bleed, a time at which a woman is most likely to not be pregnant and allows for best temporal management of contraception. Discontinuation of all methods should be done at the conclusion of a usage cycle, except in cases of medical emergencies (e.g., cardiovascular event such as myocardial infarction). *Source:* Trussell J. Contraceptive efficacy. In Hatcher RA, Trussell J, Nelson AL, Cates Jr W, Kowal D, Policar MS (eds). *Contraceptive Technology, Twentieth Revised Edition.* Valley Stream, NY: Ardent Media; 2013, pp. 69–76.

containing estradiol in lieu of EE have recently been developed and launched, though there is no current evidence that such pills differ from EE-containing pills with regard to safety or effectiveness. Indeed, all estrogen-containing regimens, regardless of the type, dose or mode of delivery of estrogen and progestin, should be considered to have similar benefits and safety concerns; that is, there is no one estrogen-containing method that should be considered to be "safer" than another. Generally speaking, COCs containing less than 50 μg of EE are considered "low-dose," and the clinical benefit(s) of using the lowest EE dose formulations (i.e, 10 to 20 μg of EE) remain unclear.

The trend in COCs has been to reduce the dose of both hormones, employ more tolerable hormonal components and reduce the number of hormone-free days during the dosing regimen. Combined oral contraceptives provide for highly effective (approximately 1% failure rate) contraception when used consistently and correctly (perfect use), though typical failure rates may be as high as 8%, mostly as result of "user failure" with the need to "take" the pill reliably to ensure optimal contraceptive and non-contraceptive benefits. In addition to their contraceptive effects and amelioration of menopausal symptoms, COCs have also been associated with a reduced risk of ovarian epithelial and endometrial cancers as well as colorectal cancer, though it is not clear if initiation of COCs during the perimenopause would exact the same disease-reducing effects as when started earlier in the reproductive years. Conversely, some studies have found an increased risk for cervical cancer among COC users, though this is likely due to increased transmission of high-risk strains of human papilloma virus (HPV) in COC users who may be less likely to use a concomitant barrier method (i.e., male condom) that would reduce the likelihood of HPV transmission.

In addition to COCs, non-oral combination methods such as the transdermal patch and vaginal ring are widely used globally. These methods also provide highly effective contraception with contraceptive and non-contraceptive characteristics similar to COCs without the need for daily, oral dosing. The transdermal patch (Ortho-Evra™; Evra™) is a once-a-week patch (3-week dosing regimen followed by a patch-free week) that provides a highly effective method of contraception (perfect-use pregnancy rate of approximately 1%). It may be a more overall effective contraceptive because of the once-weekly dosing regimen, reducing the margin for user error. A combination vaginal ring (NuvaRing™) is also available, which is self-placed at the top of the vagina, left *in situ* for 3 weeks and then removed for a ring-free week; the vaginal ring is characterized by high contraceptive efficacy and tolerability, similar to that of the transdermal patch. Continuous use (off-label) of these methods, as well as COCs, can provide a woman with a high likelihood of no withdrawal bleeding, though use of all such methods can be associated with unscheduled bleeding and spotting after several cycles of continuous use.

Transition to menopausal management

Women not exposed to pregnancy (e.g., post sterilization, not sexually active) during the perimenopause may still benefit from the use of certain contraceptives (off-label) based on the presence and severity of certain symptoms. Many of the contraceptives described here contain either a combination of an estrogen and progestin, or are progestin-only delivery systems. As discussed previously, combination methods can reduce the symptoms of vasomotor instability and provide relief from the changing bleeding patterns associated with the perimenopause. Certain progestin-only methods may provide relief from the menstrual bleeding changes associated with the perimenopause, but are not likely to provide non-bleeding symptom relief.

Such regimens can be used throughout the perimenopause in appropriately counseled and evaluated women. The onset of menopause heralds a time in which a woman is no longer able to conceive and thus does not require pregnancy prevention. However, many women entering the menopause may present with an exacerbation of the non-bleeding symptoms of the perimenopause, including hot flashes, night sweats, vaginal dryness and mood alterations. While menopausal hormone therapies might not reverse all of these menopausal-related symptoms, they can substantially reduce many of these symptoms that adversely affect a woman's health and well-being. Many of the combination contraceptive regimens, regardless of the mode of delivery, can be used during the early stages of menopause to provide both contraception and symptom control.

Conclusions

The unintended pregnancy rate among women during the perimenopause is surprisingly high, mostly as a result of profound and interrelated misperceptions: firstly, that women during their perimenopausal years are unlikely and even unable to conceive and secondly, that such women do not need to use highly effective contraception, and concerns about the safety of such methods when used by "older" women. While we are aware of the reduced, but not absent, fecundity of women during the perimenopause, there still remains reluctance by many clinicians to provide hormonal and other highly effective contraceptives to this group of women. This is possibly the result of earlier practice that recommended against the use of hormonal contraceptives by older reproductive-aged women as well as the dearth of studies specifically evaluating the clinical impact of contraception in perimenopausal women. Nonetheless, it is imperative for clinicians to understand that perimenopausal women who are sexually active and not using contraception are exposed to pregnancy and the profound maternal and fetal morbidity and mortality associated with pregnancy in older women.

In addition to pregnancy prevention, certain hormonal contraceptives can also provide important symptomatic relief to women who are beginning to experience the vasomotor instability and menstrual irregularity associated with the onset and progression of the perimenopause. While there is no age restriction to the use of any reversible contraceptive, increasing morbidity in women as they age may preclude the use of certain hormonal methods. The UK Medical Eligibility Criteria 2009 is a useful tool to determine whether a method is contraindicated dependent upon an individual woman's personal risk profile. It is based on the WHOMEC. For the healthy woman who is sexually active and may be experiencing symptoms of perimenopause, consideration of effective hormonal contraception is appropriate and warranted for pregnancy prevention and relief of symptoms, pending an assessment of her baseline health and risk for adverse clinical outcomes. Failure to do so places that woman at risk of pregnancy which may greatly complicate her personal, professional and family life as well as exposing her to an unnecessary and avoidable risk for pregnancy-related morbidity and mortality, in addition to withholding effective relief from perimenopause-associated symptoms that are likely to be increasing in frequency and severity and adversely affecting her health and well-being.

References

1. North American Menopause Society (NAMS) (year) http://www.menopause.org/for-women/menopauseflashes/menopause-101-a-primer-for-the-perimenopausal (accessed August 16, 2014).

2. Finer LB, Henshaw SK. Disparities in rates of unintended pregnancy in the United States, 1994 and 2001. *Perspect Sex Reprod Health* 2006; **38**: 90–6.

3. Baldwin MK, Jensen JT (year) Contraception during the perimenopause. *Maturitas* 2013; **76**: 235–42. doi: 10.1016/j.maturitas.2013.07.009.

4. Fritz M, Speroff L. *Clinical Gynecologic Endocrinology and Infertility*, 8th edition. Philadelphia, PA: Lippincott Williams & Wilkins; 2012.

5. Trussell J. Contraceptive efficacy. In Hatcher RA, Trussell J, Nelson AL, Cates Jr W, Kowal D, Policar MS (eds). *Contraceptive Technology, Twentieth Revised Edition*. Valley Stream, NY: Ardent Media; 2013.

6. National Cancer Institute (NCI). *Probability of Breast Cancer in American Women*; 2014. http://seer.cancer.gov/statfacts/html/breast.html (accessed August 16, 2014).

7. Hannaford PC, Selvaraj S, Elliott AM, *et al.* Cancer risk among users of oral contraceptives: cohort data from the Royal College of General Practitioner's oral contraception study. *Br Med J* 2007; **335**: 651.

Hormone replacement therapy and cancer

Franco Guidozzi

Caroline is 49, and since her periods stopped a year ago, she has suffered from debilitating menopausal symptoms, with hot flashes, vaginal dryness and mood swings. However, as both her parents died from cancer, she has so far refused HRT as she has heard that it can cause cancer.

Breast cancer

The debate about the influence of hormone therapy after menopause on breast cancer rates has resulted in a large volume of both clinical and basic research. The implication derived from the mass media is that hormone therapy can cause or increase the risk of breast cancer. Invariably this is the first question a menopausal woman wishes to discuss before she is to initiate hormone therapy, and not uncommonly, it is the point of note that she wishes to address if she is to continue with long-term usage. The etiology of breast cancer is multifactorial and is likely to involve more than just one factor when it does occur. Breast cancer will develop in about 12% of women who live to 90 years of age. The large majority of breast cancers are sporadic in nature and over 80% of breast cancers in postmenopausal women occur in women who have never taken hormone therapy. Factors that have been shown to be associated with an increased risk for breast cancer include obesity, alcohol intake, no full-term pregnancy, first full-term pregnancy > 35 years of age, never having breastfed an infant, early menarche < 12 years, late menopause > 50 years, family history of breast cancer particularly in first-degree relatives, genetic mutations (BRCA1 or BRCA2) and increased breast density. The medical literature is replete with a variety of observational studies that have shown an increase, a decrease or a null-effect on the risk for breast cancer in menopausal women receiving estrogen (E)-only therapy or estrogen and progestogen (E and P) combined therapy. The evidence from the observational studies is not consistent for an association of hormone therapy and breast cancer. The most compelling aspect from these studies is that hormone therapy acts as a promoter of breast cancer tissue and not an initiator of the disease, resulting in an increase in risk of breast cancer only being seen after 5 years of use; and that after stopping the hormone therapy, the risk rapidly returns to that observed in never-users of hormone therapy. The data suggest stimulation rather than induction of neoplasia. The Women's Health Initiative (WHI) Study initially did not find a statistically significant increase in the occurrence of invasive breast cancer in E and P combined therapy users (hazard ratio (HR) 1.26, 95% confidence interval (CI) 1.00–1.5). There was a null-effect for breast cancer in women who had never used hormone

Managing the Menopause: 21st Century Solutions, ed. Nick Panay, Paula Briggs, and Gab Kovacs.
Published by Cambridge University Press. © Cambridge University Press 2015.

therapy (HR 1.06, 95% CI 0.81–1.38), which was in agreement with the data previously published from the Collaborative Group report in women who had used hormone therapy for less than 5 years (HR 1.05, 95% CI 0.99–1.12). The overall risk of breast cancer in the WHI trial was elevated only in women who had previously used hormone therapy. Further analysis of the WHI using centrally adjudicated data and adjusted 95% CI showed that breast cancer was not significantly increased (HR 1.24, 95% CI 1.02–1.50). These data translate to four extra women developing breast cancer per 1,000 women taking combined hormone therapy for 5 years, or less than 0.1% per annum, compared with 1,000 women not taking hormone therapy. Support for the fact that it is the progestogen which is the more significant factor than estrogen in the risk for breast cancer comes from the E-only arm of the WHI, which showed an absolute reduction of eight per 10,000 person-years in the annual rate of newly diagnosed invasive breast cancers, which was not statistically significant (HR 0.77, 95% CI 0.59–1.01). A significant risk reduction was seen among women who were fully compliant with their treatment throughout the study (HR 0.67, 95% CI 0.47–0.97), which persisted after discontinuing the hormone therapy for up to 10.7 years follow-up. The level of breast cancer protection associated with E-only therapy did not vary by duration of use and among women with breast cancer diagnoses – both overall mortality and breast cancer mortality were significantly lower in the estrogen users. Fewer women died from any cause after breast cancer diagnosis than among the controls. A small increase in risk for breast cancer in lean younger women may be associated with unopposed E-only therapy. The Million Women Study reported that duration of hormone therapy is related to the incidence or occurrence of breast cancer. Both E-only and E and P therapy users had an increased risk for breast cancer but the risk decreased rapidly after stopping the therapy (at 1 year relative risk (RR) 1.03, 95% CI 0.92–1.12). Micronized progesterone and dydrogesterone in E and P combined therapy may be associated with a better risk profile for breast cancer than other synthetic progestogens. More data are still needed to determine whether mode of administration of hormone therapy may impact variably on breast cancer risk [1].

Tibolone is an analog of the progestogen, norethynedrel. After ingestion it is converted to three metabolites that provide estrogenic, progestogenic and androgenic effects. This selective tissue estrogenic activity regulator (STEAR) is effective in treating menopausal symptoms and seems to have the least likelihood of causing breast tenderness or increasing breast density. It has only been the Million Women Study that has suggested an increased risk for breast cancer (RR 1.45, 95% CI 1.25–1.67) in tibolone users, which was similar to that seen in women using E-only therapy and significantly less than that seen in women using E and P therapy within the study. This finding proved to be a surprise, and was in direct contrast to the findings of the LIFT study, a randomized placebo-controlled trial using tibolone in a fracture prevention trial where a significant reduction in invasive breast cancer was shown (HR 0.32, 95% CI 0.13–0.80) [1].

There are no data to support that testosterone hormone therapy impacts on the risk for breast cancer or for any of the gynecologic cancers.

In general, women having a first-degree relative with a history of breast cancer are at an increased risk of disease themselves, especially if the affected first-degree relative developed breast cancer before 40 years of age. A family history of a first-degree relative with breast cancer diagnosed after 50 years of age doubles the risk of breast cancer, but if the family member was diagnosed with breast cancer before 40 years of age, it increases the risk for developing breast cancer 6-fold. A second-degree relative with breast cancer increases risk slightly (RR 1.2–1.5). Even though there are only limited data, the data that are available suggest that family history does not impact negatively on risk for breast cancer if hormone therapy is taken. Family history and hormone therapy appear to have independent and no interacting effects on the risk of invasive breast cancer. Data from long-term cohort studies have not shown a further added risk with hormone therapy in those women who had a family history of breast cancer. Provided there are appropriate indications and there are no other contraindications, hormone therapy should not be withheld simply because of the family history of breast cancer.

Baseline mammographic density correlates with breast cancer risk, although this is independent of breast cancer association with hormone therapy. About 8% of the general population will have extremely dense breast tissue and their risk for breast cancer is increased (RR 1.4) compared with women with average breast density. About 39% of women will have heterogeneously dense breasts and these women have a relative risk of 1.2 for breast cancer. Screening sensitivity falls from 88% in breasts composed almost entirely of fat tissue to 62% in women with extremely dense breast tissue, whilst it is 69% in women with heterogeneously dense breasts. Digital mammography has shown to be more effective than film mammography in women with extremely dense breasts.

Endometrial cancer

Unopposed E-only therapy in a woman with an intact uterus causes endometrial hyperplasia, the precursor of most endometrial cancers, and the longer the duration of use, the greater the related increase in the risk of endometrial cancer. About 10% of women taking unopposed E-only therapy will develop complex hyperplasia after 1 year, as will 50% after 2 years and 62% after 3 years. Of importance, is the fact that this risk for endometrial cancer remains increased for many years after stopping the unopposed E-only therapy. Even after 15 years or more without estrogen therapy, there is still a significantly increased risk for endometrial cancer (RR 5.8, 95% CI 2.0–17.0), a concept directly opposite to that found with breast cancer, where the impact of E and P therapy on risk for cancer diminishes rapidly on cessation of therapy and returns to baseline by 5 years after stopping the therapy. Any estrogen therapy given to a woman with an intact uterus must therefore be accompanied by giving progestogens for 10–14 days per cycle as sequential regimens which allow monthly withdrawal bleeding, or as continuously combined regimens which avoid withdrawal bleeding, to counteract the proliferative effect of unopposed estrogen on the endometrium. Many studies have shown the beneficial effect of continuously combined E and P therapy in protecting the endometrium, particularly if used for longer than 5 years. The risk of endometrial cancer decreases significantly with increasing duration of continuous combined E and P therapy, with a 20% decrease during the first 5 years of use (odds ratio (OR) 0.8, 95% CI 0.5–1.3) and an 80% decrease if used for more than 5 years (OR 0.2, 95% CI 0.1–0.8). In contrast this is not seen with sequential E and P therapy in that the risk for endometrial cancer is not increased with short-term use, but with more than 5 years of use there appears to be an increased risk (< 5 years of use OR 1.5, 95% CI 1.0–2.2; > 5 years of use OR 2.9, 95% CI 1.8–4.6). It may therefore be prudent to change all women on sequential therapy to continuous combined E and P therapy after 5 years of use. The long-cycle E and P sequential regimen where the progestogen is given only 3-monthly to reduce the frequency of bleeding and so improve compliance is less likely to prevent endometrial hyperplasia and is therefore not suitable for long-term use. Both the WHI (HR for endometrial cancer 0.8, 95% CI 0.48–1.36) and the Million Women Study (MWS) showed that continuous combined E and P therapy protected the endometrium. The MWS showed a significant 29% decrease in the risk for endometrial cancer in women using combined hormone therapy, although this was not seen for sequential therapy. Endometrial cancer has rarely been reported in women using continuous combined E and P therapy. In the majority of such cases there commonly was a history of unopposed estrogen therapy, sequential therapy use with less than 10 days of progestogen or other risk factors such as a family history of endometrial cancer. The newer low-dose regimens containing continuous combined 0.3 mg conjugated equine estrogen and 1.5 mg of medroxyprogesterone acetate or 0.5 mg estradiol and 0.1 mg norethisterone acetate produce very acceptable bleeding profiles with no apparent evidence of endometrial stimulation as assessed by ultrasound, and at the same time providing symptom relief. The primary role for progestogen use is to prevent endometrial proliferation brought about by the estrogen, and it therefore stands to reason that if it is administered directly to the endometrial cavity it will give high local concentration of progestogen in the endometrium and lower circulating levels than if administered systemically. Intrauterine delivery of progestogen is a logical route of administration. The intrauterine system, Mirena®, delivers 20 μg of levonorgestrel per day, provides effective endometrial suppression and is a very plausible mode of delivering progestogen for continuous combined therapy in postmenopausal women.

Tamoxifen reduces the risk of developing breast cancer and of recurrences in breast cancer survivors, but it also affects the risk for developing endometrial cancer. Tamoxifen has an agonistic effect on the endometrium, increasing the risk of endometrial hyperplasia, endometrial polyps and endometrial cancer. The risk for endometrial cancer is increased significantly (RR 2.70, 95% CI 0.94–3.75), with women > 50 years of age having a greater risk compared with women < 50 years of age. Increased duration of use impacts adversely on risk. Other malignancies shown to be increased include gastrointestinal (RR 1.31, 95% CI 1.01–1.69), fallopian tube cancer, carcinosarcoma and sarcoma of the uterus.

In future, the anticipated wider use of tissue selective estrogen complex compounds (TSEC) in the treatment of menopausal symptoms hopes to avoid the use of progestogens and their role in the development of breast cancer. Bazedoxifene, a SERMS, with concomitant conjugated estrogen as the TSEC, has not been shown to cause endometrial hyperplasia or breast stimulation (no breast tenderness or increased breast density), although at the same time, it is very successful in treating vasomotor symptoms, preventing osteoporosis, reversing vulvo-vaginal atrophy, and improving sleep and quality of life [2].

Ovarian cancer

Ovarian epithelial cells express estrogen and progesterone receptors, and the receptor expression differs between normal and malignant cells. This gives reason to question whether sex hormones might have a role in ovarian carcinogenesis. The impact of hormone therapy on ovarian cancer risk has been studied in a number of different studies, including meta-analyses, pooled analyses and the WHI randomized clinical trial. The results have been less consistent than those on breast and endometrial cancer, with as many studies showing an increase in risk as there are studies that show a decrease in risk or a null effect on risk. Of the three pooled analyses published, two did not show any increase in risk (RR 1.1, 95% CI 0.9–1.4), although one study did for E-only therapy users (RR 1.7, 95% CI 1.3–2.2), whilst in the only one that analyzed the impact of E and P on risk for ovarian cancer, there was a null effect irrespective of duration of therapy use. Most of the case-control studies have detected a modest non-significant increase in ovarian cancer risk (RR 1.3 for E-only therapy and RR 2.1 for E and P therapy respectively). The magnitude of risk increased with duration of use and was detected in users of E-only therapy as well as in the women using E and P therapy. Of the five cohort studies published, two did not detect an association between hormone therapy and ovarian cancer (RR 0.9) whereas two of the others did (RR 1.3 and 1.7 respectively). In one study mortality from ovarian cancer was increased. In these studies, both the risk of ovarian cancer and the risk of dying from the ovarian cancer was related to the duration of use and increased with longer use of the hormone therapy. Of the different histologic subtypes to be affected, endometrioid adenocarcinoma shows the strongest association with hormone therapy, with mucinous adenocarcinoma being the least likely to be affected. In the WHI randomized trial, the risk for ovarian cancer in women using E and P was mildly increased after 5.6 years of follow-up (HR 1.6) compared with women using placebo. Recently, ovarian cancer risk in postmenopausal women using estradiol-progestin therapy was analyzed in a large Finnish study of over 224,000 women followed up for over 12 years. Ovarian cancer risk was not elevated in women who had used E and P therapy for less than 5 years (standardized incidence ratio (SIR) 1.21, 95% CI 1.06–1.37), and for >5 years of use the risk for ovarian cancer was similar (SIR 1.26, 95% CI 0.94–1.64). The risk did not differ between sequential or continuous E and P regimens, or between oral or transdermal E and P formulations. The risk elevations for E and P use for >5 years was only seen for serous adenocarcinoma (SIR 1.56, 95% CI 1.33–1.80). In summary, long-term E-only therapy may be associated with a small attributable risk of ovarian cancer of 0.7 per 1,000 women users for 5 years, whilst either a significantly smaller increase, or no increase at all, is seen with combined E and P hormonal therapy. The risk is so small that it is unlikely to influence prescribing habit.

The data pertaining to the impact of hormone therapy on risk for borderline tumors is sparse and only consists of case-controlled studies. The majority of the studies have not detected any association, although in one study the only significant association found was between ever-use of unopposed estrogen and serous borderline tumors (OR 2.1), whereas in women with a BMI >26 the risk was close to unity [3].

BRCA1 and BRCA2 mutation carriers

About 7–10% of ovarian cancers will have a hereditary basis, of which BRCA1 and BRCA2 are the two major susceptibility genes involved in hereditary breast and ovarian cancer. BRCA1 and BRCA2 mutation carriers have a 54–85% and 45% lifetime risk of developing breast cancer respectively and a 20–60% and 10–27% lifetime risk of developing ovarian cancer. BRCA1 mutation carriers also have a greater risk for fallopian tube and for primary peritoneal cancers and a 2–4-fold increase in colonic cancer. BRCA2 mutation carriers also have a 2–4-fold increase in malignant melanoma and pancreatic cancer. Although not as frequent, uterine serous papillary carcinoma appears to be a BRCA1-related disease. Use of the combined oral contraceptive pill is likely to decrease ovarian cancer risk, but the recommended strategy to significantly decrease the risk of breast and ovarian cancer in women with BRCA gene mutations is a bilateral salpingo-oophorectomy, and if acceptable, a total abdominal hysterectomy. Breast cancer risk is decreased by about 50% and for ovarian cancer, by about 80%. Surgical menopause in these young women invariably produces severe menopausal symptoms and although there are some non-hormonal options to treat the vasomotor symptoms, the use of E and P therapy in these women is always a topic of debate. Hormone therapy in the form of E-only or as E and P combination therapy has not been shown to be associated with any greater increase in risk for breast cancer to that which has been mentioned above and it impacts on risk in these women as it does in women who are not BRCA mutation carriers. Data comes from observational studies, and although the follow-up in these studies varies, short-term use of any type of up to 4 years does not significantly alter the protective effect of the surgery. The fact that these women require E-only therapy after their hysterectomy avoids the concerns imposed by the role of progestogens in the evolution of breast cancer [4].

Colorectal cancer

After 5.6 years of hormonal therapy, the WHI randomized trials did not show any significant impact on risk for colorectal cancer in women using E-only hormone therapy, but they did show a significant 44% decrease in risk for colorectal cancer in women taking E and P compared with those taking placebo. This was in keeping with the findings in observational studies. Three meta-analyses have reported a significantly reduced risk among E and P users (RR 0.80, 95% CI 0.74–0.86 for ever-users and RR 0.66, 95% CI 0.59–0.74 for current users). This benefit persisted for 4 years after cessation of therapy. Surprisingly though, women diagnosed with colorectal cancer on hormone therapy at the time of the diagnosis in the WHI randomized trial were likely to have more lymph node involvement and have more advanced-stage disease. Death from the disease, however, was not different between the two groups of patients. This pattern has persisted after 11.6 years of follow-up, in that fewer colorectal cancers have been diagnosed in women using E and P therapy compared with women on placebo (HR 0.72, 95% CI 0.56–0.94). Cancers at the time of diagnosis in women taking hormone therapy were at a higher stage for regional or distant disease (68.8% vs. 54%, $P = 0.003$), with a non-statistically significant higher number of deaths from the disease in the E and P therapy users compared with women using placebo (HR 1.29, 95% CI 0.78–2.11). Hormone therapy is not indicated for primary prevention of colorectal cancer.

Hereditary non-polyposis colorectal cancer, also known as Lynch syndrome, is an autosomal dominant syndrome characterized by early-onset neoplastic lesions and micro-satellite instability. Women with this syndrome have, in addition, a 40–60% lifetime risk of endometrial cancer and a 10–12% lifetime risk of ovarian cancer. Although very limited data exist, hormone therapy in these women does not increase these risks. Prophylactic hysterectomy and bilateral salpingo-oophorectomy is effective in preventing endometrial and ovarian cancer in these women [5].

Lung cancer

The observational studies have not shown a significant impact on risk for lung cancer in women using hormone therapy, with some showing an increased risk, others a decreased risk and others a null effect. The WHI clinical trial found no substantial effect of E-only therapy on lung cancer risk, although in the E and P arm, there was a small, but non-significant increase in the risk of non-small cell lung cancer as well as a significant increase in risk of death from lung cancer, particularly in women who were smokers. The increased risk was only significant in women aged 60–69 years where the absolute attributable risk was 1.8 extra cases per 1,000 users for 5 years. In women 50–59 years of age, there was no increased risk. A recently undertaken study involving 118,000 women aged 50–71 years of age and followed up for 10 years showed that neither E-only nor E and P therapy impacted adversely on risk for developing lung cancer (RR 0.97, 95% CI 0.86–1.09 and RR 1.03, 95% CI 0.90–1.17 respectively) [6].

Skin cancers

Rates of incidence of non-melanoma skin cancers and melanoma in the post hoc analyses of the WHI randomized placebo-controlled trials were similar between the women who used hormone therapy and the women who used placebo (RR 0.98, 95% CI 0.89–1.07 for non-melanoma and RR 0.92, 95% CI 0.61–1.37 for melanoma respectively). Both E-only therapy and combined E and P therapy did not affect overall incidence of non-melanoma skin cancer or melanoma. There was no evidence to support that estrogen therapy, with or without progestins, has a role in the development of skin cancer [7].

Upper gastrointestinal tract cancer

This has not been studied extensively but there is a nested case-controlled study that has shown a decrease in risk for stomach cancer in E and P therapy users (RR 0.48, 95% CI 0.29–0.79), a null effect on esophageal cancer and an increased risk for gall bladder cancer in women using hormone therapy, particularly associated with duration of use (RR 3.2, 95% CI 1.1–9.3) [8].

Hormone therapy in cancer survivors

The use of hormone therapy to treat menopausal symptoms continues to be controversial, highly emotive and challenging with regard to breast and gynecologic cancer survivors. Treatment of breast and gynecologic cancer has improved significantly during the last three decades and has resulted in an ever-increasing population of survivors who will suffer significant menopausal symptoms as a result of their surgery, irradiation, chemotherapy, or simply because of their age when the cancer was initially diagnosed. The menopausal symptoms, particularly in patients who have a surgically induced menopause, invariably are debilitating and the need for treatment is an important reality. In addition, it has been shown that hot flashes, night sweats, vaginal dryness and urinary incontinence may produce symptoms that significantly impact on the quality of life of breast cancer survivors. Clinicians are reluctant to prescribe hormone therapy because of the concern that it may lead to recurrence of the malignancy and hence curtail survival, even though they are aware that it is very likely to alleviate the menopausal symptoms.

Breast cancer

Observational data are available from nine descriptive studies reporting the outcome of about 1,700 breast cancer survivors using hormone therapy that were followed up from 6 months to 14 years. The consensus of these studies is that hormone therapy does not increase the rate of recurrence or mortality from the disease. In fact, the data support that hormone therapy in breast cancer survivors is not detrimental and appears to decrease the risk of recurrence and disease-related mortality by 40–50% respectively when compared with women not taking hormone therapy. A meta-analysis of 15 studies with 1,416 breast cancer survivors compared with 1,998 controls who were followed up for 7 years showed a significant decrease in recurrence (HR 0.5) and disease-related mortality (HR 0.3) among the hormone therapy users.

There are three randomized trials that have analyzed the impact of hormone therapy in breast cancer survivors on breast cancer recurrence and they have produced conflicting information. Two of the three trials have shown an increased risk for recurrence, but one of the trials has not shown any increased risk. In 1997, two independent randomized clinical trials, The HABITS Study (Hormonal replacement therapy After Breast cancer – Is It Safe) and the Stockholm trial were instituted to compare hormone therapy with no hormone therapy for treatment of menopausal symptoms in women treated for early-stage breast cancer. Much of the design of the studies was similar. In the HABITS Study, hormone therapy was given for 2 years and had a median follow-up of 2.1 years. About 21% were given E-only therapy, 46% combined E and P therapy, 26% sequential E and P therapy, and 6% tibolone. The study was closed prematurely because there was a significant increase in the risk for recurrence (HR 3.5, 95% CI 1.5–8.1), with about 40% of the recurrences being local, 20% in the contralateral breast and 40% were distant metastases, although there was no difference in mortality from the disease in the two arms of the trial [9]. In the Stockholm Study 22% of the women randomized to taking hormone therapy took sequential therapy, 50% took long-cycle cyclic hormone therapy and 23% took E-only therapy. These patients had a median follow-up of 4.1 years. In direct contrast to the HABITS trial, the Stockholm trial found that the risk of breast cancer recurrence was not associated with the use of hormone therapy (HR 0.82, 95% CI 0.35–1.9). Differences in the design and in the clinical characteristics of the patients in the two studies may have contributed to the differences seen in the results. In the HABITS trial there were a larger number of patients with positive lymph nodes (26% vs. 16% respectively), fewer patients received concomitant adjuvant tamoxifen therapy (21% vs. 52% respectively) and patients in the Stockholm trial did not use continuous combined hormone therapy. After an extended follow-up for both studies, namely 4 years for the HABITS trial and 10.8 years for the Stockholm trial, the findings were still very similar to the initial analyses with regard to breast cancer recurrences (HR 2.4, 95% CI 1.3–4.2 for HABITS and HR 1.3, 95% CI 0.9–1.9 for the Stockholm trial respectively) [10]. In the third study, LIBERATE trial (Livial Intervention following Breast cancer: Efficacy, Recurrence And Tolerability Endpoints), women who had been treated for breast cancer and who had vasomotor symptoms were randomized to either tibolone or placebo. In addition to this, 67% of all the patients were taking tamoxifen and 6.8% were taking aromatase inhibitors. After a median follow-up of 3.1 years, 15.2% of women taking tibolone developed a recurrence compared with 10.7% in the women taking placebo (HR 1.4, 95% CI 1.14–1.70). The increased risk was confined to women with estrogen receptor-positive breast cancers with no impact being noted in women with estrogen receptor-negative breast cancers. Most of the breast cancer recurrences in women taking tibolone were distant metastases, although there was no difference in the occurrence of local metastases or of recurrences in the contralateral breast when compared with women taking placebo [11].

The data are still controversial, but until proven differently, it is prudent not to routinely offer hormone therapy to breast cancer survivors for their menopausal symptoms. But if other possible options fail and debilitating symptoms persist, it would be plausible to offer E-only therapy to women who have had a hysterectomy, the intrauterine progestogen-containing IUS should progestogen be necessary, or topical vaginal E therapy if vulvo-vaginal atrophy and its symptoms is the prevailing complaint.

Hormone therapy in gynecologic cancer survivors

Treatment of gynecologic cancer has a significant impact on a woman's quality of life. Not only may the treatment include removal of the uterus, the core of a woman's femininity, but it may also lead to either surgical removal of the ovaries or postoperative ablation of the ovaries because of adjuvant irradiation and/or chemotherapy. These interventions will all lead to the acute onset of menopausal symptoms. About 20% of gynecologic cancer will occur in pre- or perimenopausal women, a large percentage of whom will become menopausal as a result of their treatment. There is also the large cohort of gynecologic cancer survivors who are not rendered menopausal as a result of their treatment but who will become menopausal because of natural aging. A significant number of these patients will enquire about treatment options and naturally want to know whether hormone therapy will impact on their malignancy.

Endometrial cancer

Women who present with endometrial cancer tend to have early-stage disease because the most common presenting feature is abnormal vaginal bleeding, with about 85% of patients having stage 1 or 2 disease at the time of diagnosis. Definitive data are lacking, but that which is available from observational studies does not paint a bleak picture. There are seven studies with about 330 endometrial cancer survivors, the majority of whom had stage 1 disease, although there were some women with stage 2 disease, who were given either E-only therapy or E and P therapy between 0–120 months after their treatment. These patients were followed up for between 24–168 months. There were a total of only five recurrences described in the follow-up period of the individual studies. In the only randomized study, which did not reach its accrual goal, 1,236 women were randomized to estrogen therapy after undergoing surgery. Recurrences occurred in 14 women taking hormone therapy (2.3%), 26 died as a result of their disease (4.2%), whilst eight developed a new malignancy, compared with 12 women taking placebo developing recurrences (1.9%), nine dying of their disease (3.1), whilst 10 developed a new malignancy (1.6%). The authors concluded that although the study could not definitively refute or support the safety of estrogen therapy in endometrial cancer survivors, it was important to note that the incidence and demise from the disease in users was low (RR 1.27, 95% CI 0.9–1.77). There are very few data on estrogen therapy in women with uterine sarcomas, but that which is available suggests that hormone therapy may be contraindicated in women with endometrial stromal sarcoma, but not in the other subcategories of uterine sarcomas, even though both leiomyosarcoma and endometrial stromal sarcoma express both estrogen and progesterone receptors to varying degrees.

Ovarian cancer survivors

There is a paucity of information with reference to ovarian cancer survivors and hormone therapy, but as with endometrial cancer, the available data suggest that hormone therapy does not impact significantly on disease-free interval and survival. Three observational studies involving about 135 patients with varying stages of disease were followed up between 1–150 months after having started their estrogen therapy, 0–120 months after their cytoreductive surgery. There was no difference in the rate of recurrent disease in the estrogen users compared with the women using placebo. One study published their 5-year survival of 649 ovarian cancer survivors and 150 survivors with borderline ovarian tumors according to estrogen therapy before and after diagnosis. After 5 years, 45% of women with ovarian cancer and 93% of women with borderline ovarian tumors respectively were still alive. There was no overall difference in the 5-year survival in women with ovarian cancer according to use of hormone therapy before diagnosis (HR 0.83, 95% CI 0.48–0.78), whilst analysis according to different hormonal preparations, duration, or when commenced after treatment, did not affect survival in women with ovarian cancer. A better survival was noted in those women using E-only therapy (HR 0.57, 95% CI 0.42–0.78). The only randomized study to address this concept also found that hormone therapy in ovarian cancer survivors, started about 6 weeks after surgery and followed up for a median of 4 years, did not have an adverse impact on disease-free interval or on survival compared with women taking placebo [12].

Vulval, vaginal and cervical cancer survivors

Vulval, vaginal and cervical cancers are not considered hormone dependent and therefore estrogen therapy can be given, invariably as continuous combined hormone therapy. The impact of hormone therapy on adenocarcinoma of the endocervix has not been analyzed widely, but the existing data do not show any negative impact on outcome and it appears safe to use.

References

1. Anderson GL, Chlebowski RT, Aragaki AK, et al. Conjugated equine oestrogen and breast cancer incidence and mortality in postmenopausal women with hysterectomy: extended follow-up of the Women's Health Initiative randomized placebo controlled trial. Lancet Oncol 2012; 13: 476–86.

2. Sturdee DW. Endometrial safety and bleeding with HRT: what's new? Climacteric 2007; 10: 66–70.

3. Auranen A, Heitanen S, Salmi T, Grenman S. Hormonal treatments and epithelial ovarian cancer risk. Int J Gynecol Cancer 2005; 15: 692–700.

4. Gadducci A, Biglia N, Cosio S, Sismondi P, Gennazzani AR. Gynaecologic challenging issues in the management of BRCA mutation carriers: oral contraceptives, prophylactic salpingo-oophorectomy and hormone replacement therapy. Gynecol Endocrinol 2010; 26: 568–77.

5. Simon MS, Chlebowski RT, Wactawzki-Wende J, et al. Estrogen plus progestin and colorectal cancer. Incidence and mortality. J Clin Oncol 2012; 30: 3983–90.

6. Brinton L, Schwartz L, Spitz MR, et al. Unopposed estrogen and estrogen plus progestin menopausal hormone therapy and lung cancer risk in the NIH-AARP Diet and Health Study cohort. Cancer Causes Control 2012; 23: 487–96.

7. Tang JY, Spaunhurst KM, Chlebowski RT, et al. Menopausal hormone therapy and risk of melanoma and non-melanoma skin cancers. Women's Health Initiative Randomized Trials. J Natl Cancer Inst 2011; 103: 1469–75.

8. Freedman ND, Lacey JV, Hollenbeck AR, et al. The association of menstrual and reproductive factors with upper gastrointestinal tract cancers in the NIH-AARP cohort. Cancer 2010; 116: 1572–81.

9. Holmberg L, Iverson O-E, Rudenstam CM, et al. on behalf of the HABITS Study Group. Increased risk of recurrence after hormone replacement therapy in breast cancer survivors. J Natl Cancer Instit 2008; 100: 475–82.

10. Fahlen M, Fornander T, Johansson H, et al. Hormone replacement therapy after breast cancer: 10 years follow up of the Stockholm randomized trial. Eur J Cancer 2013; 49: 52–9.

11. Kenenmans P, Bundred N, Foidart J-M, et al. on behalf of the LIBERATE Study Group. Safety and efficacy of tibolone in breast-cancer patients with vasomotor symptoms: a double-blind, randomized, non-inferiority trial. Lancet Oncol 2009; 10: 135–46.

12. Guidozzi F. Hormone therapy in gynaecologic cancer survivors. Climacteric 2013; 16: 611–17.

Hormone replacement therapy and venous thrombosis

Sven O. Skouby

Introduction

Venous thromboembolism (VTE) is a specific reproductive health risk for women. In pregnancy the relative risk of VTE is increased approximately 5-fold and in the puerperium it is increased by as much as 60-fold. Additionally, large numbers of women worldwide are exposed to an increased relative risk of VTE as a result of using combined hormonal contraception (CHC), combined oral contraceptives (COCs) or hormone replacement therapy (HRT). Even women undergoing infertility treatment may be exposed to situations of significantly increased risk of VTE [1]. Several studies have established a 2- to 4-fold increased risk of VTE for users of HRT compared with non-users [2] and comparable to the attributable risk of CHC. The risk for VTE induced by HRT is, however, higher in absolute figures because of the age factor *per se*, but is also dependent on the composition of the HRT used, since users of estrogen-only preparations have lower risk of VTE than women receiving combined estrogen-progestin preparations [3]. Also the dose and route of administration seems of importance, as women treated with transdermal HRT have lower risk of VTE than women receiving orally administered HRT, as consistently demonstrated in clinical studies [2]. Moreover, epidemiological and pharmacological factors may contribute to the precipitation of VTE among HRT users. The pharmacological alterations induced by HRT on the hemostatic system may be of particular interest [4], because HRT changes the inhibitory potential of coagulation as well as fibrinolysis significantly. Consequently, the choice of HRT may translate into clinical manifestations in thrombosis-prone individuals.

Venous thromboembolism mostly manifests in the deep veins of the leg, but may occur in other sites, such as the upper extremities, cerebral sinus, liver, and portal veins or retinal veins. Venous thrombi are composed predominately of red blood cells but also of platelets and leukocytes bound together by fibrin. Embolization occurs when parts of the clot dislodge and are transported by the blood flow, usually through the heart to the vasculature of the lungs (Figure 23.1). Major complications of VTE are a disabling post-thrombotic syndrome or acute death from a pulmonary embolus (PE) that occur in 1–2% of patients [5].

Risk factors

There are a number of risk factors for venous thromboembolism. They fit into a more contemporary and extended version of Virchow's triad (stasis, hypercoagulability, endothelial damage) and they change the hemostatic balance toward clot formation

---

Managing the Menopause: 21st Century Solutions, ed. Nick Panay, Paula Briggs, and Gab Kovacs. Published by Cambridge University Press. © Cambridge University Press 2015.

Table 23.1. Venous thrombosis: genetic and acquired risk factors.

Genetic			Acquired		
Risk factor	Prevalence	Relative risk (RR)	Risk factor	Prevalence	RR
Leiden factor V heterozygote	6%	8	Age>30 vs <30 years	50%	2.5
Leiden factor V homozygote	0.2%	64	Adiposity (BMI >25)	30%	2
Protein C insuffiency	0.2%	15	COC and HRT	30%	2–6
Protein S insuffiency	<0.1%	>10	Varicose veins	8%	2
Antithrombin III insufficiency	0.02%	50	Pregnancy	4%	8
Prothrombin 20210A	2%	3	Medical diseases	5%?	2–5
Hyper-homo-cysteinema	3%	3	Immobilization/ trauma	?	2–10

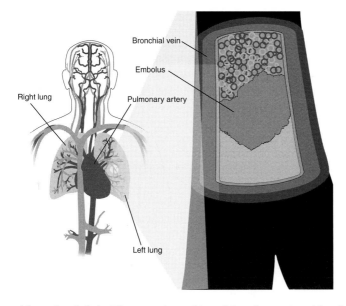

Figure 23.1. Pulmonary embolism.

(thrombophilia). This can be achieved by decreasing blood flow and lowering oxygen tension, by activating the endothelium, by activating inborn or acquired immune responses, by activating blood platelets, or by increasing the number of platelets and red blood cells, or modifying the concentrations of pro- and anticoagulant proteins in the blood. Numerous risk factors are known, which can be divided into genetic and acquired (Table 23.1).

An extended multiple-hit hypothesis implies that more than one risk factor is present at any one time. Superficial vein thrombosis combined with an acquired thrombotic risk factor increases the risk of venous thrombosis 10- to 100-fold [6], but one of the most well-known acquired risk factors is the use of exogenous sex steroids such as COCs and HRT.

Gender differences

A gender difference has been observed. The incidence rates of DVT are higher in younger women during the child-bearing years compared with men at similar age. With advancing age, however, rates are much higher in men than women. A relative risk (RR) of 1.3 in men with an age between 60 and 69 years versus women in the same age group is reported. Also the risk of recurrent venous thrombosis is 2-fold higher in men than in women [7].

Age

Venous thromboembolism has an annual incidence of 1–3 per 10,000 individuals per year (global background rate). It is uncommon in young individuals and becomes more frequent with advancing age. The risk is doubled between the ages of 20 and 40. The incidence is estimated to be approximately 5 per 10,000 per year in women in their 40s, increasing to 6–12 per 10,000 per year in women in their 50s, and is approximately 30–40 per 10,000 per year in women aged 70–80 years. For women in their 80s, the estimated annual risk is approximately 70 per 10,000 [8, 9]. Similarily in the Women's Health Initiative Study (WHI), users of combined HRT in the sixth, seventh and eighth decades of life had a 2-fold, 4-fold and 7-fold VTE risk respectively [10]. An analogous though less pronounced effect of age was seen in the estrogen-only arm of the WHI [11].

Obesity

The world is experiencing an obesity pandemic, with rates of obesity (body mass index (BMI) > 25) rising for more than two decades. Although obesity has been suggested to be a risk factor for fatal pulmonary embolism for a long time, whether obesity is an independent risk factor for pulmonary embolism or VTE has not been fully determined until recently and presented in a systematic review [12]. Investigations that reported an increased risk because of obesity have been criticized because they failed to control for hospital confinement or other risk factors and although high proportions of patients with venous thromboembolic disease have been found to be obese, the importance of the association is diminished because of the high proportion of obesity in the general population. To date, however, there is notable and consistent evidence of an association of obesity with VTE, more so in women compared with men. The risk appears to be at least double that for normal weight subjects (BMI 20–24.9) [13]. In the WHI, VTE risk increased in both overweight and obese (BMI > 30) HRT users when compared with placebo users in the normal weight group. The risk of venous thromboembolism may be additive when using HRT, and with the continuous and global rise in obesity, this interaction will become a more prevalent risk issue.

Specific risk of HRT

There are a number of different estrogen and progestin preparations in both sequential and continuous combined products. These differ according to the chemical structure of both the estrogen and the progestin component, daily dose and route of administration. The estrogen compound of combined HRT consists of either natural 17β-estradiol (E2), including estradiol valerate (E2V), or the conjugated equine estrogens (CEE). E2 can be administered orally or transdermally. CEE is synthesized from the urine of gravid mares and contains more than 30 known biologically active estrogen compounds, including mainly estrone sulfate and equilin sulfate. CEE is always orally administered. A recent study demonstrated that CEE and E2, administered alone, were associated with different risks of major thrombotic events. Compared with current use of oral E2, current use of oral CEE was associated with a doubling of the risk of DVT [14]. The association of VTE risk with the different pharmacological classes of progestogens has not been elucidated in detail, despite many clinical and epidemiologic investigations. Progestogens include both progesterone, the physiologic molecule synthesized and secreted by the ovary, and synthetic compounds named progestins, which are derived from either progesterone (pregnanes and 19-norpregnanes) or testosterone (19-nortestosterone). To date the only desired effect in relation to HRT is endometrial protection [15]. An indirect comparison within the WHI clinical trials showed that the association of estrogens plus progestogens was more thrombogenic than unopposed estrogens. Indeed, compared with placebo, the VTE risk was doubled in the estrogen plus progestogen clinical trial and not significantly elevated among HRT users in the estrogen-alone clinical trial. Similarly, the Women's International Study of long-Duration Oestrogen after Menopause (WISDOM) trial has provided a direct comparison of the effect of CEE alone and CEE plus medroxyprogesterone (MPA) on VTE risk among postmenopausal hysterectomized women [3]. Results showed that users of CEE plus MPA had a doubling in thrombotic risk compared with women treated by CEE alone [16]. While MPA may have a thrombogenic effect among postmenopausal women using estrogens, micronized progesterone could be safe with respect to thrombotic risk [3]. The effects of the different types of progestogens on VTE risk has to be further investigated.

Tibolone, a testosterone-derived progestin, has estrogenic, progestogenic and androgenic properties, and can be used alone for treatment of climacteric symptoms. All available studies, although limited in types and number, show that tibolone is not associated with an increased risk of VTE [3,17].

Route of administration

In most investigations of the relationship of venous thromboembolism and HRT, the route of hormone administration has been primarily oral. It has been proposed that orally administered estrogen may exert a prothrombotic effect through the hepatic induction of hemostatic imbalance, as has been observed with COCs. The prothrombotic effect is possibly related to high concentrations of estrogen in the liver due to the "first-pass" effect. Studies that compared oral and transdermal estrogen administration have demonstrated that transdermally administered estrogen has little or no effect in elevating prothrombotic substances and may have beneficial effects on proinflammatory markers, including C-reactive protein, prothrombin activation peptide and antithrombin activity. Also, in contrast to oral estrogen, transdermal estrogen may also have a suppressive effect on tissue plasminogen activator antigen and plasminogen activator inhibitor activity [2]. Most of the clinical data correlating HRT route of administration and VTE risk has come from the EStrogen and THromboEmbolism Risk (ESTHER) Study Group. They have demonstrated that oral but not transdermal estrogen is associated with a 4-fold increased VTE risk. In addition, they noted that norpregnane progestogens may be thrombogenic, whereas micronized progesterone and pregnane derivatives appear safe with respect to thrombotic risk [18]. Similar results were reported elsewhere and of particular importance, in women who were stratified for weight and the presence of prothrombotic mutations [2].

Smoking

No interaction between smoking and HRT was found in the WHI clinical trial [10], although smoking itself is a weak risk factor for incident VTE. Smoking further increases the risk of VTE in women using CHC [19].

Length of use

It is now generally accepted that the risk of VTE in users of HRT decreases with length of use. There is a marked increased risk in thrombosis during the first year of use with the odds ratio as high as 8 ("the timing effect") [20]. This is likely to be caused by the presence of prothrombotic/thrombophilic abnormalities in these women, as has been shown for COCs. In several studies, a high risk was observed for users of HRT who had coagulation abnormalities, such as APC resistance, increased levels of D-Dimer or high F IX levels. In women who carry the Factor V Leiden mutation there is a 15-fold increased risk of venous thrombosis, analogous to what has been observed for COCs. No such synergy has been demonstrated for carriers of prothrombin 20210A who use HRT. Apart from type and route of administration, comparisons of the thrombosis risks between HRT regimens must therefore also account for length of use and ensure that new users of one agent are truly being compared with new users of another agent. With time, the risk of thrombosis decreases, but always remains higher than non-users. This risk disappears during the first months after stopping treatment.

Thrombophilia

Thrombophilia is a term used to describe a group of conditions in which there is an increased tendency, often repeated and over an extended period of time, for excessive clotting. These include inherited conditions, based on a demonstrated genetic mutation such as factor V Leiden, protein C and S deficiencies, antithrombin deficiency and prothrombin 20210A mutations (which may be suspected on family history); or an acquired condition such as lupus anticoagulant/antiphospholipid or anticardiolipin antibody syndrome, which can occur alone as a manifestation of an autoimmune disorder, or as part of a syndrome such as systemic lupus erythematosus. The presence of an inherited thrombophilia is a major modifier of thrombosis risk in users of both CHC and HRT. However, to qualify, all hereditary thrombophilic defects as similarly strong risk factors might be questioned. The absolute risk of venous thrombosis in factor V Leiden heterozygous carriers is estimated as being 0.15 per 100 person-years, whereas in antithrombin-, protein C-, or protein S-deficient persons, these estimates range from 0.7 to 1.7 per 100 person-years, indicating a considerably higher degree of risk. Risk estimates for thrombophilic women using HRT are less precise compared with estimates performed in CHC users, because fewer women on HRT have been included in the types of retrospective studies that are informative for this situation. In principle the known relative risks for the various thrombophilias should be multiplied by the HRT baseline risk in the relevant age category. The route of administration as well as the progestin component has been clearly shown to modulate/decrease the risk. In general, women known to be carriers of a thrombophilia, or with a positive first-degree family history of venous thrombosis, should be advised not to take oral HRT. However, as part of the shared decision-making process, the gynecologist should weigh the risks against the benefits when prescribing HRT and counsel the patient accordingly, taking into consideration the possible thrombosis-sparing properties of trans-dermal administration and tibolone.

Women with a personal history of venous thrombosis

There is consensus that HRT should not be prescribed to women with a history of venous thrombosis. In one trial women with a history of previous thrombosis were randomized to HRT vs. placebo; this trial was stopped due to a rate of thrombosis of 8.5% per year in the estrogen arm vs. only 1% in the placebo arm. Factor V Leiden heterozygosity was not associated with a significantly increased risk of DVT, most likely because of the limited population size and short follow-up. However, the combined group of individuals either hetero- or homozygous for factor V Leiden or who instead had anticardiolipin antibodies at baseline, had an increased risk of VTE recurrence. The investigators also found that HRT significantly changed the levels of multiple parameters of fibrinolysis and of endogenous anticoagulants, in a procoagulant direction. For example, levels of D-Dimer significantly increased in those taking HRT and remained stable in those on placebo. Similarly, levels of anticoagulant proteins antithrombin, protein C and TFPI decreased significantly in the HRT group and did not change in the placebo group [21].

Biological mechanism of HRT-induced thrombosis risk

Oral HRT has very similar effects on coagulation and fibrinolysis variables as use of CHC. Estrogens have many different effects on hemostasis, lipids and inflammatory risk markers. The changes in the coagulation system include increases in the levels of procoagulant factors VII, X, XII and XIII, and reductions in the anticoagulant factors protein S and antithrombin. These changes predict a change toward a more procoagulant state which is confirmed in studies examining global tests, such as activated protein C (APC) resistance or global coagulation capacity measured with the thrombin generation test (TGT). With increased levels of coagulation factors VII, IX, X, XII and XIII and reduced levels of the natural anticoagulants protein S and antithrombin, the overall effect is a prothrombotic shift in the hemostatic balance [22] (Figure 23.2). Epidemiologic studies have shown that high levels of many of these factors are thrombotic risk factors. It is currently unclear how these effects are brought about at the molecular level of the estrogen receptor. It is likely that these effects at the cellular level are also under genetic control which translates to the described thrombophilia conditions above, and therefore some women appear to be more sensitive to the effect of estrogens than other women. The estrogen-induced changes in fibrinolysis are less straightforward. Estrogen use enhances the fibrinolytic activity in plasma. The main enzyme in fibrinolysis is plasmin, which dissolves the fibrin clot, producing fibrin degradation products such as D-Dimers (Figure 23.2). Levels of plasminogen-activator inhibitor 1 (PAI-1) are decreased while tissue plasminogen activator (tPA) increases. The decreased concentration and activity of PAI-1 and the increased plasma levels of tPA and plasminogen during HRT use are, however, at least partially counteracted by elevated thrombin-activated fibrinolysis inhibitor (TAFI). It is, however, not clear whether the effects of estrogens on fibrinolysis parameters have clinical implications, since there is no firm evidence that changes in the fibrinolytic system affect the risk of venous thrombosis. The hemostatic effects are due to the effect of estrogen on liver synthesis of these proteins. In contrast to ethinyl estradiol (EE) in CHC, where there is a direct chemical action on the liver, it is rather a first-pass effect, which is seen for estradiol

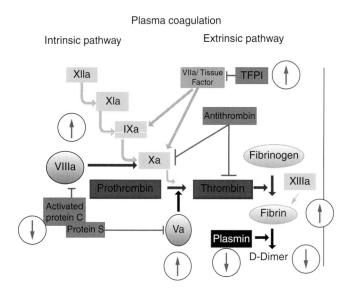

Figure 23.2. Thrombophilic impact of hormone replacement therapy.

in HRT. Although existing data indicate that women on combined oral estrogen/progestogen are more at risk of VTE compared with the risk of unopposed estrogen at this point, available data are inconclusive, especially in relation to the different types and doses of progestogens [23, 24]. The ESTHER Study was the first to establish a differential association of DVT risk with the different progestogen subgroups irrespective of the route of estrogens administration [17]. Little impact has been found from use of tibolone compared with CEE/MPA [18].

Several tests have been proposed as surrogate markers of thrombotic risk. A correlation has been demonstrated between the risk of venous thrombosis and activated protein C (APC) resistance determined with the thrombin generation-based assay. Prothrombin, protein S and tissue factor pathway inhibitor (TFPI) are considered to be the major determinants of the thrombin generation-based APC resistance test. The plasma levels of these proteins are affected by CHC, which might account for increased APC resistance. Apart from these tests we have also looked at factor VII-activating protease (FSAP). FSAP is a plasma serine protease with potential roles in the regulation of coagulation and fibrinolysis and therefore with an association to both venous and arterial thrombosis formation. A similar impact on FSAP activity and antigen levels were detected with COCs containing from 20 to 50 µg EE [25]. However, like any surrogate endpoints, it is not clear how these laboratory markers correlate with absolute thrombotic risk with clinical use of estrogen and to date these markers have not been prospectively verified. As DNA sequencing becomes more available and less expensive, testing for a limited number of mutations in the future might enable clinicians to identify women at particularly high risk for VTE.

Conclusion

Hormone replacement therapy is known to increase the risk of DVT and pulmonary embolism, though the absolute risk for a given patient is very small. The risk of DVT appears to be greatest soon after the initiation of HRT and returns to the baseline level after discontinuation. There are inconsistent data about whether estrogen-only or combined estrogen-progestin HRT products are associated with similar VTE risk. There is compelling evidence for a differential effect of estrogens according to route of administration, with blood coagulation activation and hypercoagulability state among oral estrogen users and definite hemostatic balance among transdermal estrogen users. This difference depends on neither the estrogen compound nor the daily dose. Retrospective analyses suggest that transdermal HRT is not as prothrombotic as oral HRT, though this has not been evaluated in randomized clinical trials.

Some, but not all, clinical studies have suggested that progestogens could be an important determinant of thrombotic risk, but no clear effect of the different progestogens on hemostasis has been highlighted.

Increasing age and weight further promote HRT's VTE risk. Some studies have investigated whether prothrombotic combinations may increase HRT's DVT risk. However, no benefit to screening prospective HRT users has been described, yet. Advanced proteomic and genomic studies may hold promise in the future for better elucidating which HRT users are at highest risk for VTE. Presently, physicians and prospective HRT users should discuss the potential risks and benefits for the individual patient, acknowledging there is no way to fully mitigate the risk of VTE. Shared decision-making is mandatory and the clinician should weigh the risks against the benefits when prescribing HRT and counsel the patient accordingly, taking into consideration the possible thrombosis-sparing properties associated with the route of adminstration and the preparation.

Clinical case

Claudia is 48 and she has experienced significant perimenopausal symptoms since her periods became irregular 12 months ago. She would like to try HRT, but her sister had a pulmonary embolus following a flight from Australia to the UK. She is worried about having a venous thromboembolic event, and she has heard that HRT will increase the risk.

Expert opinion

There is a relevant history of a first-degree relative having a thrombosis following a long-haul flight.

Action to take

Structured analysis including:
    Other family members with a history of VTE.
    Previous use of exogenous hormones.
    Gynecologic history and outcome of previous pregnancies.
    Medication.
    Chronic diseases.
    Sedentary lifestyle.
    Smoking.
Clinical examination.
    Calculate BMI.
    Blood pressure.
    Superficial thrombophlebitis.
    Pelvic congestion (fibroids or otherwise detected by ultrasonography).

Conclusion

Shared decision taking is mandatory.

No indication for thrombophilia screening.

Offer low-dose combined HRT, preferably using a transdermal preparation.

Tibolone is an option for women who are postmenopausal (more than 1 year since LMP or over the age of 54).

Review at 3 months.

References

1. Chan WS, Dixon ME. The "ART" of thromboembolism: a review of assisted reproductive technology and thromboembolic complications. *Thromb Res* 2008; **122**: 289–90.

2. ACOG Committee Opinion no. 556. Postmenopausal estrogen therapy: route of administration and risk of venous thromboembolism. *Obstet Gynecol* 2013; **121**: 887–90.

3. Canonico M, Plu-Bureau G, Scarabin PY. Progestogens and venous thromboembolism among postmenopausal women using hormone therapy. *Maturitas* 2011; **70**: 354–60.

4. Canonico M. Hormone therapy and hemostasis among postmenopausal women: a review. *Maturitas* 2014; **21**: 753–62.

5. Rosendaal FR. Venous thrombosis: a multicausal disease. *Lancet* 1999; **353**: 1167–73.

6. Roach RE, Lijfering WM, van Hylckama Vlieg A, *et al.* The risk of venous thrombosis in individuals with a history of superficial vein thrombosis and acquired venous thrombotic risk factors. *Blood* 2013; **122**: 4264–9.

7. Anderson FA, Wheeler HB, Goldberg RJ, *et al.* A population-based perspective of the hospital incidence and case-fatality rates of deep vein thrombosis and pulmonary embolism. The Worcester DVT study. *Arch Intern Med* 1991; **151**: 933–8.

8. White RH. The epidemiology of venous thromboembolism. *Circulation* 2003; **107**: 14–8.

9. Tsai AW, Cushman M, Rosamond WD, *et al.* Cardiovascular risk factors and venous thromboembolism incidence: the longitudinal investigation of thromboembolism etiology. *Arch Intern Med* 2002; **162**: 1182–9.

10. Cushman M, Kuller LH. Prentice R, *et al.* Estrogen plus progestin and risk of venous thrombosis, *JAMA* 2004; **292**: 1573–80.

11. Curb JD, Prentice RL, Bray PF, *et al.* Venous thrombosis and conjugated equine estrogen in women without a uterus. *Arch Intern Med* 2006; **166**: 772–80.

12. Ageno W, Becattini C, Brighton T, Selby S, Kamphuisen PW. Cardiovascular risk factors and venous thromboembolism: a meta-analysis. *Circulation* 2008; **117**: 93–102.

13. Alman-Farinelli MA. Obesity and venous thrombosis: a review. *Semin Thromb Hemost* 2011; **8**: 903–7.

14. Smith NL, Blondon M, Wiggins KL, *et al.* Lower risk of cardiovascular events in postmenopausal women taking oral estradiol compared with oral conjugated equine estrogens. *JAMA* 2014; **174**: 25–31.

15. Skouby SO, Jespersen J. Progestins in HRT: sufferance or desire? *Maturitas* 2009; **62**: 371–5.

16. Smith NL, Heckbert SR, Lemaitre RN, *et al.* Esterified estrogens and conjugated equine estrogens and the risk of venous thrombosis. *JAMA* 2004; **292**: 1581–7.

17. Skouby SO, Sidelmann J, Nilas L, Gram J, Jespersen J. The effect of continuous combined conjugated equine estrogen plus medroxyprogesterone acetate and tibolone on cardiovascular metabolic risk factors. *Climacteric* 2008; **11**: 489–97.

18. Canonico M, Oger E, Plu-Bureau G, *et al.*; Estrogen and Thromboembolism Risk (ESTHER) Study Group. Hormone therapy and venous thromboembolism among postmenopausal women: impact of the route of estrogen administration and progestogens: the ESTHER study. *Circulation* 2007; **115**: 840–5.

19. Blondon M, Wiggins KL, Van Hylckama Vlieg A, *et al.* Smoking, postmenopausal hormone therapy and the risk of venous thrombosis: a population-based, case-control study. *Br J Haematol* 2013; **163**: 418–20.

20. Eisenberger A, Westhoff C. Hormone replacement therapy and venous thromboembolism. *J Steroid Biochem Mol Biol* 2014; **142**: 76–82.

21. Hoibraaten E, Qvigstad E, Arnesen H, *et al.* Increased risk of recurrent venous thromboembolism during hormone replacement therapy – results of the randomized, double-blind, placebo-controlled estrogen in venous thromboembolism trial (EVTET). *Thromb Haemost* 2000; **84**: 961–7.

22. Reitsma PH, Versteeg HH, Middeldorp S. Mechanistic view of risk factors for venous thromboembolism. *Arterioscler Thromb Vasc Biol* 2012; **32**: 563–8.

23. Conard J, Basdevant A, Thomas JL, *et al.* Cardiovascular risk factors and combined estrogen-progestin replacement therapy: a placebo-controlled study with nomegestrol acetate and estradiol. *Fertil Steril* 1995; **64**: 957–62.

24. Lobo RA, Bush T, Carr BR, Pickar JH. Effects of lower doses of conjugated equine estrogens and medroxyprogesterone acetate on plasma lipids and lipoproteins, coagulation factors, and carbohydrate metabolism. *Fertil Steril* 2001; **76**: 13–24.

25. Sidelmann JJ, Skouby SO, Kluft C, *et al.* Plasma factor VII-activating protease is increased by oral contraceptives and induces factor VII activation in-vivo. *Thromb Res* 2011; **128**: e67–72.

Fertility and premature menopause

Anthony J. Rutherford

Sheila is 35, and has been on the combined oral contraceptive pill since the age of 18. She has now stopped the pill, and when her periods did not return after 3 months, consulted her general practitioner. A blood test has shown that she has a very high level of follicle stimulating hormone in her blood, and her physician explains that she has undergone a "premature menopause," and will not be able to conceive. She is referred to you for an expert opinion.

Introduction

Premature ovarian insufficiency is a relatively uncommon presentation for secondary amenorrhea, occurring in around 1% of women between 30 and 40 years of age [1]. This diagnosis is a devastating psychological blow to a young woman who may not have started her family. Physiologically, the implication of the very high levels of FSH is that the ovaries have no follicles that are responsive to FSH, resulting in a low estradiol level, and a subsequent lack of negative feedback to the hypothalamus. A careful history is important to rule out important concurrent disease, which may have implications for her general health. It is also essential to consider the whole patient and her needs, not just her fertility. Although the general practitioner is likely to be correct with the diagnosis, the implication that there is no chance of conception is wrong, as there remains a small chance of spontaneous ovulation, and the possibility of conception, which occurs in approximately 11% of women. This chapter will touch on the pertinent features in the initial assessment, advice about her general health and social well-being, but most importantly focus on her fertility options.

Initial assessment and diagnosis

Premature ovarian insufficiency (POI) is a devastating diagnosis for young women and it is essential that the diagnosis is confirmed as soon as possible and the news delivered in an empathetic manner. Premature ovarian insufficiency can be defined operationally as 4 months of amenorrhea and a raised FSH on two occasions. As Sheila already has had one FSH test, this test should be repeated along with a serum estradiol to confirm hypogonadism [1]. An outline of the other investigations that should be routinely performed is listed in Table 24.1. Although pelvic ultrasound is a useful tool in determining Sheila's pelvic anatomy for guidance on fertility, it is of no diagnostic use in POI, as ovarian follicles may still be evident. Pragmatically in up to 90% of patients no clear-cut cause will be identified.

Managing the Menopause: 21st Century Solutions, ed. Nick Panay, Paula Briggs, and Gab Kovacs. Published by Cambridge University Press. © Cambridge University Press 2015.

Table 24.1. Causes of premature ovarian insufficiency.

Idiopathic	No obvious cause found in up to 90%
Genetic aberrations	X chromosome mutations e.g. FMR-1 gene X chromosome defects Turner's syndrome Trisomy X Balanced X chromosome translocations X chromosome partial deletions Autosomal chromosome mutations, e.g. SALT (galactosemia), FSHR
Autoimmune	Up to 20% have a history of autoimmune disease Adrenal insufficiency Hypothroidism Autoimmune Polyglandular Syndrome I and III
Iatrogenic	Treatment of malignant disease and severe benign ovarian disease Radiotherapy Chemotherapy Severe endometriosis
Toxins and viruses	Further clarification required Mumps Cigarette smoking Heavy metals, pesticides, solvents

Sheila's assessment should always start with a detailed history, with particular reference to a family history of POI. Approximately 2–6% of spontaneous POI is associated with pre-mutations in the fragile site mental retardation 1 gene (FMR-1 gene). This is the gene responsible for the fragile X syndrome, which is the most common cause of familial mental retardation. If there is a positive family history of early ovarian insufficiency, then up to 14% of POI will be associated with pre-mutations of the FMR-1 gene. Where such a mutation is found, then referral for genetic counseling and further family studies are important due to the risk of family members having a child with mental retardation. Although there are other established rare genetic causes of POI involving mutations in genes found on the X and autosomal chromosomes, in the absence of specific symptoms extensive screening is not justified outside a research setting [2].

In contrast to those women who present with primary amenorrhea, where up to 50% may have a chromosomal abnormality, in women like Sheila presenting with secondary amenorrhea, the karyotype is generally normal. Although a proportion of women with Turner's mosaic can have a normal puberty and spontaneous menstruation, the majority will develop ovarian failure well before their 30s. Of course, this could be masked in a woman on the oral contraceptive pill for a prolonged period of time. Other chromosomal anomalies associated with POI include trisomy X, X chromosome deletions, and balanced translocations involving the X and autosomal chromosomes.

A history of any significant autoimmune disease points to a possible immunological cause of POI, with the most common association being thyroid autoimmunity. Autoimmune lymphocytic oophoritis accounts for approximately 4% of women with POI, and stands as a marker for other types of steroidogenic cell autoimmunity such as adrenal insufficiency, which can have potential fatal consequences if left undetected. There is

Table 24.2. Diagnostic assessment of premature ovarian insufficiency.

Endocrine	Follicle stimulating hormone, luteinizing hormone and estradiol Thyroid function tests
Karyotype	Turner's syndrome, Turner's mosaic, Trisomy, Balanced translocation
DNA	Fragile X pre-mutation
Autoimmune	Adrenal autoantibodies
Pelvic ultrasound scan	Not for diagnostic purposes but essential to assess treatment options

a good correlation between the presence of adrenal cortex autoantibodies, detected by immunofluorescence and POI. The POI usually pre-dates the adrenal insufficiency. Although anti-ovarian antibodies have been reported in POI, their routine detection is of limited value. The gold standard for the diagnosis of autoimmune POI is an ovarian biopsy, but due to the lack of any therapeutic benefits from identifying this condition it should not be used in routine clinical practice.

Other causes of POI may be evident from the history, with a list of the more common causes of POI outlined in Table 24.1. Iatrogenic ovarian failure can occur after therapeutic chemotherapy or radiotherapy for malignant disease, or after extensive ovarian surgery for benign or malignant disease. Uterine embolization, used to treat uterine fibroids, has been associated with POI by compromising the ovarian blood supply. A severe mumps infection has been considered to be a cause of POI, similar to the impact seen in men who develop mumps orchitis. The putative role of environmental toxins and cigarette smoking is not firmly established.

Management

Although Sheila was initially referred for fertility treatment, it is important that her overall reproductive and psychological health is considered. This includes advice on the use of adequate hormone replacement therapy (HRT) in the longer term to maintain her bone mass, and to prevent sexual dysfunction, as well as treating the vasomotor symptoms associated with estrogen deficiency. In younger women, hormone replacement can be provided from the use of the combined oral contraceptive pill or more conventional biphasic HRT. However, psychologically in a woman recently diagnosed with POI presenting with infertility, the use of the combined oral contraceptive pill may seem counterintuitive. This would prevent the small but recognized chance of spontaneous pregnancy seen in 5–10% of women with POI. Furthermore, recent evidence has suggested that the use of biphasic conventional HRT, mimicking a more normal endocrine environment, may have a more beneficial uterine effect, helping create a thicker endometrium [3]. The unfortunate media hype surrounding the risks of long-term HRT, and in particular breast cancer, need to be carefully managed, and the true risks in premature ovarian failure need to be explained to avoid lack of compliance. The lack of ovarian androgens may cause a noticeable decrease in libido and an additional small dose of testosterone replacement has been shown to be helpful [4]. This can be administered transdermally as a gel. It is important to monitor for adverse side effects of androgens such as hirsutism, acne and changes in the HDL cholesterol. A full discussion on the choice of HRT is beyond the scope of this chapter; please refer to Chapters 17 and 25.

Associated medical disorders, which may have been found on the initial assessment, should be addressed to ensure that pregnancy is safe and outcome optimized. These include normalization of endocrine disorders such as thyroid and adrenal dysfunction. Women with Turner's syndrome often have cardiac and renal abnormalities, and need to have a cardiac assessment of their aorta due to the high risk of coarctation. Appropriate psychological support is essential with referral to a trained counselor, not only for support following the diagnosis but also to talk through the implications of egg donation.

Fertility treatment

Sheila has a small chance of natural ovulation and spontaneous pregnancy, estimated to be between 5% and 10%. Reassuringly, if a spontaneous pregnancy does occur, the risk of miscarriage is no greater than women with normal ovarian function. Although numerous interventions have been attempted to increase the likelihood of spontaneous ovulation, including a short-term course of the oral contraceptive pill (pill rebound), HRT, steroids and gonadotropin-releasing hormone agonists (GnRHa), there is no substantiated evidence that any of these are better than expectant management. One small study suggested that the use of GnRHa in combination with gonadotropins with high-dose steroid therapy may be beneficial in women with POI and a normal karyotype, but much larger studies are needed confirm this potential benefit [5]. It is impossible to predict if Sheila's spontaneous ovulation will return, although normalization of serum endocrinology can occur as disease levels fluctuate. Ovarian tissue cryopreservation is a possible option for women who are about to lose their ovarian function through ablative chemotherapy, but it has no role to play in Sheila's case as her oocyte numbers are already depleted at the time of diagnosis. The best option for pregnancy is egg donation, which is discussed in detail in the following section.

Egg donation

Egg donation allows the patient to carry and deliver her husband's genetic child. Although the child is not genetically linked, the woman is responsible for the child's existence, nurturing the embryo from conception to delivery, and in the UK, her name is recorded as the mother on the child's birth certificate. The use of egg donation has increased substantially as a treatment option in Europe, almost doubling from 13,609 in 2008 [6] to 25,187 in 2010 [7].

Regulation

The regulations governing egg donation vary substantially around the world. In the UK, where *in vitro* fertilization (IVF) treatment has been closely regulated by the Human Fertilisation and Embryology Authority (HFEA) since 1991, information on donors, including a description of themselves, their ethnic group, marital status, the number and gender of their current children, their physical characteristics, details of screening tests and medical history as well as a goodwill message for potential children, are held by the HFEA. A change in the HFEA Act saw anonymity removed from all gamete donation from April 1, 2005. Since that time, at the age of 18 a child can contact the HFEA and be provided with identifying information about their genetic origins, including contact information. The

HFEA will inform the donor that a request has been received, prior to releasing information. This loss of anonymity did not receive uniform approval, and there was a fall off in those coming forward as egg donors in 2006, although this has now recovered almost completely [8]. Furthermore, in a recent survey, up to 34% of recipients travel overseas for egg donation to avoid the anonymity rules [9]. Donors who donated prior to 2005 can apply to the HFEA to remove anonymity. However, no donor has the legal right to contact their donor-conceived child, although they can find out how many children were born as a result of their donation.

Egg donors in the UK have to be under the age of 36, unless there are exceptional documented reasons to use older women, such as known donation. Donors are encouraged to allow the clinic to verify their medical and psychological history with their general practitioner. When selecting donors, clinics need to take into account the implications of the donation for the donor's family and her future fertility. Donors can put conditions on the use and storage of their gametes, but these need to be compatible with the Equality Act 2010. Donors and recipients need to be aware that the donors can withdraw their consent to the use of their gametes and to the use of embryos created from their gametes at any stage in the treatment process. It is therefore mandatory that all gamete donors and recipients are provided with the opportunity to receive appropriate implications counseling. In the UK, couples are encouraged to reveal to their donor-conceived child their genetic origins. The emphasis placed on telling the child following egg donation relates to the extensive psychological literature outlining the experiences of adopted children and their perceived need to find out about their genetic origins.

Source of egg donors

Egg donors in the UK are recruited from two clear groups. The first are women who donate altruistically, principally to help others, responding to stories in the media or who have friends or family who have had difficulty conceiving. The recipient can use a family friend or relative directly, or by agreeing to donate to others, allowing the recipient access to the "donor pool," in a cross-over arrangement. A common example is a sister donating to the other sister, although recent evidence suggests that this can at times prove difficult, as ovarian insufficiency may unknowingly be unearthed in the sibling [10]. Altruistic donors account for less than half (43% in 2010) of all UK donors [7]. Ethically, altruistic donors are showing an unselfish concern for the welfare of others, and make the donation voluntarily without payment in return, or compensation. From the child's perspective it is known that the donor's motives are hugely relevant, and that those donating altruistically are likely to be more committed, rather than those donors potentially donating for monetary gain, as the latter are less likely to think about the long-term consequences. In 2012, the HFEA changed the rules on compensation, and now UK donors can be paid reasonable expenses up to the value of £750. This encouraged some to come forward where the primary motive is monetary gain rather than altruistic donation.

The second, and largest, group of donors in the UK is those who receive benefit in kind, including free or subsidized fertility treatment by donating a proportion of their gametes during their own fertility treatment. Egg-sharing started in the UK nearly 20 years ago and now accounts for 57% of all UK donors in 2010. In these circumstances, patients who require *in vitro* fertilization (IVF) or intracytoplasmic sperm injection (ICSI) treatment, donate a set number of their oocytes to a recipient. Careful selection is essential to ensure that the donor will produce sufficient oocytes to make the process worthwhile for both parties. In general, if the assessment ultrasound suggests that the donor will not produce sufficient oocytes, clinics usually favor canceling the recipient cycle. It is not allowed by law to continue with the cycle and donate all the oocytes to the recipient, then the donor start a fresh cycle for her own use. This process known as "egg giving" was outlawed by the HFEA [8]. It is essential the clinic have a clear policy of whether a charge will apply if this situation were to occur. Egg-sharers mainly consist of women not eligible for NHS-funded treatment, often as their partners have had children in previous relationships. Research has shown that in comparison to altruistic donors the chance of a successful outcome is similar, and that both the donor and the recipient have an equal chance of a successful outcome [11]. However, there is some evidence that some unsuccessful egg-sharing donors feel regret in the knowledge that another couple may become the parents of a child genetically related to them [12]. The full extent of the implications of the change in the UK regulations with anonymity on those unsuccessful egg-sharing donors will not be known until 2023 when the first child is 18 and is able to trace their genetic parent.

The major drawback of egg donation in the UK has been the shortfall in egg donors, and as a consequence many patients now choose to travel overseas.

Recruitment of donors overseas is variable, and some countries like Sweden manage almost entirely on altruistic donation. However, those countries, which incidentally perform the majority of egg donation in Europe, pay their donors a financial incentive to donate. The largest exponent in Europe is Spain who performed 12,928 cycles in 2010. Other countries within Europe performing a large number of cycles include the Czech Republic (2,365), Russia (2,147), the UK (1,891) and Belgium (1,412). In some countries such as Turkey, egg donation is not permitted on religious grounds, and as a result services have developed in neighboring states or provinces where the rules permit, such as Northern Cyprus, which now has a flourishing egg donation program. Across the world, egg donation programs are well developed in North America, with payment of donors established practice. In 2007 the American Society of Reproductive Medicine recommended a limit on the payment to donors to $50,00, and no more than $10,000 could be justified [13]. A recent survey of agencies and clinics offering egg donor matching and donation respectively in the USA demonstrated that these guidelines are being flaunted. Furthermore, many of these agencies and clinics are paying additional amounts for certain characteristics [14]. Paid oocyte donation has potential concerns, and there is a risk that where money is involved donors may be encouraged to donate three or more times, which may ultimately have an impact on their own health and fertility.

Screening of egg donors

Assessment of egg donors includes a very careful medical and social history with specific reference to any current or past physical conditions that may have a bearing on a future child. People with a known gene, chromosomal or mitochondrial abnormality that may cause serious physical or mental disability, and those who have a personal history of a transmissible infection are excluded. Clearly lifestyle issues such as diet, weight and smoking are important in those considering donation. A thorough psychological assessment, with implications counseling is essential, and considered mandatory in the UK. Only those who successfully complete this phase of the assessment are then subject to laboratory testing.

Table 24.3. Donor screening tests.

Infection screen	Cervical swab
	Gonorrhea
	Chlamydia
	Serology
	HIV
	Hepatitis B
	Hepatitis C
	Syphillis
	Cytomegalovirus
Genetic screen	Karyotype
	Gene testing
	Cystic fibrosis
	± dependent on ethnicity – hemoglobinopathies, sickle cell trait
Blood group	
Fertility tests	Baseline pelvic ultrasound
	Antral follicle count
	Anti-Müllerian hormone (AMH)
	Endocrinology
	Follicle stimulating hormone, luteinizing hormone, estradiol day 1 to 5 of menses

Laboratory testing focuses on three aspects: the donor's natural fertility, a transmissible infection screen and a simple genetic screen. The latter will be modified according to their ethnicity. The standard tests recommended in the UK are outlined in Table 24.3. The infection screen is performed contemporaneously with the time the donor will donate, and will be repeated should the donation process happen on more than one occasion. As a fresh embryo transfer takes place there is a small but largely hypothetical risk of a donor being infected with HIV despite screening negative for HIV antibody. However, modern fourth generation tests which test for both the antibody and antigen address this potential issue [15].

Donor matching

When donor gametes are employed, most couples are keen to have a donor that closely matches their physical characteristics and their ethnicity. Physical features such as height, build, hair, skin and eye color of both partners are recorded. Blood group is often matched such that the conceived child's blood group could have arisen from the parents, to preserve the desire for anonymity. In the UK, where most clinics offering egg donation perform less than 100 cycles per annum, the choice is extremely limited, particularly for certain ethnic groups. The advent of successful oocyte cryopreservation using vitrification techniques has led to the development of egg donor banks, which potentially offer greater choice of matching for prospective donors. The large egg donation programs in southern Europe and North America offer a wider choice of donor, and as a result can provide a closer physical match.

Recipients are carefully screened for common transmissible infections, similar to the donor infection screen. Cytomegalovirus is a relatively common infection that can cause a mild flu-like illness in an adult, but if a woman is infected in early pregnancy can cause a similar spectrum of fetal abnormalities to rubella infection. Recipients found to be CMV-negative are generally matched with like donors that are CMV-negative. However, the risk of reactivation of a CMV infection using donor eggs is theoretical only, and where all other parameters match, an informed couple may select to use a CMV-positive donor.

Cycle programming

In the majority of egg donor programs the aim is to perform a fresh embryo transfer, usually achieved using freshly obtained oocytes. When the donor has her oocytes collected the recipient needs to have a well-developed endometrium completely in phase to maximize the chance of implantation. The best way of achieving synchrony is to ensure that once the donors are screened they are kept on the oral contraceptive pill, which in combination with a short antagonist stimulation cycle makes the process of donor–recipient coordination relatively straightforward. In Sheila's case where she is amenorrhoeic, programming simply involves manipulating her HRT, stopping it 7–10 days before starting endometrial stimulation. In women that continue to menstruate, most clinicians surveyed use a method to suppress residual ovarian function [16], which include the oral contraceptive pill (22%), GnRH agonists, either alone (37%) or with the contraceptive pill (40%), and more recently GnRH antagonists [17]. There is no convincing evidence that pre-programming improves the endometrium or the clinical pregnancy rate, but may reduce the risk of canceling the cycle [18]. The GnRH agonists are started in the late luteal phase in regular cycling women, or on day 1 in women with irregular cycles, and continued until the onset of the progesterone (Figure 24.1).

Endometrial development

The options for stimulating endometrial development include oral, transdermal, vaginal and intramuscular estrogen, with the majority of clinicians (86%) choosing the oral route [16]. The recipient starts estrogen a couple of days before the donor starts ovarian stimulation, with the dose increased gradually to mimic the rise in estrogen seen in natural cycles (from 2 mg going up to 8 mg). Endometrial development is assessed by ultrasound on day 12 of stimulation. The thickness of the endometrium does have a bearing on outcome, with optimal clinical pregnancy rates where the endometrium has a trilaminar appearance and measures 9–13 mm. Nevertheless, acceptable pregnancy rates are achieved where the endometrium is between 5–8 mm and 13–18 mm. If endometrial thickness remains less than 8 mm, the dose of estrogen is commonly increased and/or changed to include a transdermal preparation. In addition, tocopherol, pentoxyphyline and Viagra have also been used, but none of these as adjunct therapies have been shown to have convincing evidence of benefit [19].

Progesterone is started once the date of the donor's oocyte recovery is confirmed, administered either orally, transvaginally, intramuscularly (IM) or using a subcutaneous route. Surprisingly, the intramuscular route is favored by most clinicians (74%), compared with the transvaginal (23%) and oral alternatives (3%). Despite this preference there is no evidence

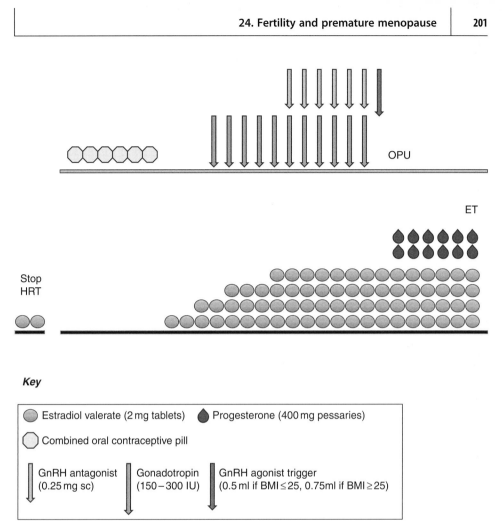

Figure 24.1. Diagram of Sheila's and her donor's coordinated treatment plan.

that any one preparation is better than the other in terms of clinical pregnancy or live birth rates. From a patient perspective, the transvaginal route would appear kinder. The dose of progesterone is generally higher than that used to support the luteal phase after conventional IVF, from 100 mg daily by IM injection, to 800–1200 mg transvaginally. The time the progesterone is started in relation to the donor's oocyte recovery is important and does influence outcome. Starting the progesterone on the day of the egg collection or the day after gives better pregnancy rates than starting the progesterone the day before the egg collection [18].

Egg collection and embryo transfer

The number of oocytes each recipient will receive will vary dependent on the number of oocytes produced by the donor, and whether those are split with other recipients. This will usually lie between 5 and 10. On the day of the donor's oocyte recovery, the recipient's partner produces his sperm sample. Under normal circumstances, the method of fertilization employed should reflect the quality of the semen sample, as there is no evidence that ICSI improves the live birth rates where the sperm sample is normal [20]. However, in reality ICSI is employed in over 55% of cases [15]. Fertilization rates are generally around 70%, providing the recipient with between three and seven early cleavage stage embryos.

The timing of the embryo transfer and the number of embryos transferred are important in determining the outcome. As the implantation rate per embryo transferred is likely to be high due to the young age of the donor, transferring two embryos will substantially increase the risk of multiple births. To reduce this risk, many countries have adopted a policy of selecting the single best embryo for transfer. Statistical modeling has shown that replacing a single embryo on day 3 will reduce the overall clinical pregnancy rate, whereas this fall is not as evident when a single embryo is selected for transfer at the blastocyst stage, on day 5 [21]. Surplus good-quality embryos that reach the blastocyst stage are cryopreserved for future use, to give the couple the chance of a genetically similar sibling. Unlike sperm donation, where sperm can be stored to help expand the family in the future, most egg donors will not go through the process of donation again, and therefore the frozen embryos may be the couple's only chance of a child with similar genetic lineage.

As the recipient has no functioning corpus luteum, the pregnancy has to be sustained by hormone replacement until the placental tissue is functional, which usually occurs around 8 weeks' gestation. Most clinicians play safe and continue both estrogen and progesterone supplements until 10–12 weeks gestation [16].

Success rates

Live birth rates throughout the world mirror the success rates seen in infertile populations, and vary from 30% to 50%. In the UK there has been a steady improvement in live birth rates following egg donation, with the latest statistics showing a rate of 30.8% [8]. Repeat treatment cycles offer a similar chance of conception, such that cumulative pregnancy rates after three attempts of 87% are possible [22]. Although high success rates are available to those traveling to overseas programs, many countries have no restrictive regulation, such that multiple embryos can be transferred. Unfortunately this has translated to a substantial increase in higher-order multiple pregnancies in women over 40, which is almost certainly as a result of egg donation, using overseas egg donation programs [23]. It is imperative for those clinicians thinking about referring or helping women to travel overseas, that there is a clear dialog outlining a commitment to reduce the number of embryos transferred to minimize multiple births. Although Sheila is only 35, many of the patients seen with ovarian insufficiency are over 40, and potentially at increased risk of obstetric complications.

Cost

Rules and regulations vary so much across the world, that it is impossible to give an accurate assessment of the cost of treatment to the patient. In the UK, a nulliparous 35-year-old presenting with POI could attract NHS funding for up to three full treatment cycles. If no state funding is available, the cost of self-funding treatment varies considerably, ranging from around €8,000 to €12,000 in Europe, and $17,000 to $30,000 in North America.

Summary

The diagnosis of premature ovarian insufficiency at the age of 35 in a nulliparous woman like Sheila has far-reaching consequences psychologically, physically and from a personal perspective, with plans for a balanced family life seemingly thrown into disarray. Careful assessment and support, treating the patient as a whole, can help women like Sheila achieve their ambition of family life.

References

1. Nelson LM, Covington SN, Rebar RW. An update: spontaneous premature ovarian failure is not an early menopause. *Fertil Steril* 2005; **83**: 1327–32.

2. Goswami D, Conway GS. Premature ovarian failure. *Hum Reprod Update* 2005; **11**: 391–410.

3. O'Donnell RL, Warner P, Lee RJ, *et al.* Physiological sex steroid replacement in premature ovarian failure: randomized crossover trial of effect on uterine volume, endometrial thickness and blood flow, compared with a standard regimen. *Hum Reprod* 2012; **27**: 1130–8.

4. Somboonporn W, Davis S, Seif MW, *et al.* Testosterone for peri and postmenopausal women (review). *Cochrane Database Syst Rev* 2005; **4**: CD004509.

5. Badawy A, Goda H, Ragab A. Induction of ovulation in idiopathic premature ovarian failure: a randomized double-blind trial. *Reprod Biomed Online* 2007; **15**: 215–19.

6. Ferraretti AP, Goossens V, de Mouzon J, *et al.*; European IVF-monitoring (EIM) Consortium, for European Society of Human Reproduction and Embryology (ESHRE). Assisted reproductive technology in Europe, 2008: results generated from European registers by ESHRE. *Hum Reprod* 2012; **27**: 2571–84.

7. Kupka MS, Ferraretti AP, de Mouzon J, *et al.*; The European IVF-monitoring (EIM) Consortium, for the European Society of Human Reproduction and Embryology (ESHRE). Assisted reproductive technology in Europe, 2010: results generated from European registers by ESHRE. *Hum Reprod* 2014; **10**: 2099–113.

8. www.HFEA.gov.uk.

9. Shenfield F, de Mouzon J, Pennings G, *et al.*; The ESHRE Taskforce on Cross Border Reproductive Care. Cross border reproductive care in six European countries. *Hum Reprod* 2010; **25**:1361–8.

10. Sung L, Bustillo M, Mukherjee T, *et al.* Sisters of women with premature ovarian failure may not be ideal ovum donors. *Fertil Steril* 1997; **67**: 912–16.

11. Oyesanya OA, Olufowobi O, Ross W, Sharif K, Afnan M. Prognosis of oocyte donation cycles: a prospective comparison of the in vitro fertilization – embryo transfer cycles of recipients who used shared oocytes versus those who used altruistic donors. *Fertil Steril* 2009; **92**: 930–6.

12. Ahuja KK, Simons EG, Mostyn BJ, Bowen-Simpkins P. An assessment of the motives and morals of egg share donors: policy of 'payments' to egg donors requires a fair review. *Hum Reprod* 1998; **13**: 2671–8.

13. Ethics Committee of the American Society for Reproductive Medicine. Financial compensation of oocyte donors. *Fertil Steril* 2007; **88**: 305–9.

14. Keehn J, Holwell E, Abdul-Karim R, *et al.* Recruiting egg donors online: an analysis of in vitro fertilization clinics and agency websites' adherence to American Society for Reproductive Medicine guidelines. *Fertility and Sterility* 2012; **98** (4): 995–1000.

15. Seem DL, Lee I, Umscheid CA, Kuehnert MJ; United States Public Health Service. PHS guideline for reducing human immunodeficiency virus, Hepatitis B virus, and hepatitis C virus transmission through organ transplantation. *Public Health Rep* 2013; **128**: 247–343.

16. Weissman A. *Oocyte Donation Survey.* IVF-Worldwide.com/survey/oocyte-donation/results-oocyte-donation.html.

17. Huang JYJ, Tomer S, Kligman I, Cholst I. The use of gonadotropin releasing hormone antagonist for ovarian suppression in donor egg recipients. *Fertil Steril* 2011; **96**: S280–1.

18. Glujovsky D, Pesce R, Fiszbajn G, *et al.* Endometrial preparation for women undergoing embryo transfer with frozen embryos or embryos derived form donor oocytes. *Cochrane Database Syst Rev* 2010; **1**: CD006359.pub2.

19. Gutarra-Vilchez RB, Bonfill Cosp X, Glujovsky D, Urrútia G. Vasodilators for women undergoing assisted reproduction. *Cochrane Database Syst Rev* 2012; **7**: CD010001.

20. Bhattacharya S, Hamilton MP, Shaaban M, *et al.* Conventional in-vitro fertilization versus intracytoplasmic sperm injection for the treatment of non male factor infertility: a randomised controlled trial. *Lancet* 2001; **357**: 2075–99.

21. Roberts SA, McGowan L, Hirst MW, *et al.*; towardSET Collaboration. Reducing the incidence of twins from IVF treatments: predictive modelling from a retrospective cohort. *Hum Reprod* 2011; **26**: 569–75.

22. Budak E, Garrido N, Soares SR, *et al.* Improvements achieved in an oocyte donation program over a 10-year period: sequential increase in implantation and pregnancy rates and decrease in high-order multiple pregnancies. *Fertil Steril* 2007; **88**: 342–9.

23. Office of National Statistics (year) *Births in England and Wales by Characteristics of Birth 2, 2011.* www.ons.gov.uk/ons/rel/vsob1/characteristics-of-birth-2–england-and-wales/2011/sb-characteristics-of-birth-2.html.

The risk-benefit analysis of hormone replacement therapy in the menopause

Tatijana Nikishina and Tim Hillard

The hormone replacement therapy (HRT) risk-benefit profile has been the subject of considerable analysis over the past decade and has been at the center of the debate that has polarized opinion between those who advocate the use of HRT and those who oppose it. Whilst there is broad agreement around some of the key benefits of HRT there is considerable difference about the interpretation of the risks in taking it. Recent revised data from the Women's Health Initiative (WHI) and other randomized clinical trials since the publication of WHI together with various authoritative position statements have helped to clarify some of the uncertainties and provide more robust evidence for clinical decision-making.

The available evidence suggests that HRT should be offered to well-informed peri- or early postmenopausal women to control moderate-to-severe menopausal symptoms, as the benefits outweigh the risks in otherwise healthy women in this age group [1, 2]. However an individualized and rational approach to commencing HRT is important, as the risk-benefit balance will differ for each woman. There is currently less evidence for the widespread use of HRT for long-term chronic disease prevention [1–3], although again the balance between potential benefits and risks will differ from individual to individual.

There are a number of factors which can influence an individual's risk-benefit ratio (Table 25.1).

This chapter aims to review the current evidence for the benefits and risks of HRT as a guide to clinical decision-making.

Benefits of HRT

For young, healthy menopausal women (below the age of 60) with bothersome symptoms the benefits of HRT generally outweigh the risks. However the risk-benefit profile for a particular woman is not static, therefore regular clinical reviews are necessary.

We will briefly discuss the main known benefits of HRT; many of these are discussed in more detail elsewhere in the book.

Vasomotor symptoms

Vasomotor symptoms – often described as hot flashes and night sweats – affect 60–80% of menopausal women to some extent [4]. The severity of these symptoms peaks in the late perimenopause and early postmenopause, but there is a large individual and ethnic variation in their prevalence, severity, frequency and duration (mean of 5–10 years) [5].

Managing the Menopause: 21st Century Solutions, ed. Nick Panay, Paula Briggs, and Gab Kovacs.
Published by Cambridge University Press. © Cambridge University Press 2015.

Table 25.1. Factors influencing an individual's risk-benefit ratio for hormone replacement therapy.

> Relevant personal or family history
> Lifestyle (weight, diet, exercise, smoking and alcohol use)
> Severity of menopausal symptoms
> Age and time of HRT initiation in relation to onset of menopause ("critical therapeutic window")
> Type of HRT (combined or estrogen only)
> Dose of HRT preparation
> Route of HRT administration
> Length of HRT use

A Cochrane review reported a 75% reduction in the frequency and an 87% reduction in severity of hot flashes in HRT users [4]. As these symptoms can be debilitating in a significant proportion of women, managing them effectively should have an important positive impact on their quality of life. Although this seems obvious, clear data on the benefits of HRT on quality of life are lacking, primarily because randomized placebo-controlled trials of symptomatic women are not considered ethical in many countries.

The addition of progestogen to estrogen as part of HRT did not show any change in results. The lowest effective estrogen dose should be used and increasingly lower and lower doses have proven to be effective [5].

Urogenital symptoms

The prevalence of vulvo-vaginal atrophy among postmenopausal women is around 27% [5].

Topical vaginal estrogen therapy provides effective symptom relief and improvement in the cytological composition and physiology of the vaginal epithelium [2, 4]. Vaginal estrogens are also effective in reducing the number of episodes of recurrent urinary tract infections in postmenopausal women.

Topical vaginal estrogens have minimal systemic absorption and are considered safe. They are not associated with the risks associated with HRT discussed later. Systemic HRT preparations offer no therapeutic advantages over low-dose local estrogens in the management of atrophic vaginitis in the menopause, indeed meta-analyses suggest that bladder symptoms such as sensory urgency respond better to topical rather than systemic preparations [4].

Thus for women with just urogenital atrophy and no other symptoms, there is no advantage in taking systemic HRT. Women taking topical vaginal estrogen preparations should be reassured of their safety and that there is no requirement to take additional progestogens.

Female sexual function

Sexual dysfunction is common amongst postmenopausal women and its correction can lead to improved quality of life for women and their partners.

Systemic and topical HRT improves the superficial and sometimes deep dyspareunia associated with vulvo-vaginal atrophy in postmenopausal women [2, 4]. Restoring libido is altogether a more complex challenge. For some women correction of underlying menopausal symptoms and improvements in sleep and mood can all have a positive impact. The addition of testosterone therapy has been shown to improve sexual desire and satisfaction in surgically and naturally menopausal women [2, 4].

Mood and depression

Peri- and postmenopause are associated with an increase in mood and depressive disorders. Estrogen interacts with mood-regulating brain mechanisms through a number of neurotransmitters and the serotonin system [6]. Recent RCTs have shown significant beneficial associations between HRT and mood; 68–80% of women using estrogen-only HRT reported decreased mood symptoms, compared with only 20–22% of women using placebo [6].

Both estrogen-only and combined preparations improve depressive symptoms in menopause when compared with placebo. Use of HRT has also been associated with a significant improvement in sleep quality [4]. For some women the additional progestogen can have a negative impact on these symptoms. This may vary with the type, dose and route of progestogen so careful selection of combination therapy is required.

Osteoporosis and fractures

Declining estrogen levels in the menopause are strongly associated with bone density loss and osteoporotic fractures [4]. Hormone replacement therapy is effective in preventing bone loss and reducing the incidence of all osteoporotic fractures in the menopause [7]. A Cochrane review indicates a 30% reduction in osteoporotic fractures (hip, vertebrae and overall) among women taking estrogen-only or combined HRT compared with placebo [8].

Hormone replacement therapy should be considered one of the first-line choices of therapy in postmenopausal women below the age of 60 with a significant fracture risk and for those women with premature ovarian insufficiency. Coincidentally, these particular groups of women are also the most likely to suffer from menopausal symptoms. Initiating HRT after the age of 60 for the sole purpose of osteoporosis prevention is not recommended as a first-line therapy although it may still be effective.

The protective effect of HRT on bone mineral density may remain for a variable length of time after cessation of therapy before an inevitable gradual decline in bone density occurs [8], emphasizing the importance of ongoing bone conservation strategies.

Degenerative arthritis

Estrogen has a regulatory role in the metabolism of cartilage [7]. In menopause, the decrease of estrogen levels is associated with thinning of intervertebral discs and osteoarthritic joint changes. Most of these changes occur in the first 5 years after the menopause [4].

Timely hormone replacement initiation can have a protective effect on intervertebral discs and articulated joint cartilage. In the WHI Study, women treated with estrogen alone had significantly lower rates (RR 0.84, 95% CI 0.70–1.00) of arthroplasty than those in the placebo group [4]. These benefits, however, were not evident in the WHI continuous combined HRT arm. It seems likely that progestogens neutralize the chondroprotective actions of estrogen; further studies are necessary to explore this.

Skin

Estrogens play an important role in skin physiology. The hypoestrogenic state of the menopause accelerates age-related skin changes (thinning and dryness of the skin, increase in the number and depth of wrinkles, decrease in skin elasticity).

Several randomized, double-blind, placebo-controlled trials have shown a 30% increase in dermal thickness in postmenopausal women after 12 months of estrogen therapy, as well as an overall increase in collagen content and a decrease in facial wrinkling.

Cognition

Estrogen receptors are widespread in the central and peripheral nervous systems and estrogens facilitate autonomic regulation and cognitive functions. Early untreated surgical menopause is associated with an increased incidence of dementia and other neurologic conditions.

The impact of HRT on cognitive function depends on the woman's age and timing of HRT initiation. Several studies have revealed cognitive benefits of HRT if commenced around the time of menopause, i.e., during a "critical therapeutic window" period. Early HRT initiators have demonstrated improved memory, stronger global cognition and executive function [6]. A recent observational study has shown a 30% reduction of Alzheimer's disease risk in women who initiated HRT within 5 years of menopause and used it for ≥ 10 years [6]. Later HRT initiation, as in the WHI Study, does not appear to have the same positive effect, indeed may even have a negative effect.

Further well-designed trials are necessary to explore the neuro-protective effects of various HRT preparations and their potential use in prevention of neurodegenerative conditions.

Cardiovascular disease

Cardiovascular disease is the leading cause of death in women over 50 years of age worldwide. Considerable evidence suggests that atherosclerotic changes are delayed by estrogen – whether endogenous in the premenopause, or exogenous in the form of HRT after the onset of menopause.

Estrogens are associated with reduction in endothelial injury, as well as plaque formation through lowering total and LDL cholesterol and raising HDL cholesterol levels.

Observational studies have shown a 40% decrease in cardiovascular disease rates, as well as cardiovascular disease-related and all-cause mortality rates, in women who commenced HRT in early menopause vs. non-users [9]. A "critical therapeutic window" theory can be applied here as the cardio-protective effect was not observed in women starting HRT after the age of 60 (Table 25.2). A more recent 10-year randomized trial of women receiving HRT started early after menopause showed that the HRT group had a significantly reduced risk of mortality, heart failure and stroke compared with the untreated group [2].

Current evidence suggests that estrogen-only regimens may offer greater cardio-protection than combined regimens, and a transdermal route of administration may provide further additional benefit of lowering the blood pressure and preventing atherosclerotic plaque rupture and thrombosis as compared with oral estrogen preparations [9]. Treatment seems to be duration dependent and becomes effective after at least 6 years of use.

More research is needed on the role of cardiovascular effects of progestogens in combined HRT preparations.

Table 25.2. Relative risk (RR) for cardiovascular events by age and time since onset of menopause in the WHI Study.

	CEE	CEE + MPA
Age (years)		
50–59	0.63	1.29
60–69	0.94	1.03
70–79	1.13	1.48
Time since menopause (years)		
<10	0.48	0.88
10–19	0.96	1.23
≥20	1.12	1.66

CEE, conjugated equine estrogens; MPA, medroxyprogesterone acetate.

Type II diabetes

Type II diabetes is a multifactorial condition with an increased incidence in the mid-life. Decline in estrogen levels during menopause transition and HRT may play a role in insulin sensitivity; however, insufficient evidence is currently available [4]. A large RCT indicated a lower incidence (by 7.5 cases per 1,000 women per 5 years of use) of type II diabetes among women using combined HRT in comparison with the placebo group [4]. The effects of HRT may depend on baseline metabolic status and abdominal obesity, and women with larger waist circumferences are more likely to benefit from HRT use [4].

Colorectal cancer

Epidemiologic studies have consistently shown up to a 20% reduction in colon cancer incidence in ever-users of HRT compared with never-users [4]. The WHI randomized trial reported a decrease in risk in women taking combined HRT; the absolute risk decreased from 9 per 1,000 in the control group to 6 per 1,000 in the HRT group [8]. Estrogen-only therapy did not have any effect on the risk of colorectal cancer [7] and there are no current data on the effects on colorectal cancer of non-oral preparations. Despite these consistent observations there is no clear explanation as to why HRT should lower colon cancer risk, and HRT should not be used solely for the prevention of colon cancer.

Other benefits

Long-term estrogen therapy appears to reduce the risk of nuclear lens opacities that form the cataract by 60–80%. A small absolute reduction in the risk of developing glaucoma has been reported in some studies.

Estrogen seems to protect the teeth and reduce edentia (RR 0.6), possibly through preserving jaw bone density.

Hormone replacement therapy users may also have a reduced incidence of stomach cancer (RR 0.48, 95% CI 0.29–0.79) [7].

Risks of HRT

Breast cancer

The potential risk of breast cancer associated with HRT remains one of the principal reasons for anxiety among patients and health-care professionals about prescribing HRT.

Women should be reassured that the absolute increase in breast cancer risk associated with HRT use is small, and is overall less than the increase in risk associated with obesity, nulliparity or consumption of three alcoholic drinks per day (Table 25.3).

The WHI reported a RR of 1.26 (95% CI 1.02–1.56) after a mean of 5.6 years of continuous combined HRT use, which is less than a 0.1% increase in risk per year [8]. This equates to 4–5 extra breast cancers/1,000 women over 5 years' usage. A more recent but smaller Danish study did not find any significant increase in breast cancer with 10 years of HRT usage [2].

Among women taking unopposed estrogen there has been a non-statistically significant decrease in the risk of breast cancer at 10.7 years follow-up in the WHI Study (RR 0.78, 95% CI 0.63 – 0.96) [8]. It has been hypothesized that estrogen causes apoptosis of breast cancer cells [4] and the available data point to the progestogen component being responsible for the small increase in breast cancer risk seen with combined HRT. Not all progestogens have the same effect; data such as those from the French EPIC Cohort suggest that whilst the nortestosterone derivatives are associated with a small increase in breast cancer risk, the natural progesterone-based preparations are not [4].

Breast cancer is relatively common in the menopausal age group. At the time of initiation of HRT, a proportion of women harbor a "reservoir" of occult undiagnosed breast tumors. Combined results from studies in women of all ages indicate that this could be the case in 0–14.7% of women. It is likely that HRT promotes the growth of these pre-existing lesions to a level at which they are detected and therefore diagnosed earlier in HRT users than in non-users. Thus newly detected breast cancers in the RCTs could be either *de novo* tumors, or pre-existing tumors promoted by HRT use, which can affect the outcome data [4]. This may also explain why women diagnosed with breast cancer on HRT seem to have a better outcome than those not [4].

Table 25.3. Comparison of relative risk (RR) for different breast cancer risk factors.

Breast cancer risk factors	RR of breast cancer
No HRT	1.0
Combined HRT (E + P)	1.26
More than 5 years of HRT use	1.35
Unopposed estrogen (E-only)	0.78
Aged >50 with a BMI >35	2.0
Alcohol ≥2 units per week	1.5–2.0
Early menarche (<12 years)	1.3
Late menopause (>55 years)	1.2–1.5
First pregnancy after the age of 30	1.9
Combined oral contraceptive pill use in the past 10 years	1.07–1.24

Cardiovascular disease

The beneficial cardio-protective effects of HRT in women under the age of 60 are discussed above. For women starting HRT after the age of 60 there appears to be an increased risk of cardiac events during the first few years of use (HR 1.47, 95% CI 1.12–1.92) [3]. However, other data suggest that cardiac morbidity declines in a population of older healthy women after taking HRT for 2 years (HR 0.79, 95% CI 0.67–0.93) [3]. Estrogen is a potent vasodilator and it is hypothesized that when HRT is initiated in women with established coronary disease, estrogen may promote atherosclerotic plaque rupture and thrombosis [9]. This effect seems to be dose dependent and may not be seen with lower doses.

Thus these potential risks should be borne in mind when weighing up the risks and benefits in women wishing to start HRT over 60, and low or ultra-low doses should be used, at least initially.

Stroke

Stroke is the second leading cause of mortality among females worldwide. Its incidence peaks in the postmenopause and is associated with hypertension, obesity and other factors. In the WHI trial, estrogen use with or without progesterone increased the risk of stroke by about one third (RR 1.31, 95% CI 1.02–1.68 with medroxyprogesterone acetate (MPA) and RR 1.37, 95% CI 1.09 – 1.73 without MPA) [4]. This relative risk seems to be independent of age at HRT initiation. As stroke incidence increases with age but RR remains constant, the absolute risk also appears to increase with age. Among women <60 years of age the excess risk related to HRT use approximates 1 case per 1,000 women per 5 years of use, whereas in women >60 years of age the risk is 4.5 cases per 1,000 women per 5 years of use [4]. This small increase in risk maybe route dependent, possibly mediated by an increased thrombotic tendency, as observational studies suggest no increase in stroke risk with low-dose transdermal preparations [2, 7].

Venous thromboembolism

Because of its background prevalence and potentially serious consequences, the risk of venous thromboembolism (VTE) is one of the most important factors in the risk-to-benefit equation of HRT. The absolute risk of thromboembolism for any individual will depend on co-existent risk factors, such as age, obesity, immobility and presence of thrombophilia.

The estimated HRT-related thromboembolic events in women aged 50–59 years approximate to 2 per 1,000 per 5 years of use of unopposed estrogen, or 5 per 1,000 per 5 years of use of combined HRT [4]. The risk of thromboembolism in women taking oral HRT seems to be higher in the first years of use [7]. These risks may be magnified in women with co-existent risk factors and thrombophilias. However, the route of estrogen administration, as well as the dosage and type of progestogen may also influence the risk by avoidance of hepatic first-pass metabolism. Case-control studies estimate an adjusted RR of 0.9 (95% CI 0.4–2.1) for thromboembolic events in transdermal estrogen users vs. placebo [4]. Micronized progesterone or pregnane derivatives have also been associated with a lower thromboembolic risk than other progestogens used in HRT [3]. Thus for women with co-existent risk factors for VTE, the non-oral routes are preferable. For those with a very high risk e.g. factor V Leiden, even transdermal estrogens are associated with a significantly increased risk. In such women with very severe symptoms, HRT may be prescribed in conjunction with thromboprophylaxis.

Ovarian cancer

Eighty percent of ovarian cancers occur in women after the age of 50. Some observational studies reported a RR of 1.6 (95% CI 1.2 – 2.0) with estrogen-only HRT with a 7% increase in risk per year of use, with the risk declining to average population risk 2–4 years after cessation of therapy [4]. However these results have not been consistently reproduced and the WHI trial observed a non-significant RR of 1.58 (95% CI 0.77–3.24) for continuous combined HRT vs. placebo [4]. In women with epithelial ovarian cancer, studies have either shown no difference or an improvement in survival rate with the use of HRT [2].

Endometrial cancer

Ninety percent of endometrial cancers develop after the age of 50. Unopposed estrogen therapy has long been associated with a dose- and duration-dependent increase in risk of premalignant and malignant endometrial conditions. Estrogen-only HRT used for 10 years increases the risk of endometrial cancer by 9.5 times. The risk tends to persist for many years after cessation of therapy, with an RR of 1.9 12 years after stopping estrogen compared with non-users [4]. The addition of cyclical or continuous progestogen eliminates the increased risk. Combined HRT regimes do not increase endometrial cancer risk in RCTs and observational studies. The WHI, for example, quote an RR of 0.81 (95% CI 0.48–1.06) in the continuous combined HRT arm versus placebo [4]. Continuous progestogen regimens are associated with a lower risk than sequential ones and it is recommended that women change to a no-bleed preparation once clearly postmenopausal.

Other gynecologic cancers

There is no evidence that HRT increases the risk of other gynecologic cancers such as cervix or vulva [2]. Equally a history of such a cancer does not preclude the use of subsequent HRT if appropriate.

Lung cancer

The WHI reported a small overall increase in death from non-small cell lung cancer with HRT use compared with placebo (RR = 1.87, 95% CI 1.22–1.88) [4]. This was not seen in women in the 50–59 age group, was more pronounced in smokers and was not seen in the estrogen-alone arm. Epidemiologic studies have not identified any association between HRT and lung cancer.

Gallbladder disease

Both estrogen-only and combined HRT increase the risk of gallbladder disease (cholecystitis and cholelithiasis) and cholecystectomy. The WHI showed a gallbladder disease or surgery hazard ratio (HR) of 1.67 in the estrogen-alone arm and an HR of 1.59 in the combined HRT arm when compared with the non-users [4]. The risk tends to persist for many years after HRT cessation and may be altered with the type and dose of estrogen as well as the route of administration. Transdermal estrogen preparations are associated with a significantly lower gallbladder disease risk. Shorter duration of HRT use also minimizes this risk.

Conclusion

Careful counseling about the risks and benefits of HRT is essential prior to commencing treatment, and an annual reappraisal of the individual risk-benefit profile thereafter should be conducted to ensure the safest effective management of symptoms. Most women seeking hormone therapy are in their late 40s or early 50s and are likely to use HRT for a few years only, so it is important that the relevant figures for the risks and benefits pertinent to that age group are used to aid the consultation (Table 25.4).

For the majority of healthy postmenopausal women below the age of 60 with moderate-to-severe menopausal symptoms, the benefits will outweigh the risks. Hormone replacement therapy commenced in this "critical therapeutic window" period will also provide additional protective cardiovascular and cognitive benefits, as well as osteoporosis prevention. For women who have premature ovarian insufficiency (POI) the potential benefits are such that the risk-benefit balance is likely to be heavily in favor of taking HRT [2, 4, 7]. Women who have been hysterectomized and only require estrogen therapy are likely to have a more beneficial risk analysis at all ages than those who require combined therapy.

Women over the age of 60 or those who wish to continue to use HRT longer term should not be denied treatment provided there is careful consideration and discussion about the potential risks. The absolute risks of many relevant conditions such as breast cancer, cardiovascular disease, stroke and thromboembolism increase with age. However, provided women make a well-informed choice, HRT can still be initiated or continued. It is important to distinguish between the risks of starting HRT over 60 (as reported in the WHI) and continuing HRT into the 60s, which would appear to have fewer risks, particularly with regard to cardiovascular disease. For this group of patients, using lower or ultra-low doses, using the transdermal route, and minimizing or eliminating the progesterone

Table 25.4. Number of excess benefit or risk cases per 1,000 women for 5 years of combined estrogen and progesterone (E+P) or unopposed estrogen (E-only) use in women starting hormone replacement therapy between the ages of 50–59 years.

Benefits and risks(+/- cases per 1,000 women per 5 years)	50–59 years old E + P	50–59 years old E-only
Coronary heart disease	−0.9	−3.8
Fractures	−4.9	−5.9
Breast cancer	+6.8	−1.5
Type II diabetes	−11	−11
Colorectal cancer	−1.2	N/A
Stroke	+1.0	+1.2
Thromboembolism	+5	+2
Cholecystitis	+9.6	+14.

component may all help reduce the potential risk. Careful documentation of the discussion should be made and regular reappraisal of benefits vs. risks is advised 6–12-monthly.

Over the last few years many of the high-profile concerns about the safety of HRT raised by the WHI and other studies around that time have been addressed and put into context. Women deserve an honest evaluation of the risks and benefits associated with any treatments to help them maintain their quality of life through the menopause and to prevent the long-term consequences of the menopause. Further research is needed to develop an individual evidence-based calculator model for the risk-benefit equation taking into account all the relevant variables which would help guide both women and their health-care professionals.

References

1. Manson JE. Current recommendations: what is the clinician to do? *Fertil Steril* 2014; **101**: 916–21.

2. Panay N, Hamoda H, Arya R, Savvas M. The 2013 British Menopause Society & Women's Health Concern recommendations on hormone replacement therapy. *Menopause Int* 2013; **19**: 59–68.

3. MacLennan AH. HRT: a reappraisal of the risks and benefits. *Med J Australia* 2007; **186**: 643–6.

4. Santen RJ, Allred DC, Ardoin SP, *et al.* Postmenopausal hormone therapy: an Endocrine Society Scientific statement. *J Clin Endocrinol Metab* 2010; **95 Suppl. 1**: S7–66.

5. Al-Safi ZA, Santoro N. Menopausal hormone therapy and menopausal symptoms. *Fertil Steril* 2014; **101**: 905–15.

6. Fischer B, Gleason C, Asthana S. Effects of hormone therapy on cognition and mood. *Fertil Steril* 2014; **101**: 898–904.

7. Sturdee DW, Pines A, Archer DF, *et al.* on behalf of the International Menopause Society Writing Group. Updated IMS recommendations on postmenopausal hormone therapy and preventive strategies for midlife health. *Climacteric* 2011; **14**: 302–20.

8. Marjoribanks J, Farquhar C, Roberts H, Lethaby A. (2102) Long term hormone therapy for perimenopausal and postmenopausal women. The Cochrane Collaboration Group. http://onlinelibrary.wiley.com/dBreast cancer is oi/10.1002/14651858.CD004143.pub4/pdf.

9. Harman SM. Menopausal hormone treatment cardiovascular disease: another look at an unresolved conundrum. *Fertil Steril* 2014; **101**: 887–97.

Premature ovarian insufficiency: hormonal aspects and long-term health

Nick Panay

Sheila is 35, and has been on the combined oral contraceptive pill since the age of 18. She has now stopped the pill, and when her periods did not return after 3 months, she consulted her general practitioner. A blood test has shown that she has a very high level of follicle stimulating hormone (FSH). Her physician explains that she has undergone a "premature menopause," and will not be able to conceive. She is referred to you for an expert opinion.

Introduction

"Premature menopause" or more accurately "premature ovarian insufficiency" (POI) remains poorly understood and under-researched [1]. It describes a syndrome consisting of early cessation of menses, sex steroid deficiency and significantly elevated levels of the pituitary hormones, follicle stimulating hormone (FSH) and luteinizing hormone (LH) in women below the age of 40. Premature ovarian insufficiency can be primary (spontaneous POI) or secondary (induced by radiation, chemotherapy or surgery). Controversy persists over nomenclature with terms such "premature menopause" and "premature ovarian failure" still in usage.

Etiology and symptoms

Causes of spontaneous POI include idiopathic (no known cause), genetic, autoimmune and infective. The typical presentation of spontaneous POI is complete cessation of menses in a woman younger than 40 years, which may or may not necessarily be accompanied by other symptoms. These symptoms may not be typically vasomotor in nature and include mood disturbances, loss of energy and generalized aches and pains. Data indicate [2] that the next most disturbing aspect of POI, after the loss of fertility, is the adverse impact on sexual responsiveness and other psychological problems.

In Sheila's case, it is possible that she had reduced ovarian reserve for a number of years, eventually leading to ovarian insufficiency. Her ovarian status and any resulting symptoms would have been masked by many years of contraceptive pill usage. There is an argument that women such as Sheila who wish to defer pregnancy until later in their reproductive years should have their ovarian reserve checked, so that they do not "miss the fertility boat" without knowing it. However, dealing with declining ovarian reserve is confusing and controversial. Sheila could have some of her oocytes collected and stored, but the whole area of "social fertility preservation" is contentious, with limited success. Furthermore, if

Managing the Menopause: 21st Century Solutions, ed. Nick Panay, Paula Briggs, and Gab Kovacs.
Published by Cambridge University Press. © Cambridge University Press 2015.

collecting oocytes from a woman with low anti-Müllerian hormone (AMH) levels, the number suitable for freezing will be further limited.

Women also have to understand that having their ovarian reserve tested is by no means a guarantee of long-term fertility/ability to achieve pregnancy; neither is oocyte/embryo freezing.

This discussion is covered in greater detail in Chapters 2 and 24.

Incidence

Premature ovarian insufficiency has been estimated to affect about 1% of women younger than 40, 0.1% under the age of 30 and 0.01% of women under the age of 20. However, as cure rates for cancers in childhood and young women continue to improve it is likely that there will be more women with POI. Data from Imperial College, London suggest that the incidence of POI may be significantly higher than originally estimated. Islam and Cartwright [3] studied 4,968 participants from a 1958 birth cohort. They found that 370 (7.4%) had either spontaneous or medically induced POI. Smoking and low socioeconomic status were predictive of POI, and poor quality of life. The incidence of POI also appears to vary according to the population studied. It appears to be significantly higher, around 20%, in some Asian populations (personal communication from the Indian Menopause Society).

Long-term health issues

In the past, the focus of medical care has been on improving survival rates. Very little attention has been given to the maintenance of quality of life in the short term and to the avoidance of the long-term sequelae of POI. One of the main reasons for this has been the bias of economic expenditure and medical endeavor to the prolongation of life (e.g. cancer treatments) rather than towards optimizing quality of life in cancer survivors. Should this trend continue, we are in danger of creating a population of young women who have been given back the gift of life, but left without the zest to live it to its full potential. Maintenance of postmenopausal health is also of paramount importance if we are to minimize the economic impact on society in this and future generations.

Life expectancy

Premature ovarian insufficiency has been associated with 50% higher mortality compared with menopause at age 52–55. A large prospective cohort study demonstrated significantly increased all-cause mortality in those with menopause before 40 years after adjustment for confounding factors (hazard ratio [HR] 1.4), and life expectancy was reduced by 2 years compared with women with menopause between 50 and 54 years. The Mayo Clinic Cohort Study of Oophorectomy and Aging demonstrated that mortality was significantly higher in women who had prophylactic bilateral oophorectomy before the age of 45 years (HR 1.67). This increased mortality was however limited to those who did not receive HRT up to the age of 45 years, therefore suggesting that estrogen may have a protective role.

Cardiovascular disease

An association between early menopause and increased mortality from cardiovascular disease has been established for many years. There is an estimated 80% increase in risk of mortality from ischemic heart disease in those with menopause before 40 years compared with those with menopause at 49–55. The risk of ischemic heart disease is more pronounced in never-users of HRT. The Danish Nurses Cohort Study showed that the risk of ischemic heart disease was greater after a surgical menopause rather than spontaneous POI. This mechanism is probably due to the profound loss of ovarian hormones resulting in insulin resistance, reduced arterial compliance and atherosclerosis.

Osteoporosis

The detrimental effects of declining estrogen levels on bone density in menopausal women have long been recognized. Women with POI have significantly lower bone density compared with controls. Both spontaneous and iatrogenic early menopause result in lower bone mineral density compared with controls and this is associated with a significantly higher fracture risk.

Cognition

The Mayo Clinic Cohort Study of Oophorectomy and Aging has shown an increased risk of cognitive impairment in women having premenopausal oophorectomies and that this risk increases the younger it is performed. There is some evidence from the same study that HRT may reduce this risk. Definitive conclusions regarding the risk of cognitive impairment in POI cannot yet be drawn due to a lack of data in women under the age of 40 and in those with non-surgical etiologies.

Integrated care of women with POI

Women such as Sheila with POI require integrated care to address physical, psychosocial and reproductive health, as well as preventative strategies to maintain long-term health. However, there is an absence of evidence-based guidelines for diagnosis and management. Premature ovarian insufficiency is a difficult diagnosis for women to accept, especially when it occurs before child-bearing has been completed and a carefully planned, sensitive approach is required when informing the patient of the diagnosis. A dedicated multi-disciplinary clinic separate from the routine menopause clinic will provide Sheila with ample time and the appropriate professionals to meet her emotional needs at such a traumatic time. At the West London Menopause Centres we have restructured our services to create dedicated clinics for POI patients.

Counseling should include explanation that remission and pregnancy can still occur in women with spontaneous or medical POI. Specific areas of management include the provision of counseling and emotional support, diet and nutrition supplement advice, hormone replacement therapy and reproductive health care, including contraception and fertility issues. There is an urgent need for large-scale, long-term randomized prospective studies to determine the optimum routes and regimens of hormone replacement therapy. Outcome measures should include relief of short-term symptoms such as vasomotor, urogenital and psychosexual issues, and the long-term effect on cardiovascular, cognitive and skeletal health.

Assessment/investigations

As a minimum, the initial investigation of patients presenting with absent or infrequent menses include exclusion of pregnancy, measurement of serum FSH, estradiol, prolactin, androgens and thyroid hormones. If FSH is in the menopausal range ($> 40\,IU/mL$) in a

Table 25.1. Premature ovarian insufficiency: key investigations.

Detailed history	Especially for family history of early menopause
Hormone profile	FSH and LH elevated > 40 on two occasions 4–6 weeks apart, estradiol, thyroid function and prolactin
Autoimmune screen	Anti-thyroid, anti-adrenal
Karyotyping and genetic analysis	Especially in < 30 years or family history
Pelvic ultrasound	To assess antral follicle count
DXA	Baseline bone mineral density
Anti-Müllerian hormone	To assess ovarial reserve

FSH, follicle stimulating hormone; LH, luteinizing hormone; DXA, dual energy X-ray absorptiometry.

woman younger than 40, the test should be repeated a minimum of 4 weeks later for confirmation, as levels can fluctuate. Estradiol levels also fluctuate and results should be interpreted in conjunction with FSH. Sheila should not be definitively informed that she has had a premature menopause before a repeat test has been performed to confirm the diagnosis.

Evaluation of other hormones of ovarian origin, such as inhibin B and AMH, and the ultrasonographic estimation of the antral follicle count can also be used to assess ovarian reserve, but these are not essential in making the diagnosis. Some studies suggest that the precise age of menopause transition can be predicted through the use of these biomarkers; this requires confirmation, especially in POI, and is discussed in greater detail in Chapter 2.

It is essential that a detailed personal and family history is taken from patients such as Sheila. There is often a family history of spontaneous POI in first-degree relatives (around 30–40% of cases). Karyotyping and fragile X testing for the FMR-1 gene mutation will detect the most common genetic causes of spontaneous POI (Turner's syndrome and fragile X syndrome), but these constitute the minority of causes of spontaneous POI. In the long term, the polygenic inheritance of risk for spontaneous POI is likely to be unraveled and banks of genes will be tested to give an individual the precise risk of POI.

It has been estimated that 20% of women with POI have associated autoimmune thyroid disease and 3% have autoimmune adrenal disease; it is therefore important that thyroid and adrenal antibodies are checked and if present, further tests of thyroid and/or adrenal function should be carried out. In view of the increased long-term risk of osteoporosis, a baseline dual energy X-ray absorptiometry (DXA) bone density scan should be carried out and repeated every 2–5 years depending on the results. Table 25.1 summarizes the key investigations in POI.

Counseling and emotional support

Women diagnosed with POI such as Sheila go through a very difficult time emotionally. The condition has been associated with higher than average levels of depression. Loss of reproductive capability is a major upsetting factor and this does not depend on whether the woman has already had children or not. Women with POI have also been shown to have decreased sexual well-being and are less satisfied with their sex lives, suffering from reduced arousal, less frequent sexual encounters and increased pain. The age of diagnosis plays an important role, with younger women more likely to develop complex psychosexual impairment. Psychological and psychosexual help should be offered to help patients cope with the emotional sequelae of POI. Adequate information should be given in a sensitive manner, including information about national self-support groups for POI, such as the Daisy Network in the UK (www.daisynetwork.org.uk).

Contraception

Since spontaneous ovarian activity can occasionally resume, consideration should be given to appropriate contraception in women not wishing to become pregnant. Sheila should not have been informed definitively that she could not conceive. Fertility aspects are covered later on in this chapter, but if pregnancy is not desired then effective contraception needs to continue for 2 years following diagnosis. Although standard oral contraceptive pills are sometimes prescribed, they contain synthetic steroid hormones at a greater dose than is required for physiologic replacement and so may not be ideal. Low-dose combined pills may be used to provide estrogen replacement and contraception, although they seem to be less effective in the prevention of osteoporosis and induce less favorable metabolic changes. There is also the option of using the newer combined oral contraceptives (COCs) containing "natural estrogen", which also have reduced hormone-free intervals. Data are awaited from two randomized studies of the COC vs. HRT which will give more information on the impact on risk markers in women with POI. If a COC is used for estrogenic support, the hormone-free interval should be omitted or shortened to avoid resurgence of cyclical menopausal symptoms. The levonorgestrel-releasing intrauterine system (LNG-IUS) may also be offered in those who choose HRT and require contraception.

Hormone replacement therapy

Young women with spontaneous POI have pathologically low estrogen levels compared with their peers who have normal ovarian function. The global consensus on hormone therapy [4] and updated 2013 British and International Menopause Society recommendations [5, 6] state that for women with POI, systemic hormone therapy is recommended at least until the average age of the natural menopause (51 years).

Hormone therapy is required not only to control vasomotor and other symptoms of the menopause, but also to minimize risks of cardiovascular disease, osteoporosis and possibly Alzheimer's disease, as well as to maintain sexual function. There is no evidence that the results of the Women's Health Initiative Study (a study of much older women) apply to this younger group. Hormone replacement therapy in POI patients is simply replacing ovarian hormones that should normally be produced at this age. It is of paramount importance that these young women understand this in view of the recent negative media publicity on HRT.

The aim is to replace hormones as close to physiologic levels as possible. In our experience, the choice of HRT regimen and the route of administration vary widely among patients. In the absence of better data, treatment should therefore be individualized according to choice and risk factors. If Sheila wishes to use a treatment which is regarded as being the "gold standard" given current evidence, she should be guided towards the use of "body identical" hormone replacement with transdermal estradiol and micronized natural progesterone. Initially, a cyclical regimen should be commenced to avoid unscheduled bleeding but after a year or two, she can be switched to a continuous combined "no bleed" regimen.

It should be remembered that young women with POI will often require higher levels of estrogen than those women who have gone through a natural menopause, in order to fully control their symptoms and achieve good bone mineralization. Transdermal 100 µg estrogen patches or double the normal therapeutic dose of estradiol gel are physiologic for this age group, typically achieving mid-follicular estradiol levels of 300–400 pmol/L. Concomitant use of vaginal estrogen may also be required to fully control urogenital atrophy symptoms.

Where libido and vitality are a problem, testosterone should be replaced at female physiologic levels. There is often a need for this in surgically menopausal women who lose 50% of their androgen production following bilateral oophorectomy. Although there is an absence of licensed androgenic preparations, "off-label" use of down-titrated doses of male transdermal testosterone gel appears to be efficacious and safe. At a typical dose of 0.5–1.0 mL of testosterone gel applied daily to the lower abdomen or inner thigh, side effects such as hirsuitism and acne are uncommon and reversible on cessation/reduction of treatment. Testosterone levels should be kept to a maximum free-androgen index of 6.0% (total testosterone × 100/sex hormone binding globulin).

To complement the role of HRT for the long-term prevention of osteoporosis, supplementary intake of adequate dietary calcium (1,000 mg/day), and vitamin D (800–1,000 IU/day) should be encouraged, as should weight-bearing exercise. The use of complementary therapies and non-estrogen-based treatments such as bisphosphonates, strontium ranelate or raloxifene for the prevention of osteoporosis in women with POI has not been studied.

Fertility

Women with POI are not necessarily sterile unless surgically menopausal. There is however only a 5% chance of spontaneous conception. Hence, women for whom fertility is a priority, such as Sheila, should be counseled to consider assisted conception by *in vitro* fertilization (IVF) using donor eggs or embryos. Future advances in the research of activation of remaining oocytes or of stem cells may make it possible for some women with POI to achieve pregnancy with their own oocytes. Until such a time, oocyte/embryo donation remains the only real chance for these women to achieve pregnancy by assisted conception, though only 50% would accept this due to personal or cultural reasons. Another option that should be discussed is adoption. These issues are considered in greater detail in Chapter 24.

Registry of POI

We urgently need to determine the scale of the POI problem, initially by the trawling of data from all clinics that manage women with POI. The data will undoubtedly demonstrate extreme variations in management and deficiencies will emerge. Armed with this information, Departments of Health can then be petitioned to provide appropriate funding for the setting up of multidisciplinary units for the management of the particular psychological and physical needs of women with POI. In the absence of data from prospective randomized controlled trials, there is a need for high-quality observational studies. There have been calls for a database/registry to provide this information [7, 8].

Individual centers generally do not see sufficient women with POI to gather observational or RCT data to give meaningful results on disease characterization and long-term outcomes. Cooper *et al.* [8] make the point that fragmented research leads to fragmented patient care. Without definitive research, we are left to advise women with POI using inappropriate postmenopausal practice guidelines that are based on a different patient population.

The potential benefits of such a database are many. It could be used to create not only an information database, but also a global biobank for genetic studies, with an ultimate goal of defining the specific pathogenic mechanisms involved in the development of POI, e.g. unraveling the polygenic inheritance mechanism. The database would also have the potential to define and characterize the various presentations of POI along the lines of the STRAW + 10 Guidelines for natural menopause [9]. The STRAW + 10 collaborators in their recent paper state that special groups such as POI warrant urgent attention for staging of reproductive aging. It could also be used to further refine the role of biomarkers such as AMH to precisely predict the course and timing of natural and early ovarian insufficiency.

There is a pressing need to determine long-term response to interventions such as the COC and hormone therapy compared with those not receiving treatment. This is particularly important in women with rare causes and hormone-sensitive cancers where randomized trials are unlikely to ever be performed. Regarding treatment, questions which urgently need to be answered include: does the type of HRT matter; "body identical" vs. other types of HRT; oral vs. transdermal estrogen; dosage of estradiol, progesterone vs. retro progesterone vs. androgenic progestogens and impact of androgens, on both short-term quality of life and long-term outcomes. A database will also give the opportunity for the role of unproven fertility interventions in POI to be studied, such as dehydroepiandrosterone (DHEA), and the use of ultra-low dose HRT and the COC to suppress FSH levels to facilitate ovulation of any remaining oocytes.

As is the case with a number of other centers, we have been collecting data from our cohort of women with POI for a number of years (over 500 subjects to date). The next step is to amalgamate these data with those of our colleagues globally. We have already had verbal agreement from more than 30 international experts in POI who would be willing to contribute to such a database. An online website has been designed as the portal for all those health professionals involved in managing POI who wish to register their interest to collaborate (https://poiregistry.net). All collaborators will have the opportunity to offer their views on the ultimate database structure and data entry fields before real-time data entry commences in late 2015.

Conclusion

Premature ovarian insufficiency is associated with significant morbidity and mortality, which will vary depending on the age of diagnosis and the underlying etiology. There is an urgent need for standardized terminology and evidence-based guidelines upon which to establish the diagnosis and manage this difficult condition. Women such as Sheila have unique needs that require special attention. Multidisciplinary care is vital to address all facets of her care including psychosocial and psychosexual aspects. The long-term consequences of her premature estrogen deficiency can be positively influenced via hormone replacement, but optimization of delivery methods and regimens requires further research. We hope that the development of an international POI database will ultimately lead to better understanding of the condition and the development of truly evidence-based guidelines for the strategic optimization of health in POI.

References

1. Panay N, Fenton A. Premature ovarian failure: a growing concern. *Climacteric* 2008; **11**: 1–3.

2. Singer D, Mann E, Hunter MS, Pitkin J, Panay N. The silent grief: psychosocial aspects of premature ovarian failure. *Climacteric* 2011; **14**: 428–37.

3. Islam R, Cartwright R. The impact of premature ovarian failure on quality of life: results from the UK 1958 Birth Cohort. Paper presented at the *ESHRE*, Stockholm, June 2011, Abstract 0–270.

4. de Villiers TJ, Gass ML, Haines CJ, *et al.* Global consensus statement on menopausal hormone therapy. *Climacteric* 2013; **16**: 203–4.

5. Panay N, Hamoda H, Arya R, Savvas M; British Menopause Society and Women's Health Concern. The 2013 British Menopause Society & Women's Health Concern recommendations on hormone replacement therapy. *Menopause Int* 2013; **19**: 59–68.

6. de Villiers TJ, Pines A, Panay N, *et al.*; International Menopause Society. Updated 2013 International Menopause Society recommendations on menopausal hormone therapy and preventive strategies for midlife health. *Climacteric* 2013; **16**: 316–37.

7. Panay N, Fenton A. Premature ovarian insufficiency: working towards an international database. *Climacteric* 2012; **15**: 295–6.

8. Cooper AR, Baker VL, Sterling EW, *et al.* The time is now for a new approach to primary ovarian insufficiency. *Fertil Steril* 2011; **95**: 1890–7.

9. Harlow SD, Gass M, Hall JE, *et al.*; STRAW +10 Collaborative Group. Executive summary of the Stages of Reproductive Aging Workshop +10: addressing the unfinished agenda of staging reproductive aging. *Climacteric* 2012; **15**: 105–14.

Male menopause – similarities and differences with the female menopause

Malcolm E. Carruthers

Ian is a 43-year-old surgeon. For the last couple of years he has noticed loss of his early morning erections and libido, loss of enthusiasm for his work, increasing difficulty in concentration, brain fog and feeling tired all the time.

Alarmed by these symptoms, and his abilities as a surgeon, he went to his general practitioner, who couldn't find anything wrong with him, but because Ian had read an article suggesting these symptoms might be due to the "male menopause," he had a testosterone level done, which the lab reported as within the lower limits of normal.

Increasingly desperate he went to a private clinic where after taking a full history, particularly focusing on symptomatology, and further blood tests, the specialist considered that a trial of a testosterone skin gel was fully justified.

Within 2 weeks, he was feeling better, and within a month his symptoms had entirely cleared and stayed away over the next 3 months while he felt clear-headed and could function normally in bed and at work.

Then his wife had a good idea – since the treatment obviously worked so well, why shouldn't he get it under the NHS. He went back to his general practitioner, who was impressed with his improved condition, but said he couldn't prescribe testosterone without the sanction of the local endocrinologist. After a 2-month delay, the patient saw the local specialist in endocrinology and diabetes who said he was too young to have "hypogonadotrophic hypogonadism" as shown by his original normal testosterone level, and that he should come off treatment for 6 months so that he could then be "properly investigated."

What should he do, and would you like him to operate on you if he decides to come off testosterone treatment?

The typical story is of a man in middle age who gradually loses his drive, strength, energy and enthusiasm for life and love. An all-enveloping mental and physical tiredness descends on him, often for no apparent reason. He changes from being a positive, optimistic, outgoing person who it is good to be around, to a negative, pessimistic, depressed bear with a sore head, and it is increasingly difficult to live or work with him. At work he is seen to have "Gone off the Boil," and no amount of encouragement or urging will improve his performance. At home, family relations tend to become increasingly strained, and social life and activities dwindle and wilt. His sexual life is usually a disaster area, with loss of libido, intermittent failures to achieve an erection, leading to performance anxiety and eventually complete impotence. This creates a vicious downward spiral of failing function in both boardroom and bedroom.

Managing the Menopause: 21st Century Solutions, ed. Nick Panay, Paula Briggs, and Gab Kovacs. Published by Cambridge University Press. © Cambridge University Press 2015.

When, after ignoring or denying this identikit pattern of symptoms for months or even years, the quietly desperate man goes to see a doctor, he comes across the second, medically approved, cover story. "So you feel tired, dispirited, exhausted and your sex life is non-existent – It's your age – I feel like that too – What do you expect? – What do you mean your wife had the same symptoms when she went through the menopause and she got hormones from her gynecologist which revitalized her so much that you can't keep up? – There's no such thing as the male menopause or male hormone replacement therapy – Forget it, and take these antidepressants – It'll make us both feel better."

You will be relieved to hear that the *surgeon* mentioned in the opening case history decided that the benefits to his improved ability to carry out his professional duties and save his social and married life, made it imperative for him to continue on testosterone replacement therapy (TRT).

Why is the loss denied?

Even if dignified with the medical title of Andropause, as it is known in Europe, it is still an unacceptable threat to their macho self-image. It is seen as the end of their lives as potent males, as leaders and as lovers.

One American author, Gail Sheehy, who has written an excellent book on the female menopause entitled *The Silent Passage*, described the male menopause in an article in *Vanity Fair* as the "Unspeakable Passage." While women are willing to discuss with each other, and with their medical advisors, their menopausal symptoms and the use of hormone replacement to alleviate them, men are remarkably reluctant to turn to either unless desperate [1].

Some feminists delight in using the term as a put-down for any man showing any signs of weakness, ineffectiveness or any difficulty in coping with life generally. At cocktail parties someone will say "You must meet Jill – She's divinely menopausal and is looking radiant after her hormone treatment." No one would dare to introduce husband Jack in similar terms, however good the results of his hormone treatment. Firstly he is unlikely to have told even his closest friend, and secondly he would almost certainly serve a knuckle sandwich to anyone suggesting he had needed such treatment. It is the joke that is no joke, when it happens to you. If cancer is the unmentionable "Big C," the male menopause is the even more inadmissible "Big M."

Also, even in men who have greatly improved on the treatment with testosterone, it is difficult to get them to talk to reporters or appear on television for fear of being thought weak or being ridiculed by their friends or relatives. It is often the many "hammer blows of fate" involving living life to the full as a man, which cause this condition. Anything that puts a man down, whether it is loss of partner or job, can put his testosterone activity down, both by suppressing its synthesis and increasing production of hormones such as cortisol, adrenaline and noradrenaline which antagonize its action.

Testosterone resistance

This is where the concept of "testosterone resistance" comes in and explains why there is virtually no correlation between symptoms, their relief by treatment and testosterone levels. Like insulin in adult-onset diabetes, as well as an absolute reduction with age causing an absolute deficiency, there can be a relative deficiency of testosterone due to an increase in the binding protein sex hormone binding globulin (SHBG), drug effects, defects in the androgen

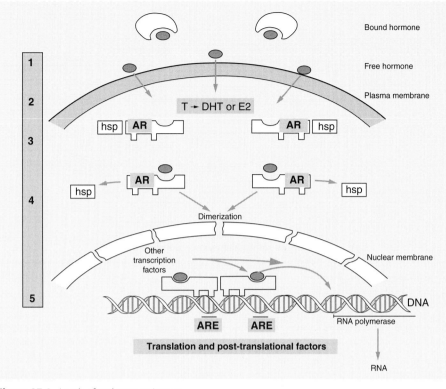

Figure 27.1. Levels of androgen resistance.
Source: Carruthers M. *J Sex Med* 2008; 5: 998–1012.

receptors, or interference with its action lower in the metabolic chain (Figure 27.1) [2]. It can also lead to the common failure to diagnose testosterone deficiency because of the invalidity of the concept of a "normal" testosterone level.

Consequences of androgen deficiency

Partly modulated by one of the factors in testosterone deficiency, SHBG, testosterone, dihydrotestosterone and estrogen all act on multipotent stem cells, and modify their differentiation into the progenitor cells forming and renewing the three types of muscle cell, vascular endothelium, osteoblasts, neurons and hematoblast. The consequences of testosterone deficiency can be seen in Figure 27.2.

This explains why testosterone deficiency can contribute to atrophy of smooth muscle, skeletal muscle and cardiac failure. Further, there is vascular damage and promotion of atherosclerosis due to lack of epithelial cells to repair the vascular endothelium. There may also be anemia due to underactivity of the hematoblasts, together with polycythemia, while a rise in hemoglobin is a regular feature of TRT.

There is evidence that reductions of neural progenitor cells occur, and the resulting decrease in neurogenesis may contribute to Alzheimer's disease, Parkinsonism and the "brain fog" often seen in testosterone-deficient patients, which clears when they go on TRT.

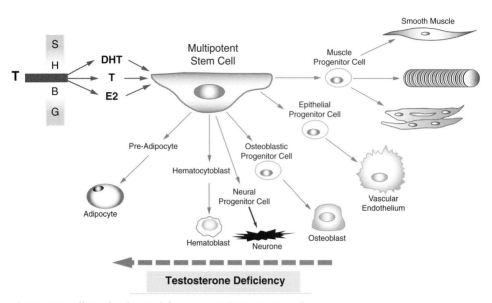

Figure 27.2. Effects of androgen deficiency on multipotent stem cells.
Source: Carruthers, Trinick, Jankowska, Traish 2007.

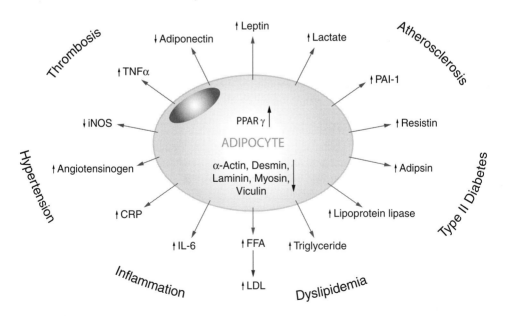

Figure 27.3. The adipocyte – the "axis of evil."
Source: Carruthers, Trinick, Jankowska, Traish 2007.

At the same time, with testosterone deficiency there is a tendency to favor adipocyte production and activity, at the expense of other cells in the body, which has widespread effects that make it the "axis of evil," by the mechanisms seen in Figure 27.3. This sets the scene for the onset of the "metabolic syndrome" with abdominal obesity, diabetes, hyperlipidemia and hypertension.

More reasons for the opposition to TRT

Despite all the above scientific evidence speaking loudly of the benefits for TRT, there are still many in the medical profession who say that is a rare condition which can safely be ignored.

Sometimes even the most macho of males can suffer from it. Logically, there should be no shame attached, but emotionally there often is. Fortunately there are an increasing number who are willing to stand up and be counted, and they greatly help recognition of the condition and its treatment by doing so.

Also, detractors of TRT point out that the number of testosterone estimations being ordered by physicians prescribing it is not rising at the same rate as its usage. But if you go by diagnosis on history, signs and symptoms, together with monitoring of symptomatic response, then the situation is similar to that in prescription of HRT based on history, symptom and the clinician's opinion, not on laboratory measures of estrogens.

Why has testosterone had such a bad press?

Firstly, there is the public perception of testosterone as the hormone responsible for undesirable male traits such as aggression and hypersexuality. My experience is that in practice there is no evidence that treatment with this hormone will "bring out the beast" in men, and turn them into rapacious monsters as portrayed in the film "Wolf," by Jack Nicholson, but this fear holds many menopausal men back from being treated, who unlike him cannot claim to have "retained my testosterone longer than most males."

Also, reports of the abuse of anabolic steroids by athletes and bodybuilders, together with deliberately exaggerated horror stories of their physical and psychological dangers, have appeared in the newspapers at increasingly frequent intervals over the last 30 years. As testosterone is the basic compound from which all the other anabolic steroids are derived, it is the most important part of this "pharmacological arms race," as well as being the hormone used to treat the male menopause, and therefore by association it has suffered a very bad press.

In the USA, partly because a prominent Senator's son overdosed on anabolic steroids, and because national athletics heroes such as Ben Johnson have been disgraced by taking them, there seems to be a "witch-hunt" going on which has turned the minds of politicians, drug companies, doctors and even the Food and Drug Administration (FDA) against testosterone [3].

Especially in the USA, doctors do what they are taught to do, paid to do and not likely to be sued for doing. At present, testosterone treatment doesn't fall under any of these headings. This has limited the range of testosterone preparations available and made them much more difficult for American doctors to prescribe because they are regarded as dangerous drugs. This means a lot more paperwork has to be filled in if you need to keep stocks and prescribe them, and you are more likely to be sued for mega-bucks if any possible side effects are experienced by the patients. Ambulance-chasing lawyers are advertising for patients who think they may have had any of a range of conditions following even the briefest course of testosterone treatment, inviting them to sue their doctors.

To make things worse, by some inverted logic, the drug regulatory body in the USA, the FDA, allows the most poisonous of the many preparations which can be taken by mouth, methyl testosterone, to be prescribed. This is in the mistaken belief that even athletes, let alone doctors, know that it is toxic to the liver and heart, and therefore won't obtain it illegally and abuse it. Of course, a few athletes and bodybuilders will be naive enough to use it anyway. The majority are more knowledgeable about it than most doctors, and read the detailed manuals which are put out largely by mail order on this subject. They then get supplies of safer preparations from other countries, especially Mexico, that caters on a large scale for this illicit market.

A report as recently as 2014 found that in Canada methyl testosterone was still the most commonly prescribed form of TRT [4], even though it has been taken off the market in most European countries and Australia.

When HRT was combined with an androgen, it was often methyl testosterone.

The alleged harms of HRT are extrapolated to include TRT by a curious group of nay-saying epidemiologists and endocrinologists who play on the inherent caution of the medical establishment to prevent the spread of hormonal replacement treatments for either sex. They do this by deriding any attempt to hold back the ravages of time as being "the quest for eternal youth," and preach that people should modify their lifestyle, and learn to "grow old gracefully," however incapacitating, painful, undignified and expensive to the individual and community that process may be.

Also, they base their beliefs not on the clinical experience of doctors who have expertly applied these treatments to large numbers of patients over many years, but on the application of sophisticated statistics to massive rag-bags of facts and theories gained from huge trials which assume all forms of HRT or TRT have similar endocrine effects in all subjects and can therefore be bracketed together, while largely ignoring any beneficial effects.

They also ignore the fact that very large trials generate differences between groups which may be statistically significant, but can easily be clinically insignificant. Also, it has been said that "If you torture the data long enough, it will confess to anything."

Finally, they delight in drawing conclusions from their studies which generate "myths" which they can tell to other doctors with no experience of hormone replacement to put them off prescribing the treatment.

The myths of TRT

As President John Kennedy said, "The great enemy of the truth is very often not the lie deliberate, contrived and dishonest, but the myth, persistent, persuasive, and unrealistic. Belief in myths allows the comfort of opinion without the discomfort of thought."

The first myth which has held up the introduction of TRT for over 70 years is that it might cause prostate cancer (PCa). Introduced by an American urologist called Charles Huggins on the basis of one patient whose prostate cancer appeared to worsen while he was on TRT, this idea was affirmed by the apparent regression of tumors when estrogens were given.

This fortunately did not appear to occur in practice, but it was not until 2012 that another American urologist called Abraham Morgentaler published his saturation theory of a testosterone threshold above which no further stimulation of the receptors occurred. Morgentaler also pointed out that many cases of prostate cancer presented with low levels of testosterone. More challenging still was that when he started giving TRT to patients who had been treated, there was no recurrence of their cancers [5].

A long-term study of 1,500 patients over 15 years (the UK Androgen Study – UKAS) [6] showed "The incidence of PCa during long-term TRT was equivalent to that expected in the general population. This study adds to the considerable weight of evidence that with proper clinical monitoring, testosterone treatment is safe for the prostate and improves early detection of PCa. Testosterone treatment with regular monitoring of the prostate may be safer for the individual than any alternative without surveillance."

Many men showed not only benefits in losing the symptoms of testosterone deficiency, but had improvement in "lower urinary tract symptoms," such as passing water more frequently, especially at night. This illustrates the point that TRT causes neither benign nor malignant prostate conditions, but is good for the health of the entire urinary tract.

The second myth was that TRT might contribute to cardiovascular disease. Perhaps not coincidently this myth reared its ugly head just as the prostate cancer myth was being slain. Having disposed of the myth that testosterone treatment causes prostate cancer [6, 7], those that wish to block its use have switched their line of reasoning to the mistaken idea that it contributes to cardiovascular disease [3].

That this is not so is clearly obvious to doctors who use this form of treatment with their patients suffering the classic symptoms of testosterone deficiency syndrome and related disorders. These include diabetes, obesity, metabolic syndrome, osteoporosis and even Alzheimer's disease. A range of risk factors for heart disease such as blood pressure, cholesterol, triglycerides and abdominal obesity are seen to decrease on the treatment [8, 9], and especially in diabetics there is a decrease in heart attack and mortality rates.

Undeterred by 20 years of clinical studies showing benefits to the heart and circulation, opponents base their current attacks on three studies as put forward in the *British Medical Journal*-commissioned article "Washington Brief" [3].

Also, blood levels of testosterone in the male population in many countries are showing a marked downward trend, which increases the problems of using them as a diagnostic marker of deficiency [10].

In support of the "testosterone as a cause of heart disease" theory, one article frequently cited [11] involved a cohort in which the men were old, frail and above all were overdosed.

Another article often quoted [12] is a vast retrospective study of 8,709 men from the Veterans Affairs system who were having coronary angiography between 2005 and 2011.

The problem of such large groups is that there are very few data on each patient available for detailed assessment, and that factors which are not clinically or biologically significant can and were made statistically significant. Very few had adequate and consistent treatment, and while the raw data showed a marked benefit to the treated group, by the use of "sophisticated statistics," the findings were somehow reversed, and have been heavily criticized by leading experts in the field [13, 14].

The third article in 2014 [15] had an incomparable control group. Therefore its findings should be largely discounted and not treated as sufficient evidence for changing pharmaceutical regulations.

Misled by studies such as the three above, the orthodox medical establishment and the general public are being unduly alarmed about the possibility of an unproven association between testosterone treatment and circulatory disease [16].

Most doctors interested in developing new forms of testosterone treatment have experienced the disinterest and even extreme apathy of pharmaceutical companies when approached with such ideas. Apart from the risk of litigation, particularly in the USA, the existing testosterone preparations, many of which have proved safe and successful for up to 50 years, are out of their product licenses, so that anyone can make them and profit margins are smaller. These sex hormones just aren't sexy any more. Even so, foresight would suggest the potential market is vast, and more convenient long-acting forms are urgently needed to make TRT more popular, more economic and more easily available.

Many doctors, politicians and economists argue on financial grounds that no country could afford the cost of this "His and Hers HRT," and who wants to keep an increasing number of "Golden Oldies" going anyway?

Well, that doesn't seem to make either ethical or economic sense for either sex, especially men whose active lifespan is shorter by 5–7 years at least than that of women. Recently a report from the USA [17] has made the economic case for preventing or delaying cases of heart disease, diabetes and osteoporosis-related fractures. It estimated that over a 20-year period "T deficiency may be directly responsible for approximately $190–$525 billion in inflation-adjusted U.S. health-care expenditures, and that testosterone deficiency may be a significant contributor to adverse public health."

Similarly, a Swedish doctor [18] concluded that lifelong testosterone undecanoate (TU) depot injection therapy of patients with Klinefelter syndrome and late-onset hypogonadism is a cost-effective treatment, and he suggests that such information can support clinicians in decision-making when considering appropriate treatment strategies for patients with this

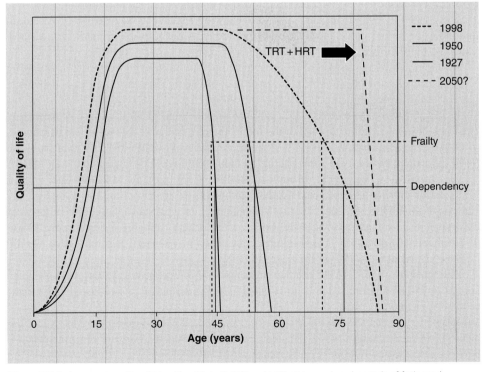

Figure 27.4. Improved quality of later life with both TRT and HRT, giving reduced periods of frailty and dependency.

condition. Other health economic theorists have also pointed out that substantial savings can be made by shortening the terminal period of frailty and dependency, and give many people's lives a happier ending (Figure 27.4).

Supporters of "Men's Lib" would say that they have up to now been sadly neglected, have a 7- or 8-year shorter life expectancy than women, and its time they had a chance of catching up in the health stakes on the last lap of life. There are many good reasons for regarding "His and Hers HRT" as an important part of the preventive medicine of the future, helping both sexes to prolong an active and enjoyable life in a "Square Wave" form, like alkaline batteries going full charge to the end!

References

1. Sheehy G. *The Silent Passage*. London: HarperCollins; 1991.

2. Carruthers M. The paradox dividing testosterone deficiency symptoms and androgen assays: a closer look at the cellular and molecular mechanisms of androgen action. *J Sex Med* 2008; 5: 998–1012.

3. Wolfe SM. Increased heart attacks in men using testosterone: the UK importantly lags far behind the US in prescribing testosterone. *Br Med J* 2014; 348: g1789.

4. Hall SA, Ranganathan G, Tinsley LJ, *et al.* Population-based patterns of prescription androgen use, 1976–2008. *Pharmacoepidemiol Drug Saf* 2014; 23: 498–506.

5. Morgentaler A. Testosterone therapy in men with prostate cancer: scientific and ethical considerations. *J Urol* 2013; 189: S26–33.

6. Feneley MR, Carruthers M. Is testosterone treatment good for the prostate? Study of safety during long-term treatment. *J Sex Med* 2012; 9: 2138–49.

7. Khera M, Crawford D, Morales A, Salonia A, Morgentaler A. A new era of testosterone and prostate cancer: from physiology to clinical implications. *Eur Urol* 2014; 65: 115–23.

8. Stanworth R, Jones T. Testosterone in obesity, metabolic syndrome and type 2 diabetes. *Frontiers Horm Res* 2009; 37: 74–90.

9. Jones TH, Arver S, Behre HM, *et al.* Testosterone replacement in hypogonadal men with type 2 diabetes and/or metabolic syndrome (the TIMES2 study). *Diabetes Care* 2011; 34: 828–37.

10. Perheentupa A, Mäkinen J, Laatikainen T, *et al.* A cohort effect on serum testosterone levels in Finnish men. *Eur J Endocrinol* 2013; 168: 227–33.

11. Basaria S, Coviello AD, Travison TG, *et al.* Adverse events associated with testosterone administration. *N Engl J Med* 2010; 363: 109–22.

12. Vigen R, O'Donnell CI, Barón AE, *et al.* Association of testosterone therapy with mortality, myocardial infarction, and stroke in men with low testosterone levels. *JAMA* 2013; 310: 1829–36.

13. Jones TH, Channer KS. Deaths and cardiovascular events in men receiving testosterone. *JAMA* 2014; 311: 961–5.

14. Traish AM, Guay AT, Morgentaler A. Death by testosterone? We think not! *J Sex Med* 2014; 11: 624–9.

15. Finkle WD, Greenland S, Ridgeway GK, *et al.* Increased risk of non-fatal myocardial infarction following testosterone therapy prescription in men. *PLoS ONE* 2014; 9: e85805.

16. Morgentaler A. Testosterone, cardiovascular risk, and hormonophobia. *J Sex Med* 2014; 11: 1362–6.

17. Moskovic DJ, Araujo AB, Lipshultz LI, Khera M. The 20-year public health impact and direct cost of testosterone deficiency in U.S. men. *J Sex Med* 2013; 10: 562–9.

18. Arver S, Luong B, Fraschke A, *et al.* Is testosterone replacement therapy in males with hypogonadism cost-effective? An analysis in Sweden. *J Sex Med* 2013; Aug 12. [Epub ahead of print]. PubMed PMID: 23937088.

Index